Brain-Targeted Drug Delivery

Brain-Targeted Drug Delivery

Editor

Flávia Sousa

MDPI • Basel • Beijing • Wuhan • Barcelona • Belgrade • Manchester • Tokyo • Cluj • Tianjin

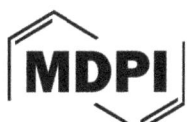

Editor
Flávia Sousa
Adolphe Merkle Institute
University of Fribourg
Fribourg
Switzerland

Editorial Office
MDPI
St. Alban-Anlage 66
4052 Basel, Switzerland

This is a reprint of articles from the Special Issue published online in the open access journal *Pharmaceutics* (ISSN 1999-4923) (available at: www.mdpi.com/journal/pharmaceutics/special_issues/brain_delivery).

For citation purposes, cite each article independently as indicated on the article page online and as indicated below:

LastName, A.A.; LastName, B.B.; LastName, C.C. Article Title. *Journal Name* **Year**, *Volume Number*, Page Range.

ISBN 978-3-0365-5282-8 (Hbk)
ISBN 978-3-0365-5281-1 (PDF)

© 2022 by the authors. Articles in this book are Open Access and distributed under the Creative Commons Attribution (CC BY) license, which allows users to download, copy and build upon published articles, as long as the author and publisher are properly credited, which ensures maximum dissemination and a wider impact of our publications.
The book as a whole is distributed by MDPI under the terms and conditions of the Creative Commons license CC BY-NC-ND.

Contents

About the Editor vii

Flávia Sousa
Brain-Targeted Drug Delivery
Reprinted from: *Pharmaceutics* **2022**, *14*, 1835, doi:10.3390/pharmaceutics14091835 1

Ghazal Naseri Kouzehgarani, Pankaj Kumar, Susan E. Bolin, Edward B. Reilly and Didier R. Lefebvre
Biodistribution Analysis of an Anti-EGFR Antibody in the Rat Brain: Validation of CSF Microcirculation as a Viable Pathway to Circumvent the Blood-Brain Barrier for Drug Delivery
Reprinted from: *Pharmaceutics* **2022**, *14*, 1441, doi:10.3390/pharmaceutics14071441 5

Asya I. Petkova, Ilona Kubajewska, Alexandra Vaideanu, Andreas G. Schätzlein and Ijeoma F. Uchegbu
Gene Targeting to the Cerebral Cortex Following Intranasal Administration of Polyplexes
Reprinted from: *Pharmaceutics* **2022**, *14*, 1136, doi:10.3390/pharmaceutics14061136 25

Farheen Fatima Qizilbash, Muhammad Usama Ashhar, Ameeduzzafar Zafar, Zufika Qamar, Annu and Javed Ali et al.
Thymoquinone-Enriched Naringenin-Loaded Nanostructured Lipid Carrier for Brain Delivery via Nasal Route: In Vitro Prospect and In Vivo Therapeutic Efficacy for the Treatment of Depression
Reprinted from: *Pharmaceutics* **2022**, *14*, 656, doi:10.3390/pharmaceutics14030656 45

Hiba Natsheh and Elka Touitou
Improved Efficiency of Pomegranate Seed Oil Administrated Nasally
Reprinted from: *Pharmaceutics* **2022**, *14*, 918, doi:10.3390/pharmaceutics14050918 67

Devon J. Griggs, Aaron D. Garcia, Wing Yun Au, William K. S. Ojemann, Andrew Graham Johnson and Jonathan T. Ting et al.
Improving the Efficacy and Accessibility of Intracranial Viral Vector Delivery in Non-Human Primates
Reprinted from: *Pharmaceutics* **2022**, *14*, 1435, doi:10.3390/pharmaceutics14071435 81

Julian S. Rechberger, Kendra A. Porath, Liang Zhang, Cody L. Nesvick, Randy S. Schrecengost and Jann N. Sarkaria et al.
IL-13R Status Predicts GB-13 (IL13.E13K − PE4E) Efficacy in High-Grade Glioma
Reprinted from: *Pharmaceutics* **2022**, *14*, 922, doi:10.3390/pharmaceutics14050922 103

Takashi Nakano, Shakila B. Rizwan, David M. A. Myint, Jason Gray, Sean M. Mackay and Paul Harris et al.
An On-Demand Drug Delivery System for Control of Epileptiform Seizures
Reprinted from: *Pharmaceutics* **2022**, *14*, 468, doi:10.3390/pharmaceutics14020468 123

Yaquelyn Casanova, Sofía Negro, Karla Slowing, Luis García-García, Ana Fernández-Carballido and Mahdieh Rahmani et al.
Micro- and Nano-Systems Developed for Tolcapone in Parkinson's Disease
Reprinted from: *Pharmaceutics* **2022**, *14*, 1080, doi:10.3390/pharmaceutics14051080 141

Junzhi Yang, Robert D. Betterton, Erica I. Williams, Joshua A. Stanton, Elizabeth S. Reddell and Chidinma E. Ogbonnaya et al.
High-Dose Acetaminophen Alters the Integrity of the Blood–Brain Barrier and Leads to Increased CNS Uptake of Codeine in Rats
Reprinted from: *Pharmaceutics* **2022**, *14*, 949, doi:10.3390/pharmaceutics14050949 . . . . **157**

Wiam El Kheir, Bernard Marcos, Nick Virgilio, Benoit Paquette, Nathalie Faucheux and Marc-Antoine Lauzon
Drug Delivery Systems in the Development of Novel Strategies for Glioblastoma Treatment
Reprinted from: *Pharmaceutics* **2022**, *14*, 1189, doi:10.3390/pharmaceutics14061189 . . . . **171**

Toshihiko Tashima
Delivery of Intravenously Administered Antibodies Targeting Alzheimer's Disease-Relevant Tau Species into the Brain Based on Receptor-Mediated Transcytosis
Reprinted from: *Pharmaceutics* **2022**, *14*, 411, doi:10.3390/pharmaceutics14020411 . . . . **209**

Marie-Laure Custers, Liam Nestor, Dimitri De Bundel, Ann Van Eeckhaut and Ilse Smolders
Current Approaches to Monitor Macromolecules Directly from the Cerebral Interstitial Fluid
Reprinted from: *Pharmaceutics* **2022**, *14*, 1051, doi:10.3390/pharmaceutics14051051 . . . . **231**

About the Editor

Flávia Sousa

Flávia Sousa is a senior researcher at Adolphe Merkle Institute (AMI) in Fribourg, Switzerland. She completed her MSc in Pharmaceutical Sciences in 2013 and achieved her PhD in Biomedical Sciences at ICBAS, University of Porto, in 2019. Her PhD was developed at I3S (Porto, Portugal) in collaboration with INL (International Iberian Nanotechnology Laboratory, Braga, Portugal), Aalborg University (Aalborg, Denmark) and Northeastern University (Boston, USA). After finishing her PhD studies, Flávia Sousa completed her first postdoctoral studies at Imperial College London, followed by a Marie Curie MINDED fellowship at IIT (Istituto Italiano di Tecnologia). In 2022, she began an independent Women in Science (WINS) research fellowship awarded by the NCCR for Bio-Inspired Materials. Her current research is focused on developing polymeric nanodelivery systems for biomolecule delivery (e.g., monoclonal antibodies, proteins, and saRNA). In the past 5 years, she has authored over 30 publications and received 8 scientific awards from different countries, acquiring over 1000 citations and yielding an H-index of 19. She has been an invited Associate Professor at IUCS, Instituto Universitario Ciencias da Saude since 2018, as a Master of Pharmaceutical Sciences and Nutrition Sciences. To date, she has taught more than 400 hours in the pharmaceutical technology, biotoxicology, nanomedicine, biotechnology, and analytical chemistry field.

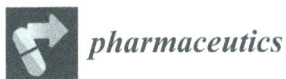

Editorial

Brain-Targeted Drug Delivery

Flávia Sousa

Adolphe Merkle Institute, University of Fribourg, Chemin des Verdiers 4, 1700 Fribourg, Switzerland; flavia.sousa@unifr.ch

At present, brain diseases affect one in six people worldwide, and they include a wide range of neurological diseases from Alzheimer's and Parkinson's diseases to epilepsy, brain injuries, brain cancer, neuroinfections and strokes. The treatment of these diseases is complex and limited due to the presence of the blood–brain barrier (BBB), which covers the entirety of the brain. The BBB not only has the function of protecting the brain from harmful substances but is also a metabolic barrier and a transport regulator of nutrients/serum factors/neurotoxins. Knowing these characteristics when it comes to the treatment of brain diseases makes it easy to understand the lack of efficacy of therapeutic drugs, resulting from the innate resistance of the BBB to permeation. To overcome this limitation, drug delivery systems based on nanotechnology/microtechnology have been wisely developed. Brain-targeted drug delivery allows targeted therapy with a higher therapeutic efficacy and low side effects because it targets moieties present in the drug delivery systems.

Brain-targeted drug delivery research is an active, rich and multidisciplinary research area, and this Special Issue aims to present the current state of the art in the field. A series of nine research articles and three review articles are presented, with authors from 10 different countries, which demonstrates the multidisciplinarity of investigations that have been carried out in this area. This Special Issue brings together the latest research from the treatment of glioblastoma (GBM) to neurodegenerative diseases and epilepsy. Furthermore, literature reviews are presented on the topics of (i) novel drug delivery systems for GBM treatment, (ii) the potential of Alzheimer's disease immunotherapy, and, lastly, (iii) current methods to detect and monitor macromolecules in the brain.

The main obstacle to treating disorders of the central nervous system (CNS) is the presence of the BBB, which hinders the delivery of therapeutics. It is well known that few small-molecule drugs can cross the BBB, and most biologic drugs cannot. As an alternative route to overcome the BBB, Kouzehgarani et al. evaluated the biodistribution of an anti-EGFR antibody in the rat brain after intra-cisterna magma injection. They show vastly greater and deeper penetration of the monoclonal antibody (mAb) into the brain parenchyma after CSF administration compared to IV administration. The authors demonstrate that circumventing the BBB via CSF microcirculation might be a strategy to improve the delivery of mAbs into the brain, achieving deep penetration of IgG-size biologics [1].

Another administration route that allows us to successfully reach the brain is the intranasal route. Intranasal administration has recently been explored by researchers because it reaches the brain, bypassing the BBB through the olfactory bulb. Petkova et al. used this strategy to enhance gene delivery to the cerebral cortex using hyaluronidase-coated glycol chitosan–DNA polyplexes (GCPH) [2]. The authors show high levels of protein expression in the brain regions upon intranasal administration of hyaluronidase-coated polyplexes. Following the same strategy of intranasal administration, Qizilbash et al. developed a naringenin-encapsulated nanostructured lipid carrier (NGN-NLC) with thymoquinone (TQ) oil to investigate the antidepressant potential of the nanosystem [3]. Their ex vivo and in vivo results show higher penetration and greater antidepressant potential from NGN-NLC compared to NGN suspension achieved by intranasal administration. Lastly,

Nathshed et al. developed a pomegranate seed oil (PSO) phospholipid oil gel for nasal administration to test its biological effect on memory and locomotor activity [4]. The results show a significant improvement in the behavior of animals when they were treated with intranasal gel compared to orally administrated oil.

Another common administration route for brain-targeted drug delivery is intracranial. To improve intracranial viral vector delivery in non-human primates (NHPs), Griggs et al. developed a new method based in bench-side convection-enhanced delivery (CED) that provides users with a hands-on CED experience. This method aims to help and guide researchers in the surgical preparations for intracranial viral delivery using CED in NHPs [5]. Indeed, other authors have used CED for the intratumoral administration of biologics. Rechberger et al. studied the effect of direct intratumoral administration of GB-13 in an orthotopic xenograph model of high-grade glioma via CED [6]. This novel peptide–toxin conjugate that binds to IL-13Rα2 was able to significantly decrease tumor size and prolong survival in both diffuse midline and high-grade glioma with high levels of IL-13Rα2, opening doors for IL-13Rα2-targeted therapy.

Focusing on intravenous administration for brain-targeted drug delivery, Nakano et al. developed hollow-gold nanoparticles tethered to liposomes (HGN-liposomes) loaded with muscimol to be released by laser or ultrasound stimulation and to inhibit neurons and suppress epileptiform seizures [7]. The combination of ultrasound stimulation and intravenous administration of HGN-liposomes suppressed seizure activity in the hippocampus, demonstrating the therapeutic potential of HGN-liposomes for controlling epileptiform seizures without continuous exposure.

Drug delivery into the brain can also be done by intraperitoneal administration. Casanova et al. developed PLGA microparticles and nanoparticles loaded with Tolcapone to improve the treatment of Parkinson's disease (PD) [8]. There is an urgent need to find new and promising therapeutic strategies to treat PD that are able to overcome the BBB. The authors demonstrate that Tolcapone-loaded PLGA nanoparticles were able to revert PD-like symptoms of neurodegeneration in an in vivo model upon intraperitoneal administration.

Undoubtedly, the BBB is essential for protecting the organ from toxins, drugs, and pathogens, serving as a highly selective semipermeable membrane of endothelial cells. Damaging the BBB can lead to serious consequences for brain homeostasis and neuronal degeneration. Yang et al. studied the impact of high-dose acetaminophen (APAP) on the integrity of the BBB, demonstrating increased paracellular permeability of the BBB as well as increased protein expression of claudin-5 in brain microvessels [9]. The authors also observed that APAP-induced paracellular "leak" contributed to increased CNS uptake of codeine, bringing awareness to the biological effects of concomitant administration of APAP with opioids.

Lastly, this Special Issue presents three review articles to provide the reader with a broad overview of brain-targeted drug delivery research. Kheir et al. reviews the literature on the development of new drug delivery systems and novel strategies for GBM treatment [10]. The authors discuss (i) current GBM traditional treatments, (ii) the role of chemokine CXCL12 and its receptor CXCR4 in GBM invasion, (iii) interstitial fluid flow in GBM, (iv) models to study GBM cell migration and (v) innovative treatments for GBM. On the other side, Toshihiko Tashima discusses the potential of Alzheimer's disease immunotherapy using intravenously administered anti-tau and anti-receptor bispecific antibodies [11]. These anti-tau and bispecific mAbs are able to induce receptor-mediated transcytosis in capillary endothelial cells of the BBB and might represent a solution for Aβ-targeting therapies. Lastly, Custers et al. reviews the literature on the current approaches to detect and monitor macromolecules in the brain directly from the cerebral interstitial fluid [12]. Direct sampling from the cerebral interstitial space can be done via a few techniques such as microdialysis, cerebral open flow microperfusion and electrochemical biosensors. The authors discuss the current limitations and advantages of each technique.

Overall, the articles in this Special Issue highlight a very active and interesting field for society since, in recent years, brain diseases are affecting more people and starting earlier.

Therefore, there is an urgent need to understanding the biological properties of the BBB and to apply that knowledge to finding new therapeutic strategies for brain diseases. I would like to thank all the authors of this Special Issue for contributing high-quality works, as well as all the reviewers who critically evaluated the articles. In addition, I would like to thank the Assistant Editor, Mr. Jaimin Tao, for his kind help.

Funding: This research received no external funding.

Conflicts of Interest: The author declares no conflict of interest.

References

1. Naseri Kouzehgarani, G.; Kumar, P.; Bolin, S.E.; Reilly, E.B.; Lefebvre, D.R. Biodistribution Analysis of an Anti-EGFR Antibody in the Rat Brain: Validation of CSF Microcirculation as a Viable Pathway to Circumvent the Blood-Brain Barrier for Drug Delivery. *Pharmaceutics* **2022**, *14*, 1441. [CrossRef] [PubMed]
2. Petkova, A.I.; Kubajewska, I.; Vaideanu, A.; Schätzlein, A.G.; Uchegbu, I.F. Gene Targeting to the Cerebral Cortex Following Intranasal Administration of Polyplexes. *Pharmaceutics* **2022**, *14*, 1136. [CrossRef] [PubMed]
3. Qizilbash, F.F.; Ashhar, M.U.; Zafar, A.; Qamar, Z.; Annu; Ali, J.; Baboota, S.; Ghoneim, M.M.; Alshehri, S.; Ali, A. Thymoquinone-Enriched Naringenin-Loaded Nanostructured Lipid Carrier for Brain Delivery via Nasal Route: In Vitro Prospect and In Vivo Therapeutic Efficacy for the Treatment of Depression. *Pharmaceutics* **2022**, *14*, 656. [CrossRef] [PubMed]
4. Natsheh, H.; Touitou, E. Improved Efficiency of Pomegranate Seed Oil Administrated Nasally. *Pharmaceutics* **2022**, *14*, 918. [CrossRef] [PubMed]
5. Griggs, D.J.; Garcia, A.D.; Au, W.Y.; Ojemann, W.K.S.; Johnson, A.G.; Ting, J.T.; Buffalo, E.A.; Yazdan-Shahmorad, A. Improving the Efficacy and Accessibility of Intracranial Viral Vector Delivery in Non-Human Primates. *Pharmaceutics* **2022**, *14*, 1435. [CrossRef] [PubMed]
6. Rechberger, J.S.; Porath, K.A.; Zhang, L.; Nesvick, C.L.; Schrecengost, R.S.; Sarkaria, J.N.; Daniels, D.J. IL-13Rα2 Status Predicts GB-13 (IL13.E13K-PE4E) Efficacy in High-Grade Glioma. *Pharmaceutics* **2022**, *14*, 922. [CrossRef] [PubMed]
7. Nakano, T.; Rizwan, S.B.; Myint, D.M.A.; Gray, J.; Mackay, S.M.; Harris, P.; Perk, C.G.; Hyland, B.I.; Empson, R.; Tan, E.W.; et al. An On-Demand Drug Delivery System for Control of Epileptiform Seizures. *Pharmaceutics* **2022**, *14*, 468. [CrossRef] [PubMed]
8. Casanova, Y.; Negro, S.; Slowing, K.; García-García, L.; Fernández-Carballido, A.; Rahmani, M.; Barcia, E. Micro- and Nano-Systems Developed for Tolcapone in Parkinson's Disease. *Pharmaceutics* **2022**, *14*, 1080. [CrossRef] [PubMed]
9. Yang, J.; Betterton, R.D.; Williams, E.I.; Stanton, J.A.; Reddell, E.S.; Ogbonnaya, C.E.; Dorn, E.; Davis, T.P.; Lochhead, J.J.; Ronaldson, P.T. High-Dose Acetaminophen Alters the Integrity of the Blood–Brain Barrier and Leads to Increased CNS Uptake of Codeine in Rats. *Pharmaceutics* **2022**, *14*, 949. [CrossRef] [PubMed]
10. El Kheir, W.; Marcos, B.; Virgilio, N.; Paquette, B.; Faucheux, N.; Lauzon, M.-A. Drug Delivery Systems in the Development of Novel Strategies for Glioblastoma Treatment. *Pharmaceutics* **2022**, *14*, 1189. [CrossRef] [PubMed]
11. Tashima, T. Delivery of Intravenously Administered Antibodies Targeting Alzheimer's Disease-Relevant Tau Species into the Brain Based on Receptor-Mediated Transcytosis. *Pharmaceutics* **2022**, *14*, 411. [CrossRef] [PubMed]
12. Custers, M.-L.; Nestor, L.; De Bundel, D.; Van Eeckhaut, A.; Smolders, I. Current Approaches to Monitor Macromolecules Directly from the Cerebral Interstitial Fluid. *Pharmaceutics* **2022**, *14*, 1051. [CrossRef] [PubMed]

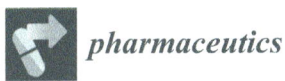

Article

Biodistribution Analysis of an Anti-EGFR Antibody in the Rat Brain: Validation of CSF Microcirculation as a Viable Pathway to Circumvent the Blood-Brain Barrier for Drug Delivery

Ghazal Naseri Kouzehgarani ⓘ, Pankaj Kumar, Susan E. Bolin, Edward B. Reilly and Didier R. Lefebvre *

AbbVie Inc., 1 N Waukegan Road, North Chicago, IL 60064, USA;
ghazal.naserikouzehgarani@abbvie.com (G.N.K.); pankaj.kumar2@abbvie.com (P.K.);
susan.bolin@abbvie.com (S.E.B.); ed.reilly@abbvie.com (E.B.R.)
* Correspondence: didier.lefebvre@abbvie.com

Citation: Naseri Kouzehgarani, G.; Kumar, P.; Bolin, S.E.; Reilly, E.B.; Lefebvre, D.R. Biodistribution Analysis of an Anti-EGFR Antibody in the Rat Brain: Validation of CSF Microcirculation as a Viable Pathway to Circumvent the Blood-Brain Barrier for Drug Delivery. *Pharmaceutics* 2022, 14, 1441. https://doi.org/10.3390/pharmaceutics14071441

Academic Editor: Flávia Sousa

Received: 28 April 2022
Accepted: 4 July 2022
Published: 12 July 2022

Publisher's Note: MDPI stays neutral with regard to jurisdictional claims in published maps and institutional affiliations.

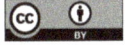

Copyright: © 2022 by the authors. Licensee MDPI, Basel, Switzerland. This article is an open access article distributed under the terms and conditions of the Creative Commons Attribution (CC BY) license (https://creativecommons.org/licenses/by/4.0/).

Abstract: Cerebrospinal fluid (CSF) microcirculation refers to CSF flow through brain or spinal parenchyma. CSF enters the tissue along the perivascular spaces of the penetrating arteries where it mixes with the interstitial fluid circulating through the extracellular space. The potential of harnessing CSF microcirculation for drug delivery to deep areas of the brain remains an area of controversy. This paper sheds additional light on this debate by showing that ABT-806, an EGFR-specific humanized IgG1 monoclonal antibody (mAb), reaches both the cortical and the deep subcortical layers of the rat brain following intra-cisterna magna (ICM) injection. This is significant because the molecular weight of this mAb (150 kDa) is highest among proteins reported to have penetrated deeply into the brain via the CSF route. This finding further confirms the potential of CSF circulation as a drug delivery system for a large subset of molecules offering promise for the treatment of various brain diseases with poor distribution across the blood-brain barrier (BBB). ABT-806 is the parent antibody of ABT-414, an antibody-drug conjugate (ADC) developed to engage EGFR-overexpressing glioblastoma (GBM) tumor cells. To pave the way for future efficacy studies for the treatment of GBM with an intra-CSF administered ADC consisting of a conjugate of ABT-806 (or of one of its close analogs), we verified in vivo the binding of ABT-414 to GBM tumor cells implanted in the cisterna magna and collected toxicity data from both the central nervous system (CNS) and peripheral tissues. The current study supports further exploration of harnessing CSF microcirculation as an alternative to systemic delivery to achieve higher brain tissue exposure, while reducing previously reported ocular toxicity with ABT-414.

Keywords: blood-brain barrier; brain targeted therapy; drug delivery; cerebrospinal fluid microcirculation; brain biodistribution

1. Introduction

Drug delivery via cerebrospinal fluid (CSF) circulation is a pathway allowing the distribution of therapeutics, either small molecules or large biologics, in brain and spinal tissue. This pathway has drawn renewed attention since the recent discovery of the brain-wide perivascular pathway for CSF and interstitial fluid exchange system [1]. For decades, CSF circulation was thought to be limited to flow through the brain ventricles and into the subarachnoid space (SAS) around both the brain and spinal tissue, only exposing contiguous tissues. Now, it is recognized that the CSF also flows through the parenchyma via a mechanism referred to as the CSF microcirculation [2]. The recent literature reported data indicating that this intraparenchymal flow can be harnessed to transport therapeutic molecules to deep regions of the brain [2].

Many biologics with great promise for the treatment of neurodegenerative diseases or tumors have poor brain uptake due to their low permeation across the blood-brain barrier (BBB) following systemic delivery [3,4]. Furthermore, their size is thought to slow transport through brain tissues [5–7]. This includes antibody-drug conjugates (ADCs) targeting epidermal growth factor receptors (EGFRs) expressed on glioblastoma (GBM) tumors [8]. As part of an ongoing effort to overcome the biodistribution challenge of tumor-treating ADCs, we report data verifying that CSF microcirculation indeed enables the brain-wide distribution of an IgG-sized antibody. Our primarily tool compound, ABT-806, is a humanized monoclonal parent antibody (mAb) of Depatuxizumab Mafodotin (Depatux-M, also known as ABT-414). Depatux-M is an antibody-drug conjugate in which the parent antibody is conjugated to a potent antimicrotubule agent, monomethyl auristatin F (MMAF). The antibody selectively binds to a unique conformation of human EGFR that is exposed due to EGFR overexpression, gene amplification, or a mutant form of EGFR with deletions of exons 2 through 7 (EGFRvIII) [9,10].

Intellance-I, a previous phase 3 clinical trial using systemic delivery of ABT-414 in GBM patients, did not provide increased survival benefits. This randomized, placebo-controlled study was conducted with intravenous (IV) administration of the ADC in newly diagnosed GBM patients [11]. According to several authors, the BBBs in these patients were not compromised enough to allow for sufficient crossing of the large-sized therapeutic [8,12]. This setback prompted us to explore whether bypassing the BBB via the CSF microcirculation pathway could lead to improved brain exposure, thereby potentially reviving interest in the use of ADCs for the treatment of EGFR$^+$ GBM tumors.

Here, we report a time course study of ABT-806 biodistribution in the brain parenchyma showing vastly greater and deeper penetration of the antibody when it was administered via the CSF vs. via the IV route. Our toxicology study indicates no toxicity in the brain or the eye, as opposed to the previously reported ocular toxicity of systemically administered ABT-414 [13,14], further suggesting the potential of the CSF microcirculation as a drug delivery pathway. Lastly, we verify that ABT-414 injected into the rat cisterna magna binds to an EGFR$^+$ GBM implant. Although the cisterna magna obviously differs from the location of orthotopic GBM xenografts, it provides a convenient location to verify and optimize the tumor penetration of ABT-414 for future efficacy studies in brain tissues.

2. Materials and Methods

2.1. Animals

Male Sprague Dawley rats were purchased from Charles River Laboratories (Wilmington, MA, USA). A total of 57 rats, 8–12-weeks of age at 300–400 g body weight, were used for intra-CSF administration (n = 18), IV dosing (n = 18), tumor inoculation (n = 12) and toxicology study (n = 9). Rats were socially housed prior to the study in an enriched environment under a 12:12 h light/dark cycle. Diet and sterile tap water were provided ad libitum. All animal studies were reviewed and approved by AbbVie's Institutional Animal Care and Use Committee (IACUC). Animal studies were conducted by an Association for Assessment and Accreditation of Laboratory Animal Care International (AAALAC) accredited program and veterinary care was available to ensure appropriate animal care.

2.2. Intra-Cisterna Magna (ICM) Cannulation Surgery

Two types of cannulation procedures were performed: acute and chronic. Acute cannulation was used in non-survival surgeries where the test articles were injected immediately after catheter implantation and animals were not subsequently recovered. Chronic cannulation was performed in survival surgeries where the cannula was fixed in place for at least 4 h for a single injection and up to 1 month for weekly injections and the animals were allowed to recover from anesthesia. The surgical technique was the same in both acute and chronic cannulation, as described below, and was adapted from Xavier et al. [15]. All injections were performed under anesthesia. IACUC guidelines were followed for both procedures.

Animals were anesthetized in a 3–4% isoflurane induction chamber. Once they achieved a surgical level of anesthesia, as confirmed by the lack of toe pinch reflexes, the surgical area was clipped of hair and prepared with a surgical disinfectant (povidone-iodine or equivalent) followed by 70% alcohol. Surgical preparation was performed in a station separate from the surgery. The surgeon wore sterile gloves and scrubs. Surgical instruments and materials were sterilized prior to use with the first rat. Between rats, instruments were sterilized by immersion in a hot bead sterilizer for 10–15 s and allowed to cool before being used on another animal.

Animals were fixed in the stereotaxic frame using ear bars and a nose cone to maintain isoflurane anesthesia at 2% during the surgery. Ophthalmic ointment was applied to avoid drying of the eyes. The animal head was tilted at an angle of 120° to the body exposing the protruding occipital crest on the back of the skull which was used as the reference point for making incisions. Using a surgical scalpel, the skin was incised approximately 1 cm along the midline to expose the neck muscles below. Two layers of muscle located underneath the skin were subsequently cut and separated at the midline by the blunt side of the scalpel and were held apart using a retractor. The last muscle layer was pulled apart using either a pair of curved forceps or two cotton tip applicators, taking care to avoid tearing of the dura membrane immediately underneath. The exposed inverted triangular structure in between the cerebellum and the medulla, covered by the translucent dura membrane, was identified as the cisterna magna (CM).

The injection was performed using a cannula made up of a beveled 27-gauge needle attached to a PE20 tubing that was connected to a Hamilton syringe, filled with sterile artificial CSF (ACSF, Tocris Bioscience, Bristol, UK). Using a syringe infusion pump, the tubing was filled with either a fluorescently conjugated ABT-806 or ABT-414 solution, ensuring that an air bubble was introduced to separate the test article and the ACSF. The needle was then inserted into the center of the cisterna magna to a depth of ~1 mm, taking care to not puncture the cerebellum or the medulla. For all surgeries, the cannula was fixed in place by dispensing a mixture of dental cement and cyanoacrylate glue onto the dura membrane. The tubing was cut to an approximate 3–5 cm in length and the end was sealed using a hemostat heated in the hot bead sterilizer. This was done to prevent any CSF leakage and to maintain the intracranial pressure [15].

2.3. Acute ICM Cannulation

Immediately after cannula implantation, a dose of 0.3 mg/kg injection was performed with a syringe pump at a rate of 0.8 µL/min to a total volume of 10–15 µL. Post-injection, the test article was allowed to circulate throughout the brain for varying times, i.e., 15 min, 30 min, 45 min, and 60 min, with the cannula remaining in place. At the end of the study and under deep anesthesia, the animal was transferred to a chamber where it was euthanized by CO_2 overdose followed by formalin perfusion and decapitation. The brain was quickly dissected and fixed by immersion in 10% formalin overnight at 4 °C. The following day, the brain was transferred to a phosphate-buffered saline (PBS) solution before it was sectioned and stained.

2.4. Chronic ICM Cannulation

For the 4 h and 24 h timepoints, following 30 min after the injection, the cannula was secured in place as described above and the skin was closed using non-absorbable sutures, wound clips, or tissue adhesive. The animal was recovered from anesthesia and was single housed in a cage to ensure that the cannula was not disturbed. At the respective timepoints, the animal was euthanized, and the brain was collected as explained above.

2.5. IV Dosing

The tail vein was used for systemic administration. The rat was made comfortable in a plastic restrainer. The syringe needle was inserted into the tail vein and a dose of either 0.3, 3 or 10 mg/kg of the test article was injected. Pressure was then applied to the site of injection to stop the bleeding. At either 4 h or 24 h post-injection, the animal was euthanized by CO_2 overdose followed by PBS perfusion and decapitation. The harvested brain was cut in half along the midline. The left hemisphere was fixed in 10% formalin overnight and transferred to PBS the next day for sectioning and immunohistochemistry, whereas the right half was snap frozen in −80 °C for subsequent pharmacokinetic analysis.

2.6. Tumor Inoculation and Dosing

The U87Mgde2,7 cell line, an in-house human EGFRvIII mutant GBM tumor cell line, was used for target engagement studies in the cisterna magna in preparation for future experiments in cortical tissues. A bolus of 0.1×10^6 cells in Spinner Modification of Minimum essential Eagle's medium (SMEM, Sigma-Aldrich, St. Louis, MO, USA) was injected into the CM via the chronic cannulation procedure at a rate of 0.8 μL/min and a total volume of 10 μL. Upon 30 min of injection, the animal was recovered and put back in the home cage. Following 24 h after tumor inoculation, a dose of 0.3 mg/kg of either fluorescently labeled ABT-806, ABT-414, or a 1:1 ratio cocktail of the fluorescent conjugates of ABT-806: ABT-414 was injected under anesthesia through the same implanted cannula. A list of these antibody conjugates is presented in Table 1. At either 30 min, 1 h or 2 h post-injection, the animal was euthanized by CO_2 overdose followed by formalin perfusion and decapitation, and the brain was collected as described above in the ICM cannulation procedure.

Table 1. List of fluorescently labeled antibodies administered in vivo.

Antibody	Specifications
ABT-806	
Type	Parental Antibody—IgG1
Toxin Conjugate	None
FL Dye Conjugate	Alexa Fluor® 555 NHS Ester (Thermo Fisher Scientific—#A20009)
FL Dye Excitation/Emission Wavelength	555/572 nm
FL Dye Extinction Coefficient	155,000 $cm^{-1}\ M^{-1}$
FL Dye Molecular Weight	981 g/mol
ABT-414	
Type	Antibody-Drug Conjugate of ABT-806—IgG1
Toxin Conjugate	Monomethyl Auristatin F (MMAF)
FL Dye Conjugate	Atto 488 NHS ester (Sigma-Aldrich—#41698)
FL Dye Excitation/Emission Wavelength	500/520 nm
FL Dye Extinction Coefficient	90,000 $cm^{-1}\ M^{-1}$
FL Dye Molecular Weight	1250 g/mol

2.7. Sectioning, Immunohistochemistry (IHC), and Imaging

Coronal brain slices were prepared at 50-μm thickness using a vibrating blade microtome (Leica, Wetzlar, DE, USA). For the biodistribution studies, the free-floating tissue slices were stained with 4′,6-diamidino-2-phenylindole (DAPI, Thermo Fisher Scientific, Waltham, MA, USA), a nuclear marker, for 4 min followed by PBS washes. Stained sections were then mounted onto glass slides and cover slipped using prolong gold mounting solution (ProLong® Gold Antifade Mountant). For the tumor studies, tissue slices were permeabilized with 0.3% (v/v) PBS-Triton X-100 (EMD Millipore, Burlington, MA, USA) and blocked with 5% Normal Goat Serum (NGS, Abcam, Cambridge, UK) for 1 h at room temperature. To confirm the identity of the implanted human tumor cells, slices were incubated with human-Lamin A+C antibody (1:250, Abcam) in 0.3% PBS-Triton and 2% NGS for 48 h at 4 °C and subsequently washed with PBS. Sections were then incubated with Alexa Fluor 488 goat anti-rabbit IgG antibody (1:1000, Invitrogen, Waltham, MA, USA) in 0.3% PBS-Triton and 2% NGS for 2 h at room temperature in the dark. DAPI was then added for 4 min, followed by PBS washes, mounting, and cover slipping as explained above [16]. Imaging was performed with the Olympus Fluoview FV1000 confocal laser-scanning microscope.

2.8. Pharmacokinetic (PK) Analysis

In the IV administration studies, the snap frozen brain hemispheres were transferred to pre-weighed low binding tubes. Upon thawing on ice, the brain samples were weighed and homogenized using a mixture of protein inhibitor cocktail (Thermo Fisher Scientific, Waltham, MA, USA) and a custom radioimmunoprecipitation assay (RIPA) buffer (Boston Bioproducts, Milford, MA, USA). The homogenates were centrifuged at 13,000 rpms for 10 min at 4 °C and the supernatants were collected and transferred into 2 mL 96-well low binding plates. The plates were sealed and were used for subsequent ligand-binding assay (LBA) analysis.

The LBA analysis was performed with an in-house MSD (Meso Scale Discovery) assay. An MSD assay is an electro-chemiluminescent where the MSD reader measures the intensity of the light generated from the plate once an electric charge is applied [17]. The samples were transferred to streptavidin plates and were blocked by adding blocking buffer for 1 h at room temperature. The samples were then incubated in a 0.1 µg/mL dilution of a biotinylated goat anti-human IgG antibody for 1 h. Prepared standards and quality controls (QCs) were made at 3 different dilutions of 1:5 resulting in 25×, 125× and 625× serial dilutions, and were then added to the plates. Following 1 h at room temperature, the samples were incubated in a 0.1 µg/mL dilution of goat anti-human IgG Sulfo TAG. After 1 h of incubation time, MSD Read Buffer was added, and plates were read using the MSD Sector Imager. The plates were washed after each step. Details of the MSD assay are provided in Table 2.

Table 2. Meso Scale Discovery (MSD)-based ligand-binding assay for pharmacokinetics (PK) analysis.

Plates
MSD std bind streptavidin plates: MA6000 96 Plate (MSD cat# L11SA-1)
2 mL 96 well polypropylene plates
Buffers
Capture Dilution Buffer: Assay Buffer
Blocking Buffer: 3% MSD Blocker A (MSD cat# R93AA-1) in 1× Phosphate Buffered Saline (PBS)
Wash Buffer: 1× PBS with 0.05% Tween-20 (Obtained from Media Lab)
Standard Dilution Buffer: Assay Buffer
Sample Dilution Buffer for the first and subsequent dilutions: Assay Buffer
Detection Dilution Buffer: Assay Buffer
Assay buffer: 1% MSD Blocker A, in 1× Tris-Buffered Saline (TTBS with 0.02% Tween-20)
Read Buffer: MSD GOLD READ BUFFER A (MSD cat# R92TG-2) is provided at the working concentration and is used at this supplied concentration without any additional dilution.
Equipment
Tecan EVO
MSD QuickPlex 120 Reader
Biotek Stacker Plate Washer
VWR Microplate Shaker
Reagents
Goat anti Human IgG Fc Biotin
Goat anti-human IgG Sulfo TAG = MSD cat # R32AJ-1
Standard Range: In Duplicate
- 25–0.102 ng/mL with 2.5 serial dilution (made with assay buffer)
- Predilute test article 1:200 in PBS by doing a 1:20 dilution (3 µL of stock/57 µL of PBS then further dilute 1:10 (5 µL of previous 1:20/45 µL of PBS)
- Add 6.47 µL of the final predilution into 143.5 µL of assay buffer to make a 2.5 µg/mL Standard
- Serial dilute top standard 1:2.5 in assay buffer 7 times
Quality Controls: In Duplicate (made with assay buffer)

Table 2. *Cont.*

- High = 1.75 µg/mL (4.53 µL of final predilution/145.5 µL of assay buffer)
- Medium = 0.350 µg/mL (1:5 dilutions from High control—20 µL high/80 µL of assay buffer)
- Intermediate = 0.070 µg/mL (1:5 dilutions from Medium control—20 µL high/80 µL of assay buffer)
- Low = 0.014 µg/mL (1:5 dilutions from Intermediate control—20 µL high/80 µL of assay buffer)

2.9. Toxicology Study

The same procedure as in chronic cannulation surgeries was carried out, except that this time, three weekly injections were performed through the same cannula under anesthesia. The treatment groups received ABT-414 at either 0.3 or 1 mg/kg dose, whereas the control group was administered AB095, a non-targeted isotype control of ABT-806, at a dose of 1 mg/kg. At each injection timepoint, a new catheter made up of a 27-gauge needle tip attached to a PE20 tubing was filled with the test article. The catheter was then quickly connected to the previously implanted cannula in the CM and the solution was injected using a syringe pump. To achieve a final injection volume of 10–15 µL, a volume of 12–17 µL was injected, thereby compensating for the residual solution in the implanted cannula. Post-injection, the test article was allowed to flow through the brain for 30 min before the needle was removed, the CM cannula was sealed, and the animal was recovered [15].

2.10. Histopathology and Immunohistochemistry

Within 48 h after the last injection, the animal was euthanized by CO_2 followed by exsanguination. A comprehensive set of tissues was collected and evaluated microscopically. This included the brain and spinal cord with meninges, eyes, heart, lungs, kidneys, liver, peripheral sciatica nerves from right and left legs, spleen, and representative sections of the gastrointestinal tract. To rule out any toxicity related to the surgical procedure of ICM delivery, a trimming scheme recommended for brain sampling in rodents for general toxicity studies was employed. This trimming scheme for brain utilizes 7 coronal sections chosen to contain major functional areas known to be targeted by proven neurotoxicants [18]. The tissue samples were fixed in 10% neutral buffered formalin for 2 days, processed to paraffin blocks, and the sections were stained with hematoxylin and eosin (H&E) for microscopic examination [19].

Vascular Endothelial Growth Factor Receptor 2 (VEGFR2) antibody, an endothelial cell marker, was used for immunohistochemical staining of liver samples from one control animal administered AB095 at 1 mg/kg and one treatment animal administered ABT-414 at 1 mg/kg. Formalin-fixed and paraffin embedded liver sections of 5 mm thickness were stained on BOND RX Automated Research Stainer (Leica Biosystems, Wetzlar, Germany). The relevant details of the IHC assay are provided in the Table 3. The slides were counterstained with hematoxylin, dehydrated in graded alcohol, cleared with xylene, and cover slipped [20].

Table 3. Immunohistochemistry assay for toxicology study.

Antibody	Vascular Endothelial Growth Factor Receptor 2 (VEGFR2)
Primary antibody	
Source	Cell Signaling
Catalog number	9698
Lot number	4
Concentration	59 µg/mL
Dilution	0.6 µg/mL (~1:100)

Table 3. *Cont.*

Antibody	Vascular Endothelial Growth Factor Receptor 2 (VEGFR2)
Incubation time	60 min
Negative control	Rabbit IgG
Source	Abcam
Catalog number	ab172730
Tissues used as positive controls	Liver
Secondary antibody	
Source	BOND Polymer Refine Detection
Catalog number	DS9800
Lot number	69657
Concentration	N/A
Dilution	RTU
Incubation time	8 min
Antigen Retrieval	ER2; pH 9; 40 min on LEICA BOND RX automated stainer
Chromogen	DAB

DAB: 3,3′-Diaminobenzidine tetrahydrochloride hydrate; RTU: Ready to Use.

2.11. Data Analysis for IHC Studies

For analysis, an average of 20–25 stained slices per animal (n = 3 animals) per experimental group were imported into ImageJ software (ImageJ, NIH, Bethesda, MD, USA). Regions of interest (ROIs) consisting of brain tissue but excluding the vasculature, were drawn around the puncta in the interstitium, representing the ABT-806 biodistribution in the brain parenchyma. Integrated density and area were calculated for each ROI. To be able to account for staining variances across brains and compare fluorescence intensity across timepoints, background ROIs were selected in areas of the image with no fluorescence. Average fluorescence was calculated for background ROIs and the following formula was used to calculate the fluorescence intensity:

$$\text{Fluorescence Intensity} = \text{Integrated density} - (\text{area of selected ROI} \times \text{mean fluorescence of background})$$

Statistical difference was calculated by analysis of variance (ANOVA) followed by Tukey's post-hoc test with significance indicated by $p < 0.05$. The sample size is indicated within the corresponding figure legends. All data are presented as mean ± standard error of mean (SEM).

3. Results

To assess whether an intra-CSF injected antibody of size 150 kDa can penetrate the brain parenchyma, we ran a time course study by injecting a fluorescently conjugated ABT-806 solution at a dose of 0.3 mg/kg into the cisterna magna of three rats per timepoint. Ex vivo tissue slices were evaluated for the extent of antibody penetration into the cortex and were compared across multiple timepoints. We found that the antibody followed the well-established route of CSF flow from the CM to the SAS surrounding the brain tissue, as observed by the continuous red color along the edges of the slices (Figure 1a). Subsequently, the antibody entered the cortex through the perivascular spaces along the large penetrating arteries that branched into arterioles. This observation matched the anatomy of these structures where smooth muscle cells form concentric rings along the arteriole lumen [21–23]. The smooth muscle cell morphology is revealed in the bottom panel under 15 min post-injection time, at which timepoint no tissue penetration was observed (Figure 1a).

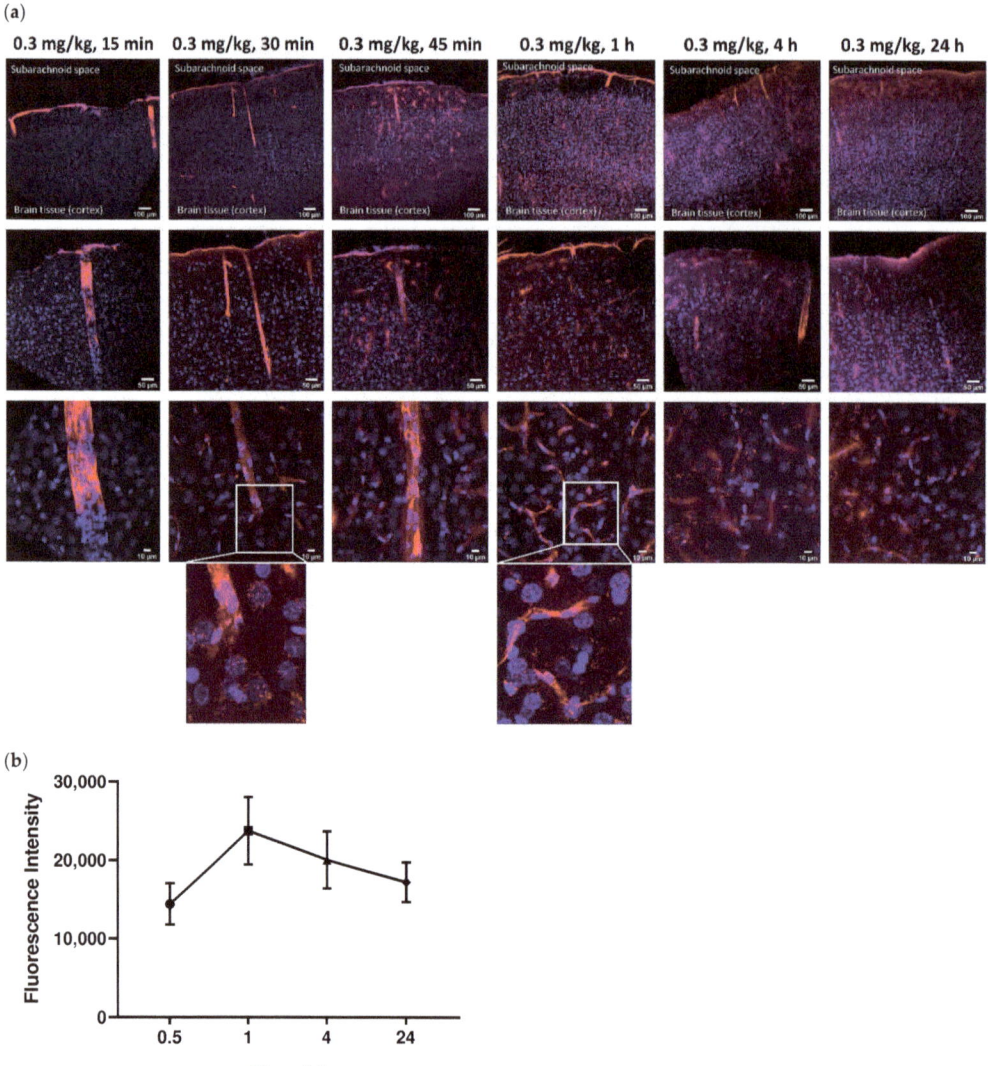

Figure 1. Intra-Cerebrospinal Fluid (CSF) Cortical Biodistribution Data. The parent IgG1 antibody penetrated the brain parenchyma within 30 min of administration into the rat cisterna magna. Representative images. (**a**) Within 15 min post-injection, at a dose of 0.3 mg/kg, intra-CSF administered ABT-806 could only be seen along the periarteriolar spaces with no tissue penetration. After 30 min, the parent antibody started penetrating the brain parenchyma via the periarteriolar spaces. More penetration was observed after 45 min and 60 min of administration with ABT-806 starting to clear out of the parenchyma via the perivenular spaces. The parent antibody continued to enter the parenchyma even after 4 h post-injection. After 24 h, ABT-806 was still present in the tissue. Blue = 4′,6-diamidino-2-phenylindole (DAPI), Red = ABT-806. (**b**) Quantification of the fluorescence intensity in the parenchyma but excluding the vasculature, indicates highest antibody concentrations at 1 h post-injection. 0.5 h: 14,437 ± 2655; 1 h: 23,750 ± 4280; 4 h: 20,063 ± 3635; 24 h: 17,245 ± 2514. $p > 0.05$. $n = 3$ animals per timepoint, average of 20–25 slices per animal per timepoint.

Within 30 min post-injection, the antibody continued to follow the path of CSF microcirculation and was released into the cortical parenchyma via the periarteriolar spaces, as observed by the red puncta near and around the cell nuclei. ABT-806 binds to a unique epitope on EGFR which is only exposed when EGFR is overexpressed or mutated [9]. Since EGFR in healthy tissue is not commonly found in the overexpressed or mutated conformation, our observation suggests non-specific binding of the antibody to the brain cells and the interstitial space (Figure 1a).

Brain harvest after 45 min and 1 h of ICM administration displayed a higher number of penetrating arteries carrying the antibody into the cortex along their perivascular spaces. Additionally, an increased number of red puncta was observed in the brain parenchyma, suggesting a greater extent of tissue penetration. Concurrently, uptake by the perivenular spaces was observed. This observation was confirmed by the anatomy of venules specified by the stellate shape of the smooth muscle cells with interwoven formations around the lumen of the vessels [21–23], noted in the bottom panel under 60 min timepoint (Figure 1a).

Interestingly, after 4 h of ICM injection, the antibody continued to enter the cortex along perivascular spaces and permeated the tissue. Although more ABT-806 was observed to be cleared via the perivenular spaces, the antibody was still present in the brain parenchyma following 24 h post-injection (Figure 1a).

Quantification of the fluorescence intensity in the parenchyma but excluding the vasculature, showed the highest antibody concentration in the cortical parenchyma at 1 h post-injection. It was noteworthy that the mAb concentration in the tissue after 24 h was still higher than that at 30 min following ICM administration (Figure 1b). However, no statistical significance was reached at any timepoint ($p > 0.05$).

In a control study aimed to compare the extent of antibody penetration with systemic administration as opposed to intra-CSF, fluorescently labeled ABT-806 was injected into the rat tail vein at three separate doses and the brains were assessed either 4 h or 24 h post-injection in three rats per experimental group. The dose of 3 mg/kg was chosen to match previous experiments showing antitumor activity at this dose after systemic administration. For bracketing purpose, both a lower and a higher dose were added to the experimental design. The 4 h and 24 h timepoints were selected according to a preliminary DMPK simulation suggesting that upon IV administration, brain concentrations peak at ~ 4 h and plateau at ~ 24 h (data not shown). Injection of a dose of 0.3 mg/kg, the same dose as administered in the ICM studies, resulted in very little red fluorescence inside the brain tissue at either 4 h or 24 h. At 3 mg/kg and 10 mg/kg doses, (10- and ~30-fold higher than administered intra-CSF, respectively), only trace amounts of antibody were visible in the brain parenchyma. This observation further confirms the low permeability of the BBB to molecules of large size when administered systemically (Figure 2a).

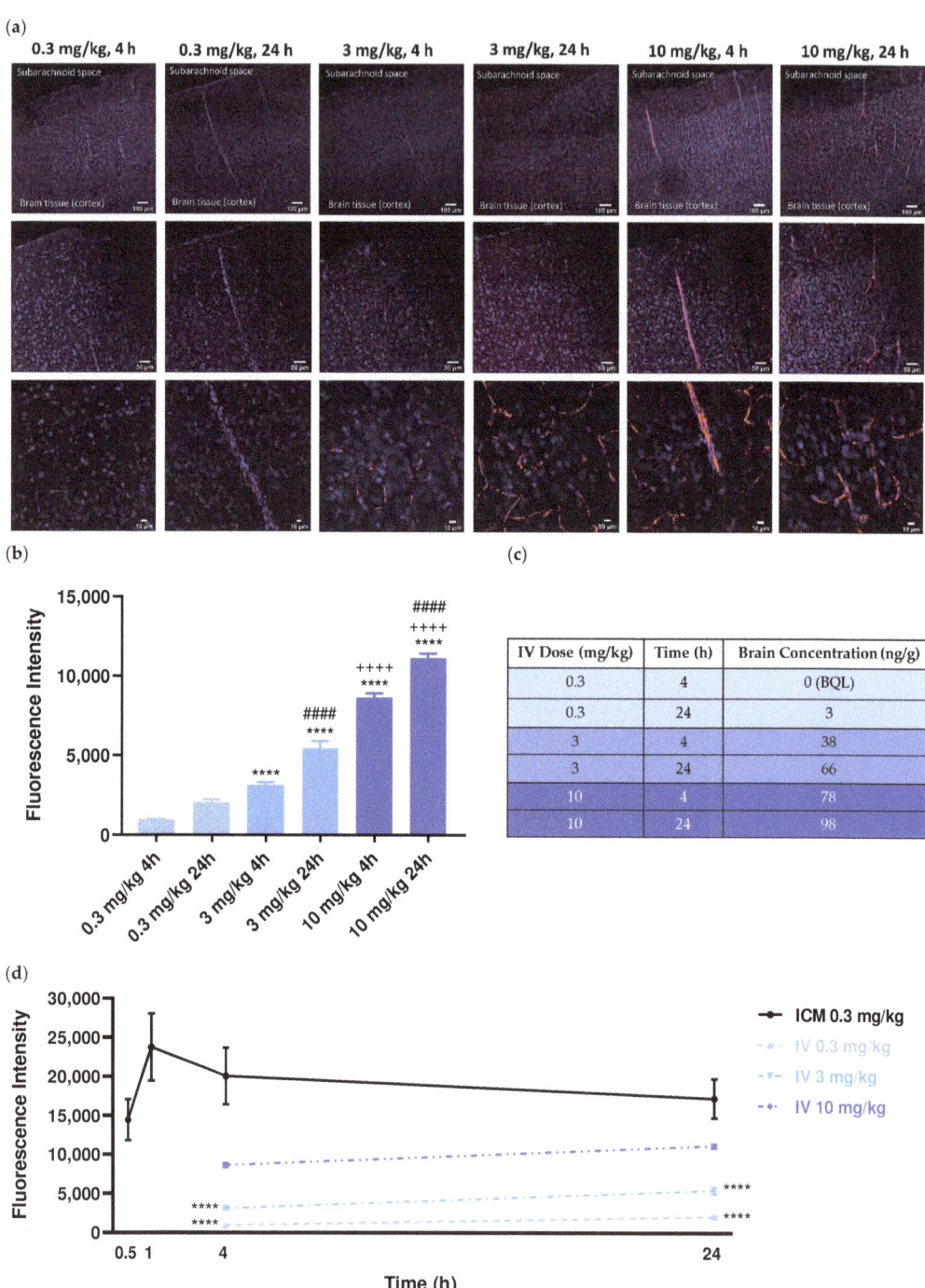

Figure 2. Intravenous (IV) Cortical Biodistribution Data. At equal dose, the tissue penetration of the parent IgG1 antibody administered via the rat tail vein was an order of magnitude lower than when administered intra-CSF. Representative images. (**a**) Upon IV delivery of ABT-806 at 0.3 mg/kg (same

dose as administered intra-CSF), the parent antibody was barely detectable in the brain tissue, both within 4 h and 24 h post-injection. Within 4 h of tail vein injection at 3 mg/kg (10-times higher than administered intra-CSF), ABT-806 was observed in trace amounts in the brain tissue. Even at 10 mg/kg, (~30-fold higher than administered intra-CSF), IV-delivered ABT-806 resulted in low penetration in brain tissue, consistent with a poorly permeable blood-brain barrier (BBB). Blue = DAPI, Red = ABT-806. (**b**) Quantification of the fluorescence intensity (vasculature excluded) displays a dose-response relationship which is also time-dependent. 0.3 mg/kg 4 h: 979.1 ± 51; 0.3 mg/kg 24 h: 2085 ± 163; 3 mg/kg 4 h: 3166 ± 180; 3 mg/kg 24 h: 5452 ± 452; 10 mg/kg 4 h: 8663 ± 272; 10 mg/kg 24 h: 11155 ± 292. **** $p < 0.0001$ vs. 0.3 mg/kg at that timepoint, ++++ $p < 0.0001$ vs. 3 mg/kg at that timepoint, #### $p < 0.0001$ vs. same dose at 4 h; One-way ANOVA, Tukey's post-hoc test. $n = 3$ animals per timepoint, average of 20–25 slices per animal per timepoint. (**c**) The IHC observation and quantification are consistent with the results from the PK analysis of IV-administered brain homogenates that are summarized in the table. BQL = Below Quantification Limit. (**d**) Comparison of the fluorescence intensity between ICM and IV administered brains indicates an order of magnitude higher exposures with intra-CSF vs. systemic administration at 0.3 mg/kg dose. **** $p < 0.0001$ vs. ICM at that timepoint; Two-way ANOVA, Tukey's post-hoc test.

Quantification of the fluorescence intensity indicated the antibody concentration to be both dose- and time-dependent. The concentration of the fluorescently labeled ABT-806 was lowest at the 0.3 mg/kg dose at 4 h and highest at the 10 mg/kg at 24 h ($p < 0.0001$) (Figure 2b). The results from the PK analysis matched our ex vivo imaging observations. The fluorescently labeled ABT-806 was non-detectable in the brain homogenate within 4 h of IV injection at 0.3 mg/kg, consistent with our finding of trace amounts of antibody in the brain slices. Upon 24 h of administration, the antibody concentration was reported at 3 ng per g of total brain homogenate weight. Higher doses of 3 and 10 mg/kg at 4 h post-injection resulted in greater brain concentrations of 38 and 78 ng/g, respectively. Furthermore, the antibody concentration was reported to increase to 66 and 98 ng/g within 24 h of injection at the two higher doses (Figure 2c).

Comparison of the fluorescence intensity between ICM and IV groups showed an order of magnitude higher antibody concentrations in the brain parenchyma following intra-CSF administration at 0.3 mg/kg. At 4 h and 24 h post ICM injections at a dose of 0.3 mg/kg, fluorescence intensity was significantly higher than that of IV administration at either 0.3 or 3 mg/kg ($p < 0.0001$). Interestingly, following 24 h after IV dosing at 10 mg/kg, the antibody concentration was still lower than that of 30 min post-ICM injection at 0.3 mg/kg (~30-fold lower dose) (Figure 2d).

To assess the extent of antibody penetration via intra-CSF administration, subcortical brain regions including the hippocampus, were analyzed ex vivo, in three animal brains per timepoint. Within 30 min post-injection, ABT-806 delivered via the cisterna magna at a dose of 0.3 mg/kg had penetrated the dentate gyrus layer of the hippocampus, including its molecular layer, subgranular zone and the hilus. The antibody presence was observed in these layers following 1 h, 4 h and 24 h after injection (Figure 3).

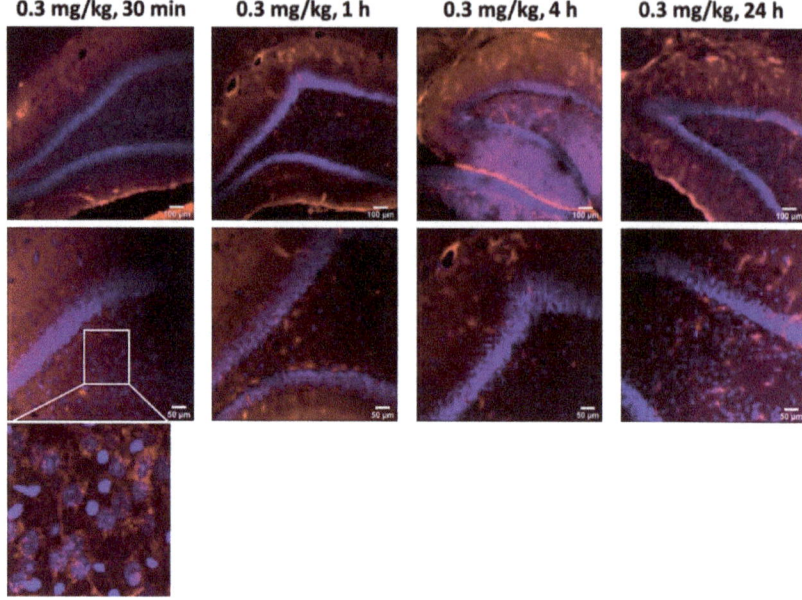

Figure 3. Intra-CSF Subcortical Biodistribution Data. The parent IgG1 antibody penetrated deep into the hippocampal parenchyma within 30 min of administration into the rat cisterna magna. Representative images. Intra-CSF delivery of ABT-806 at a dose of 0.3 mg/kg resulted in the penetration of the antibody into the deeper brain regions, including the hippocampus, as early as 30 min post injection. The antibody was still present in the subcortical regions after 24 h. Blue = DAPI, Red = ABT-806. n = 3 animals per timepoint.

Target engagement studies were performed to evaluate the in vivo binding of ABT-806 and ABT-414 to GBM tumor cells directly implanted in the cisterna magna of three rats per experimental group. The cisterna magna was chosen as a prelude to future experiments to be conducted with orthotopic implants located in the cortical or subcortical area of the parenchyma. The CM was deemed to be an "easy-to-reach" area of the brain to verify target engagement and to study the effect of ADC dilution without introducing too many variables. Efficacy is not reported here. This will be investigated in a follow-up study with orthotopically implanted GBM cells.

The injected tumor cells formed clusters within 24 h of injection and attached to the cell linings of the cisterna magna and the fourth ventricle. Within 30 min of ABT-806 administration, in vivo binding to the outer layer of the tumor cell cluster was observed. This observation suggested penetration to the core might have been hindered by receptor saturation at the tumor periphery. Deeper penetration of the parent antibody was found after 1 h (Figure 4a). To confirm the binding of the antibody to human tumor cells as opposed to rat tissue, human-Lamin A + C antibody, a nuclear envelope marker, was used for immunostaining. This antibody colocalized with DAPI, a nuclear cell marker, only in the tumor cell cluster, which further confirmed the nature of the cell cluster as human (Figure 4b). Additionally, ICM administration of ABT-414 within 24 h of tumor cell implantation in the cisterna magna resulted in in vivo binding. The extent of the ADC penetration into the core of the tumor cluster was greater after 2 h vs. 1 h (Figure 4c). To verify our receptor saturation hypothesis, we injected a 1:1 ratio mixture of ABT-806: ABT-414 through the CM cannula and assessed target engagement 2 h post-injection. We found a higher concentration of ABT-414 within the tumor cluster core, as evidenced by a brighter fluorescence intensity (Figure 4d). This finding was a confirmation that we could indeed increase ADC transport to the center of the tumor cell cluster by utilizing the parent antibody to occupy target GBM receptors at the periphery.

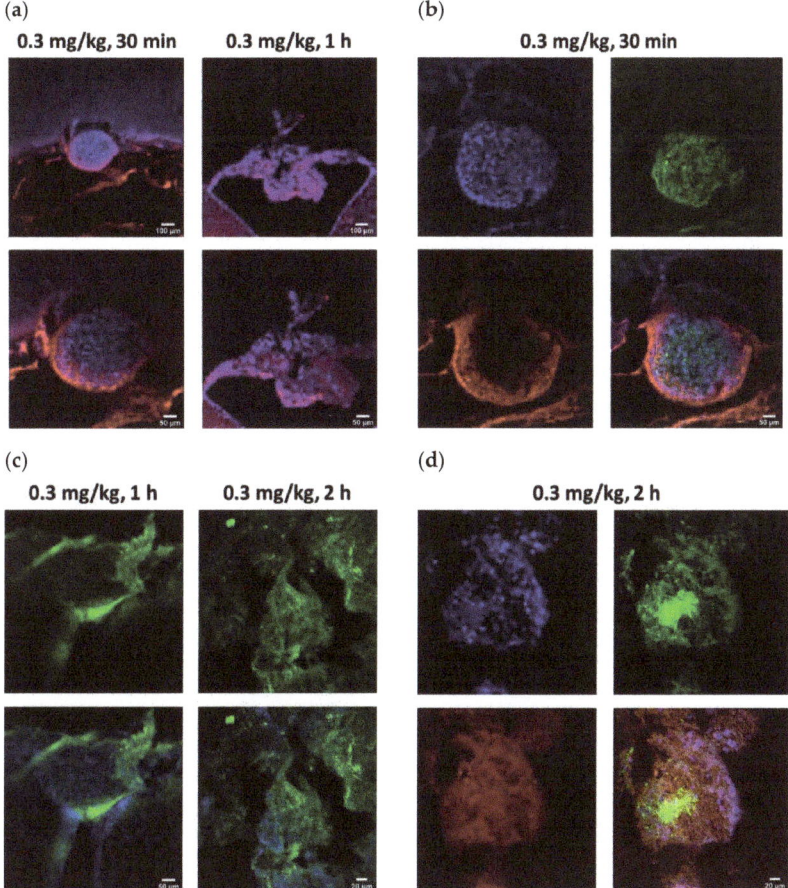

Figure 4. Target Engagement. Intra-CSF injection of U87MGde2,7 tumor cell line followed by next day intra-cisterna magna (ICM) delivery of fluorescently labeled ABT-806 or ABT-414 (FL-ABT-806 or FL-ABT-414) resulted in in vivo binding. Representative images. (**a**) FL-ABT-806 bound to tumor cells after 30 min of intra-CSF delivery. Antibody penetration was limited to the tumor periphery, as evidenced by the red color only on the outer layer of the tumor cluster. The antibody penetrated deeper into the tumor cluster 1 h post-injection, as seen by the red puncta inside. (**b**) To confirm that FL-ABT-806 bound to human tumor cells as opposed to the rat tissue, human-Lamin A + C antibody was used for immunostaining. This antibody colocalized with DAPI only in the tumor cell cluster, thereby confirming the human nature of the cells. Blue = DAPI, Red = FL-ABT-806, Green = Human-Lamin A+C. (**c**) Intra-CSF delivery of FL-ABT-414 resulted in deeper penetration into the tumor cluster 2 h vs. 1 h post-injection, as evidenced by more green puncta inside the tumor. (**d**) ICM administration of a "cocktail" with 1:1 ratio of FL-conjugates of ABT-806: ABT-414 increased penetration of FL-ABT-414 into the tumor cluster core after 2 h of injection, as seen by a higher intensity of green color inside the tumor. Blue = DAPI, Red = FL-ABT-806, Green = FL-ABT-414. $n = 3$ animals per treatment group.

The toxicology study indicated no definite microscopic findings directly related to ICM delivery in three rats per experimental group receiving either AB095 (non-specific and payload-free) or ABT-414 (target binding) antibodies. There were no microscopic changes indicative of neurotoxicity in either the brain or the spinal cord such as neuronal necrosis, gliosis, or axonal degeneration (Figure 5a). No inflammation or neuronal necrosis in the neuropil adjacent to the site of catheter placement was observed. Additionally, there were no significant microscopic findings in the eye. Emphasis was placed on evaluating cornea as corneal toxicity has been reported after intravenous administration of ABT-414 in previous nonclinical studies [24] and clinical trials [13] (Figure 5a).

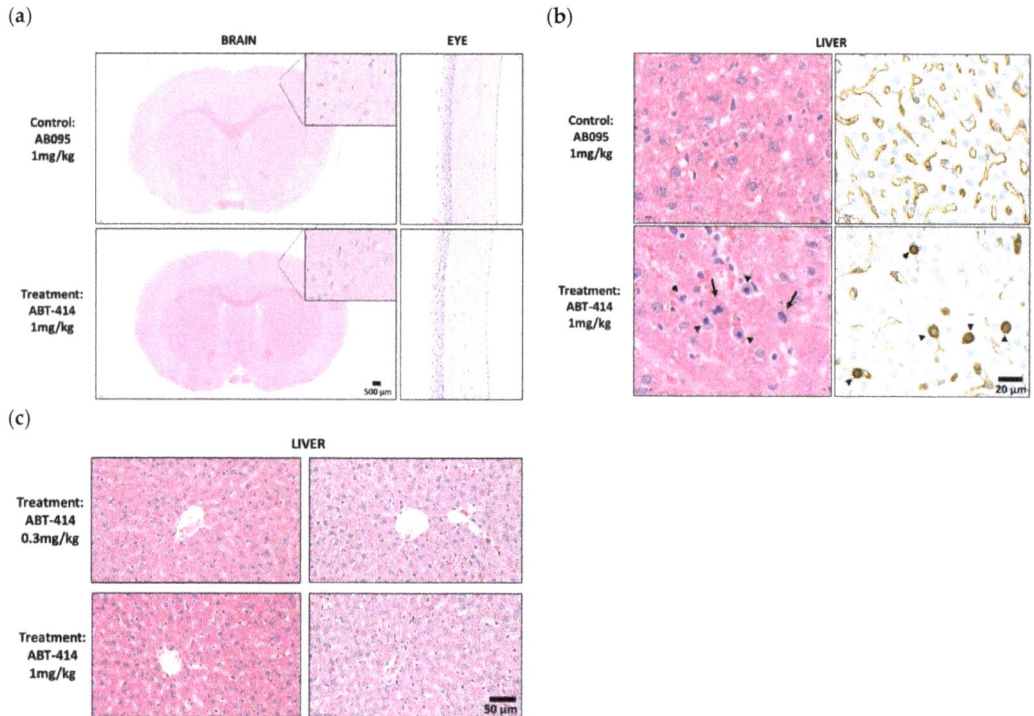

Figure 5. Toxicity Data. No toxicity was found with ICM delivery of ABT-414 in the brain. Systemic exposure was observed in the liver of one rat. Representative images of brain (left), eye (middle), and liver (right) from one control animal administered 1 mg/kg AB095 (upper panel) and one treatment animal administered 1 mg/kg ABT-414 (lower panel). (**a**) There was no toxicity in the brain (inset showing healthy neurons from the cerebral cortex) and eye (cornea). (**b**) In the liver of one animal administered 1 mg/kg ABT-414, there were increased number of mitotic figures and single cell necrosis within hepatocytes (arrows) and mitotically arrested sinusoidal cells (arrow heads) in the animal administered ABT-414 (H&E). Sinusoidal cells showed strong reactivity to Vascular Endothelial Growth Factor Receptor 2 (VEGFR2) immunostaining (arrow heads, lower right corner). In contrast, VEGFR2 staining of control rat liver tissue showed diffuse and continuous positive signal in sinusoidal endothelial cells (SECs) lining the hepatic cords (upper right corner) (IHC). (**c**) There were no microscopic liver changes associated with ICM delivery of a lower dose of ABT-414 at 0.3 mg/kg. The other two rats administered ABT-414 at 1 mg/kg did not show any microscopic findings in the liver (H&E). n = 3 animals per treatment group.

The only ABT-414-related microscopic findings were observed in the liver of a single animal at 1 mg/kg and were characterized by increased numbers of atypical mitotic figures representing metaphase arrest within hepatocytes and sinusoidal cells. The sinusoidal cells were demonstrated to be sinusoidal endothelial cells (SECs) by immunostaining with endothelial cell marker VEGFR2 (Figure 5b). These minimal liver findings were qualitatively consistent with those observed previously with intravenous administration of ABT-414 and were indicative of limited systemic exposure to the drug. However, such microscopic liver observations were not found in either the 0.3 mg/kg treatment group, nor the other two rats receiving the 1 mg/kg dose (Figure 5c).

4. Discussion

The current study verifies the feasibility of utilizing intra-CSF delivery to achieve deep brain exposure with high molecular weight biologics. This is consistent with earlier studies from Iliff et al., 2012 and 2013 [1,25,26], Yadav et al., 2017 [27], and Pizzo et al., 2018 [28] and further confirms that CSF microcirculation holds promise to deliver antibodies into deep brain regions. It is noteworthy that the molecular weight, depth of penetration and imaging resolution reported here, i.e., requisites for the delivery of molecules the size of mAbs and ADCs by bypassing the BBB, were all greater than those reported in previously published studies.

In the landmark study of CSF microcirculation discovery, Iliff et al. injected fluorescent tracers of small (759 Da and 3 kDa), intermediate (45 kDa), and large (500 kDa and 2000 kDa) molecular weight into the cisterna magna of rodents. They observed that in contrast to dyes of small or intermediate size that penetrated the interstitium within 30 min of injection, the 500 kDa and 2000 kDa tracers remained confined to the perivascular spaces [1,25,26]. While these studies were significant milestones, the feasibility of achieving similar results with a molecule in the orders of hundreds of kDa molecular weight, such as a 150 kDa antibody, remained unexplored. Additionally, tissue penetration was only reported at the level of the cortex within a 240 μm depth from the surface using in vivo two-photon confocal microscopy [1,26]. In comparison our study reports penetration within mm depths of the cortical surface. The ex vivo fluorescence distribution analysis of the whole brain slices was quantified at a 4× magnification and at 30 min post-injection timepoint only [1]. Our data span quantification up to 24 h following intra-CSF administration and at 64× magnification.

Yadav et al. performed a 6-week continuous intracerebroventricular (ICV) infusion study in non-human primates with a 56 kDa anti-BACE1 IgG antibody as well as a 150 kDa control IgG antibody. They observed uniform distribution of both antibodies throughout the brain parenchyma including both cortical and subcortical regions, not unlike what we found in our biodistribution findings. The brain concentrations were quantified using ELISA on brain homogenates as well as ex vivo fluorescence microscopy on whole brain slices at a low imaging resolution [27]. Our ex vivo analysis of brain slices increased resolution significantly. This was accomplished by drawing multiple ROIs in each brain slice only around the puncta indicative of mAb penetration while making sure to exclude the perivascular spaces, averaging the fluorescence intensity of those ROIs and correcting against the background in an average of ~70 slices per timepoint.

Pizzo et al. compared the brain penetration of a 16.8 kDa single-domain antibody (sdAb) to that of a 150 kDa IgG antibody with ICM infusion. Using ex vivo fluorescence imaging and in vivo 3D magnetic resonance imaging (MRI), they observed widespread distribution of both molecules in deep brain regions where the sdAb crossed the perivascular spaces much more easily than the full-size antibody, resulting in a four to seven-fold higher brain exposure as measured by the percentage area with antibody signal within brain slices [28]. Our research builds on Pizzo et al. work by revealing extensive mAb penetration in deep brain areas using a quantification technique with higher resolution in the brain tissue but excluding the perivascular spaces. Using punctate immunostaining as evidence for parenchymal penetration has been previously used with IV administered BBB-permeable single-domain antibodies [29].

Our study demonstrates that an intra-CSF administered antibody follows the recently established path of CSF microcirculation by flowing along the perivascular spaces before distributing itself into the interstitial space of both cortical and subcortical brain regions. Our finding of antibody penetration into the brain tissue was based on the observation of large numbers of puncta near and around the cell nuclei, suggesting non-specific binding.

Non-specific binding can result from binding of the antibody to amino acids outside of the target epitope of the antigen. This includes interactions between the antibody, serum proteins and/or endogenous molecules in the tissue that can affect the IHC detection [30]. Non-specific binding can result in high background staining which in turn, can cause the target antigen to optically appear at the incorrect location. However, such artifacts did not perturb our findings, as the antigen of interest, i.e., overexpressed or mutated EGFR, is not found in healthy brain tissues. This gives us confidence that the observed non-specific binding indicates permeation of the antibody into the interstitium.

The dose administered in our ICM administration studies was an order of magnitude lower than that administered systemically in preclinical studies and clinical trials with ABT-414 [10,11,14]. We hypothesized that by bypassing the BBB, ICM injection would give rise to higher brain concentrations of antibodies at lower doses compared to IV administration. In addition to using the same 0.3 mg/kg ICM dose, two higher doses of 3 and 10 mg/kg were selected for IV delivery to facilitate comparison with prior studies with systemic administration [10,11,14].

Quantification of the fluorescence intensity in ICM administered brain slices represents relative concentrations of ABT-806 in the parenchyma. Although semi-quantitative from the standpoint of drug concentration in the parenchyma, the preliminary PK data is remarkable in that the rates of uptake and clearance are quite high, considering that the transport of large molecules through the extracellular matrix is hindered by narrow space, high tortuosity, and potentially, by a variety of physicochemical interactions [2]. We also want to caution that this PK profile might have been affected by the anesthesia state resulting in a higher CSF flow [1,31] and/or our ex vivo analysis. It has been shown that brain perfusion and fixation can cause the perivascular spaces to collapse and significantly reduce their size compared to their natural state in vivo, resulting in the release of the material into the parenchyma [32]. However, we believe our observation is not an ex vivo procedural artifact since the uptake of the antibody by perivenular spaces could not have occurred without prior transport from the periarteriolar spaces into the interstitial fluid of the parenchyma while the animal was still alive. In addition, the drug could not have appeared in the venules as a result of CSF bulk clearance since the antibody is observed in the perivenular spaces and not in the vasculature.

The observed time- and dose- dependency in our IV delivery study is in line with previous reports of systemically administered antibodies. Lee and Tannock reported the distribution of cetuximab and trastuzumab in tumor xenografts to be both time- and dose-dependent after systemic injection. These observations were not made in the healthy brain tissue, as was the case in our study, but rather in relation to distance from blood vessels and regions of hypoxia in the tumor [33]. Later on, two review papers by Lucas et al. mentioned time and dose as factors affecting the pharmacokinetic disposition of mAbs and ADCs within tumors [34,35]. In another study, a BBB penetrating bispecific antibody of 210 kDa in size displayed time- dependent brain concentrations, expressed as percent of injected dose per gram tissue (%ID/g). The brain exposure was higher within the first 8 h post IV injection, followed by a net elimination up to 24 h [36]. This observation matches the reports on time- and dose- dependent changes in antibody turnover and clearance as a function of the half-life [37,38].

Our preliminary study of target engagement with ABT-806 and ABT-414 in ICM implanted tumors shows that both the mAb and ADC can bind to the tumor cells though intra-CSF administration. Target engagement is achieved by the binding of these compounds to the epitope of interest on the human tumor cells. Incomplete ABT-806 penetration into the tumor cluster was observed within 30 min of injection. This raises the question as to whether the kinetic of transport within the tumor was diffusion-limited or target engagement-limited. We think that the answer is a mix of both: we did observe higher antibody penetration into the tumor core by increasing the circulation time to 1 h and 2 h. We also demonstrated that a 1:1 molar mixture of ABT-806 with ABT-414 increased the occupancy of the peripheral receptors by the parent antibody, leading to increased ADC penetration in the GBM cluster core. The latter is consistent with the receptor saturation hypothesis previously reported elsewhere [39].

Our toxicology study with ICM administration of ABT-414 indicates no microscopic findings in tissues exposed to the CSF flow, i.e., the brain, spinal cord, and eyes. The minimal liver findings in one rat at 1 mg/kg are consistent with limited ABT-414 systemic exposure that matches the exit pathway of the CSF circulation through the venous system [2]. The objective of the toxicology study was primarily to evaluate potential central nervous system (CNS) effects related to ICM delivery and associated distribution in the cerebral parenchyma. We did not intend to fully characterize the systemic toxicity of ABT-414 that has been comprehensively evaluated after IV administration in monkeys and mice. Mitotic arrest with secondary apoptotic cell death has been reported with microtubule inhibitors such as auristatin and maytansinoid derivatives in a diverse set of tissues, including the liver [40,41]. Minimal to mild mitotic arrest in the absence of associated tissue structural alteration is usually considered non-adverse. In the toxicology study reported here, increased mitoses/mitotic arrest was observed only in the liver (sinusoidal cells and hepatocytes) in a single rat dosed with ABT-414 at 1 mg/kg, indicating limited systemic exposure to ABT-414. In addition, the mitotic arrest was not associated with parenchymal injury and this minimal liver finding was non adverse. Future toxicology studies should include clinical pathology parameters such as liver enzymes levels to better correlate with our microscopic findings. Collecting toxicokinetic data exploiting bioanalytical measurements from the plasma would also help further evaluate the systemic exposure achieved after ICM delivery.

The ICM cannulation procedures used throughout this study provide a relatively simple and safe pathway to access the CSF circulation in rodents. Future studies in rodents will be conducted using ICV cannulation. This is because, unlike ICM delivery, ICV is translatable to humans.

Except for patients with head and neck injuries, ICM delivery via a suboccipital puncture is not seen as routinely translatable to clinical practice due to unacceptable procedural risks of serious, or fatal, complications. These can include inadvertent injury to vascular structures and brainstem damage. An alternate ICM route has been reported requiring the adaptation of intravascular microcatheter, which can be safely navigated intrathecally under fluoroscopic guidance. This approach to ICM delivery has been used to deliver viral vectors to the brain. Despite its promise, this ICM technique has not yet reached wide adoption [42].

Two approaches to intra-CSF drug delivery are currently considered acceptable in humans: Intrathecal (IT) or ICV delivery. With CSF "near stagnant" in the lumbar area, IT delivery requires pumping a higher initial dose to reach the SAS at therapeutic levels, a precondition to sustained penetration via the microcirculation system. In contrast, ICV delivery leverages brain physiology by infusing the drug proximal to the site of CSF production, thereby allowing the drug to go with the outward flow of the CSF in the direction of the SAS [2]. Despite its invasive nature, ICV delivery in humans is gaining more acceptance, for the treatment of acute and rapidly progressing conditions. A state of the art, fully implantable ICV system is currently used in a clinical trial to treat refractory epilepsy [43]. A comprehensive review of the safety of ICV delivery by Cohen-Pfeffer et al. can be found here [44].

5. Conclusions and Future Directions

This biodistribution data combined with preliminary evidence of no toxicity raise the hope that CSF delivery might be a viable route to expose diseased brain tissues to therapeutic mAbs or ADCs. This is important because the low permeability of the BBB to mAbs renders promising therapeutics ineffective or toxic when administered systemically, as observed in past clinical trials [11,13,14]. This was quite apparent in our study of IV delivered ABT-806, where trace amounts of antibody were detected in the brain tissue.

ABT-806 and ABT-414 were used as model molecules to determine whether intra-CSF delivery holds promise for the treatment of large regions of the brain. Their choice by no means implies that they are currently viewed as lead compounds for the treatment of GBM. It is too early to conclude that therapeutic doses can be achieved through this route of administration. Nonetheless this proof-of-concept study has intriguing ramifications for the future of drug delivery in both neuro-oncology and neuroscience.

While the preliminary PK profile obtained via image analysis provides useful insight on the rate of penetration and clearance of unbound molecules, it remains only semi-quantitative. Fully quantitative PK studies are underway by ex vivo analysis of brain homogenates as well as in vivo sampling of brain tissues using microdialysis after intra-CSF administration. Should PK studies confirm that a therapeutic dose is achievable with ABT-414, we may proceed to verify efficacy against cortically implanted GBM models.

Although commonly used in rodent studies, ICM delivery would not be suitable in humans for safety reasons. Our future preclinical studies will therefore utilize the ICV route of administration. A review of suppliers has revealed that ICV technology for human use has become safer and easier to use in recent years. While systemic delivery is clearly preferable over intra-CSF delivery, the desired outcome of this research would be a future where ICV delivery would enable therapies that would otherwise be prevented or hampered by side effects when administered systemically.

If the ability of achieving deep penetration of IgG-size biologics throughout the entire brain is confirmed in higher order species, the strategy of circumventing the BBB via CSF microcirculation would also be preferred over localized drug delivery modalities such as focused ultrasounds or intraparenchymal injections, especially when diseased tissues are present throughout large regions of the brain.

Author Contributions: Conceptualization, E.B.R. and D.R.L.; Data curation, G.N.K. and P.K.; Formal analysis, G.N.K.; Funding acquisition, D.R.L.; Investigation, G.N.K.; Methodology, G.N.K., P.K. and S.E.B.; Project administration, G.N.K. and P.K.; Resources, S.E.B., E.B.R. and D.R.L.; Supervision, S.E.B. and D.R.L.; Validation, S.E.B. and D.R.L.; Visualization, G.N.K. and P.K.; Writing—original draft, G.N.K., P.K. and D.R.L.; Writing—review & editing, S.E.B., E.B.R. and D.R.L. All authors have read and agreed to the published version of the manuscript.

Funding: This research received no external funding.

Institutional Review Board Statement: The study was conducted according to the guidelines of the Association for Assessment and Accreditation of Laboratory Animal Care International and approved by AbbVie's Institutional Animal Care and Use Committee (protocol code: 2007A00086; date of approval: 26 August 2020).

Informed Consent Statement: Not applicable.

Data Availability Statement: The data that support the findings of this study are available upon reasonable request.

Acknowledgments: The authors wish to thank Magali Guffroy of AbbVie for her review of the toxicology sections; John Harlan, Enrico Digiammarino, and Matthew Ravn of AbbVie for preparing fluorescent conjugates of antibodies; Phil Krueger, Shuai Niu, Michelle L Viner, and Ian Haire of AbbVie for helping with the LBA analysis; Phuong Le of AbbVie for providing tumor cells; Kuldip Mirakhur for help with the animal research; AbbVie veterinary staff for providing support for animal care; and Ramakrishna Venugopalan and Shuhong Zhang of AbbVie for their support and funding of the project.

Conflicts of Interest: All authors are employees of AbbVie and may own AbbVie stock. AbbVie sponsored and funded the study; contributed to the design; participated in the collection, analysis, and interpretation of data, and in writing, reviewing, and approval of the final publication.

References

1. Iliff, J.J.; Wang, M.; Liao, Y.; Plogg, B.A.; Peng, W.; Gundersen, G.A.; Benveniste, H.; Vates, G.E.; Deane, R.; Goldman, S.A.; et al. A paravascular pathway facilitates CSF flow through the brain parenchyma and the clearance of interstitial solutes, including amyloid beta. *Sci. Transl. Med.* **2012**, *4*, 147ra111. [CrossRef] [PubMed]
2. Naseri Kouzehgarani, G.; Feldsien, T.; Engelhard, H.H.; Mirakhur, K.K.; Phipps, C.; Nimmrich, V.; Clausznitzer, D.; Lefebvre, D.R. Harnessing cerebrospinal fluid circulation for drug delivery to brain tissues. *Adv. Drug Deliv. Rev.* **2021**, *173*, 20–59. [CrossRef] [PubMed]
3. Banks, W.A. From blood-brain barrier to blood-brain interface: New opportunities for CNS drug delivery. *Nat. Rev. Drug Discov.* **2016**, *15*, 275–292. [CrossRef]
4. Veldhuijzen van Zanten, S.E.M.; De Witt Hamer, P.C.; van Dongen, G. Brain Access of Monoclonal Antibodies as Imaged and Quantified by (89) Zr-Antibody PET: Perspectives for Treatment of Brain Diseases. *J. Nucl. Med.* **2019**, *60*, 615–616. [CrossRef]
5. Wolak, D.J.; Thorne, R.G. Diffusion of macromolecules in the brain: Implications for drug delivery. *Mol. Pharm.* **2013**, *10*, 1492–1504. [CrossRef] [PubMed]
6. Wolak, D.J.; Pizzo, M.E.; Thorne, R.G. Probing the extracellular diffusion of antibodies in brain using in vivo integrative optical imaging and ex vivo fluorescence imaging. *J. Control. Release* **2015**, *197*, 78–86. [CrossRef]
7. Pardridge, W.M. Blood-Brain Barrier and Delivery of Protein and Gene Therapeutics to Brain. *Front. Aging Neurosci.* **2019**, *11*, 373. [CrossRef]
8. Marin, B.M.; Porath, K.A.; Jain, S.; Kim, M.; Conage-Pough, J.E.; Oh, J.H.; Miller, C.L.; Talele, S.; Kitange, G.J.; Tian, S.; et al. Heterogeneous delivery across the blood-brain barrier limits the efficacy of an EGFR-targeting antibody drug conjugate in glioblastoma. *Neuro-Oncology* **2021**, *23*, 2042–2053. [CrossRef]
9. Reilly, E.B.; Phillips, A.C.; Buchanan, F.G.; Kingsbury, G.; Zhang, Y.; Meulbroek, J.A.; Cole, T.B.; DeVries, P.J.; Falls, H.D.; Beam, C.; et al. Characterization of ABT-806, a Humanized Tumor-Specific Anti-EGFR Monoclonal Antibody. *Mol. Cancer Ther.* **2015**, *14*, 1141–1151. [CrossRef]
10. Phillips, A.C.; Boghaert, E.R.; Vaidya, K.S.; Mitten, M.J.; Norvell, S.; Falls, H.D.; DeVries, P.J.; Cheng, D.; Meulbroek, J.A.; Buchanan, F.G.; et al. ABT-414, an Antibody-Drug Conjugate Targeting a Tumor-Selective EGFR Epitope. *Mol. Cancer Ther.* **2016**, *15*, 661–669. [CrossRef]
11. ClinicalTrials.gov. Available online: https://clinicaltrials.gov/ct2/show/NCT02573324?term=ABT-414&phase=1&draw=2&rank=2 (accessed on 7 February 2022).
12. Abounader, R.; Schiff, D. The blood-brain barrier limits the therapeutic efficacy of antibody-drug conjugates in glioblastoma. *Neuro-Oncology* **2021**, *23*, 1993–1994. [CrossRef] [PubMed]
13. Parrozzani, R.; Lombardi, G.; Midena, E.; Leonardi, F.; Londei, D.; Padovan, M.; Caccese, M.; Marchione, G.; Bini, S.; Zagonel, V.; et al. Corneal side effects induced by EGFR-inhibitor antibody-drug conjugate ABT-414 in patients with recurrent glioblastoma: A prospective clinical and confocal microscopy study. *Ther. Adv. Med. Oncol.* **2020**, *12*, 1758835920907543. [CrossRef] [PubMed]
14. Van Den Bent, M.; Eoli, M.; Sepulveda, J.M.; Smits, M.; Walenkamp, A.; Frenel, J.S.; Franceschi, E.; Clement, P.M.; Chinot, O.; De Vos, F.; et al. INTELLANCE 2/EORTC 1410 randomized phase II study of Depatux-M alone and with temozolomide vs temozolomide or lomustine in recurrent EGFR amplified glioblastoma. *Neuro-Oncology* **2020**, *22*, 684–693. [CrossRef] [PubMed]
15. Xavier, A.L.R.; Hauglund, N.L.; von Holstein-Rathlou, S.; Li, Q.; Sanggaard, S.; Lou, N.; Lundgaard, I.; Nedergaard, M. Cannula Implantation into the Cisterna Magna of Rodents. *J. Vis. Exp.* **2018**, *135*, e57378. [CrossRef]
16. Abcam. Available online: https://www.abcam.com/protocols/immunostaining-paraffin-frozen-free-floating-protocol (accessed on 5 October 2020).
17. Bastarache, J.A.; Koyama, T.; Wickersham, N.E.; Ware, L.B. Validation of a multiplex electrochemiluminescent immunoassay platform in human and mouse samples. *J. Immunol. Methods* **2014**, *408*, 13–23. [CrossRef]
18. Rao, D.B.; Little, P.B.; Sills, R.C. Subsite awareness in neuropathology evaluation of National Toxicology Program (NTP) studies: A review of select neuroanatomical structures with their functional significance in rodents. *Toxicol. Pathol.* **2014**, *42*, 487–509. [CrossRef]
19. Feldman, A.T.; Wolfe, D. Tissue processing and hematoxylin and eosin staining. *Methods Mol. Biol.* **2014**, *1180*, 31–43. [CrossRef]
20. Kohnken, R.; Falahatpisheh, H.; Janardhan, K.S.; Guffroy, M. Anatomic and Clinical Pathology Characterization of Drug-Induced Sinusoidal Obstruction Syndrome (Veno-Occlusive Disease) in Cynomolgus Macaques. *Toxicol. Pathol.* **2022**, *50*, 13–22. [CrossRef]
21. Ushiwata, I.; Ushiki, T. Cytoarchitecture of the smooth muscles and pericytes of rat cerebral blood vessels. A scanning electron microscopic study. *J. Neurosurg.* **1990**, *73*, 82–90. [CrossRef]
22. Armulik, A.; Genove, G.; Betsholtz, C. Pericytes: Developmental, physiological, and pathological perspectives, problems, and promises. *Dev. Cell* **2011**, *21*, 193–215. [CrossRef]
23. Hartmann, D.A.; Underly, R.G.; Grant, R.I.; Watson, A.N.; Lindner, V.; Shih, A.Y. Pericyte structure and distribution in the cerebral cortex revealed by high-resolution imaging of transgenic mice. *Neurophotonics* **2015**, *2*, 041402. [CrossRef] [PubMed]
24. Loberg, L.I.; Henriques, T.A.; Johnson, J.K.; Miller, P.E.; Ralston, S.L. Characterization and Potential Mitigation of Corneal Effects in Nonclinical Toxicology Studies in Animals Administered Depatuxizumab Mafodotin. *J. Ocul. Pharmacol. Ther.* **2022**. [CrossRef] [PubMed]
25. Iliff, J.J.; Lee, H.; Yu, M.; Feng, T.; Logan, J.; Nedergaard, M.; Benveniste, H. Brain-wide pathway for waste clearance captured by contrast-enhanced MRI. *J. Clin. Investig.* **2013**, *123*, 1299–1309. [CrossRef] [PubMed]

26. Iliff, J.J.; Wang, M.; Zeppenfeld, D.M.; Venkataraman, A.; Plog, B.A.; Liao, Y.; Deane, R.; Nedergaard, M. Cerebral arterial pulsation drives paravascular CSF-interstitial fluid exchange in the murine brain. *J. Neurosci.* **2013**, *33*, 18190–18199. [CrossRef] [PubMed]
27. Yadav, D.B.; Maloney, J.A.; Wildsmith, K.R.; Fuji, R.N.; Meilandt, W.J.; Solanoy, H.; Lu, Y.; Peng, K.; Wilson, B.; Chan, P.; et al. Widespread brain distribution and activity following i.c.v. infusion of anti-beta-secretase (BACE1) in nonhuman primates. *Br. J. Pharmacol.* **2017**, *174*, 4173–4185. [CrossRef]
28. Pizzo, M.E.; Wolak, D.J.; Kumar, N.N.; Brunette, E.; Brunnquell, C.L.; Hannocks, M.J.; Abbott, N.J.; Meyerand, M.E.; Sorokin, L.; Stanimirovic, D.B.; et al. Intrathecal antibody distribution in the rat brain: Surface diffusion, perivascular transport and osmotic enhancement of delivery. *J. Physiol.* **2018**, *596*, 445–475. [CrossRef]
29. Farrington, G.K.; Caram-Salas, N.; Haqqani, A.S.; Brunette, E.; Eldredge, J.; Pepinsky, B.; Antognetti, G.; Baumann, E.; Ding, W.; Garber, E.; et al. A novel platform for engineering blood-brain barrier-crossing bispecific biologics. *FASEB J.* **2014**, *28*, 4764–4778. [CrossRef]
30. Buchwalow, I.; Samoilova, V.; Boecker, W.; Tiemann, M. Non-specific binding of antibodies in immunohistochemistry: Fallacies and facts. *Sci. Rep.* **2011**, *1*, 28. [CrossRef]
31. Xie, L.; Kang, H.; Xu, Q.; Chen, M.J.; Liao, Y.; Thiyagarajan, M.; O'Donnell, J.; Christensen, D.J.; Nicholson, C.; Iliff, J.J.; et al. Sleep drives metabolite clearance from the adult brain. *Science* **2013**, *342*, 373–377. [CrossRef] [PubMed]
32. Mestre, H.; Mori, Y.; Nedergaard, M. The Brain's Glymphatic System: Current Controversies. *Trends Neurosci.* **2020**, *43*, 458–466. [CrossRef]
33. Lee, C.M.; Tannock, I.F. The distribution of the therapeutic monoclonal antibodies cetuximab and trastuzumab within solid tumors. *BMC Cancer* **2010**, *10*, 255. [CrossRef] [PubMed]
34. Lucas, A.T.; Price, L.S.L.; Schorzman, A.N.; Storrie, M.; Piscitelli, J.A.; Razo, J.; Zamboni, W.C. Factors Affecting the Pharmacology of Antibody-Drug Conjugates. *Antibodies* **2018**, *7*, 10. [CrossRef]
35. Lucas, A.T.; Robinson, R.; Schorzman, A.N.; Piscitelli, J.A.; Razo, J.F.; Zamboni, W.C. Pharmacologic Considerations in the Disposition of Antibodies and Antibody-Drug Conjugates in Preclinical Models and in Patients. *Antibodies* **2019**, *8*, 3. [CrossRef]
36. Faresjo, R.; Bonvicini, G.; Fang, X.T.; Aguilar, X.; Sehlin, D.; Syvanen, S. Brain pharmacokinetics of two BBB penetrating bispecific antibodies of different size. *Fluids Barriers CNS* **2021**, *18*, 26. [CrossRef] [PubMed]
37. Ryman, J.T.; Meibohm, B. Pharmacokinetics of Monoclonal Antibodies. *CPT Pharmacomet. Syst. Pharmacol.* **2017**, *6*, 576–588. [CrossRef]
38. Ovacik, M.; Lin, K. Tutorial on Monoclonal Antibody Pharmacokinetics and Its Considerations in Early Development. *Clin. Transl. Sci.* **2018**, *11*, 540–552. [CrossRef]
39. Lu, G.; Nishio, N.; van den Berg, N.S.; Martin, B.A.; Fakurnejad, S.; van Keulen, S.; Colevas, A.D.; Thurber, G.M.; Rosenthal, E.L. Co-administered antibody improves penetration of antibody-dye conjugate into human cancers with implications for antibody-drug conjugates. *Nat. Commun.* **2020**, *11*, 5667. [CrossRef]
40. CDER. Blenrep NDA/BLA Multi-Disciplinary Review and Evaluation. Available online: https://www.accessdata.fda.gov/drugsatfda_docs/nda/2020/761158Orig1s000MultidisciplineR.pdf (accessed on 8 June 2022).
41. Poon, K.A.; Flagella, K.; Beyer, J.; Tibbitts, J.; Kaur, S.; Saad, O.; Yi, J.H.; Girish, S.; Dybdal, N.; Reynolds, T. Preclinical safety profile of trastuzumab emtansine (T-DM1): Mechanism of action of its cytotoxic component retained with improved tolerability. *Toxicol. Appl. Pharmacol.* **2013**, *273*, 298–313. [CrossRef]
42. Taghian, T.; Marosfoi, M.G.; Puri, A.S.; Cataltepe, O.I.; King, R.M.; Diffie, E.B.; Maguire, A.S.; Martin, D.R.; Fernau, D.; Batista, A.R.; et al. A Safe and Reliable Technique for CNS Delivery of AAV Vectors in the Cisterna Magna. *Mol. Ther.* **2020**, *28*, 411–421. [CrossRef]
43. Cook, M.; Murphy, M.; Bulluss, K.; D'Souza, W.; Plummer, C.; Priest, E.; Williams, C.; Sharan, A.; Fisher, R.; Pincus, S.; et al. Anti-seizure therapy with a long-term, implanted intra-cerebroventricular delivery system for drug-resistant epilepsy: A first-in-man study. *EClinicalMedicine* **2020**, *22*, 100326. [CrossRef]
44. Cohen-Pfeffer, J.L.; Gururangan, S.; Lester, T.; Lim, D.A.; Shaywitz, A.J.; Westphal, M.; Slavc, I. Intracerebroventricular Delivery as a Safe, Long-Term Route of Drug Administration. *Pediatr. Neurol.* **2017**, *67*, 23–35. [CrossRef] [PubMed]

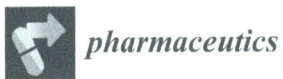

Article

Gene Targeting to the Cerebral Cortex Following Intranasal Administration of Polyplexes

Asya I. Petkova [1,2], Ilona Kubajewska [1,2], Alexandra Vaideanu [1], Andreas G. Schätzlein [1,2] and Ijeoma F. Uchegbu [1,2,*]

1. UCL School of Pharmacy, 29–39 Brunswick Square, London WC1N 1AX, UK; asya.petkova.15@ucl.ac.uk (A.I.P.); i.kubajewska@ucl.ac.uk (I.K.); a.vaideanu@ucl.ac.uk (A.V.); a.schatzlein@ucl.ac.uk (A.G.S.)
2. Nanomerics Ltd., Northwick Park and St. Mark's Hospital, Y Block, Watford Road, London HA1 3UJ, UK
* Correspondence: ijeoma.uchegbu@ucl.ac.uk

Abstract: Gene delivery to the cerebral cortex is challenging due to the blood brain barrier and the labile and macromolecular nature of DNA. Here we report gene delivery to the cortex using a glycol chitosan—DNA polyplex (GCP). In vitro, GCPs carrying a reporter plasmid DNA showed approximately 60% of the transfection efficiency shown by Lipofectamine lipoplexes (LX) in the U87 glioma cell line. Aiming to maximise penetration through the brain extracellular space, GCPs were coated with hyaluronidase (HYD) to form hyaluronidase-coated polyplexes (GCPH). The GCPH formulation retained approximately 50% of the in vitro hyaluronic acid (HA) digestion potential but lost its transfection potential in two-dimensional U87 cell lines. However, intranasally administered GCPH (0.067 mg kg^{-1} DNA) showed high levels of gene expression (IVIS imaging of protein expression) in the brain regions. In a separate experiment, involving GCP, LX and naked DNA, the intranasal administration of the GCP formulation (0.2 mg kg^{-1} DNA) resulted in protein expression predominantly in the cerebral cortex, while a similar dose of intranasal naked DNA led to protein expression in the cerebellum. Intranasal LX formulations did not show any evidence of protein expression. GCPs may provide a means to target protein expression to the cerebral cortex via the intranasal route.

Keywords: nose to brain delivery; gene therapy; polyplexes; hyaluronidase; glycol chitosan

1. Introduction

Delivering intravenously injected macromolecules, such as genes, to the brain is severely hampered by the blood brain barrier (BBB) [1] While the BBB is a major obstacle when delivering macromolecules to the brain, the delivery of genes to the brain is further hampered by the fact that gene delivery nanoparticles (NPs) are rapidly cleared from the circulation due to the interaction between the positively charged NPs and the negatively charged plasma proteins and erythrocytes. These electrostatic interactions result in aggregation, opsonization and subsequent clearance of the particles from the body [2].

Intranasal administration is used to treat nasal epithelium infections or conditions such as nasal congestion, rhinorrhoea and rhinosinusitis [3]. More recently, the potential of intranasal delivery to ensure transport through the olfactory bulb to the brain, bypassing the BBB, has been explored for a variety of molecules [4–7]. Additionally, the intranasal delivery route has other advantages such as ease of administration, non-invasiveness, rapid onset of action, a relatively large and permeable surface area and avoidance of the first-pass hepatic metabolism. Intranasally administered insulin has shown promise in alleviating the symptoms in both Alzheimer's disease type (AD-type) dementia and non-AD-type dementia in clinical trials, resulting in improvement of memory, cognitive functions and attention [8–10]. In parallel with these exciting clinical results, there are also a number of studies in animal models describing the promise of intranasally administered lectin, for the treatment of obesity, and oxytocin, as a treatment option for depression [11–14] In terms of gene delivery, the intranasal route was first used for the delivery of a reporter plasmid to the brain. A 30mer peptide with PEGylated lysine residues was shown to deliver a green fluorescent protein (GFP) DNA, resulting in GFP expression in multiple brain regions, predominantly in the frontal cortex [15]. Similarly, intranasally administered PEI and chitosan-coated superparamagnetic iron oxide nanoparticles (SPIONs) were shown to deliver a reporter plasmid coding for a red fluorescent protein (RFP) to the cortex and hippocampus of rats. Intranasally delivered NPs formed by DNA coding for glial cell line-derived neurotrophic factor (GDNF) complexed with polyethylene glycol (substituted with lysine residues) showed peak expression in the rat striatum a week after administration and neuroprotective action in a rat model of Parkinson's disease (PD) [16]. Similarly, a self-assembling electrostatic complex between an antisense RNA against a microRNA (miR-21) associated with inhibition of pro-apoptotic genes and a peptide delivered intranasally to mice bearing intracranial tumours showed a significant decrease in the tumour volume a week post administration of the NPs [17]. Furthermore, miR-21 levels were reduced, while the expression of pro-apoptotic genes such as PTEN and PDCD4 was induced by the NPs.

Nose to brain delivery is well-documented in humans [18] and has been reviewed recently [19]. Molecules transported via the intranasal route of administration after mucociliary clearance reach the interior of the nasal cavity where the respiratory, olfactory neuronal networks and blood vessels are accessible [20,21]. The neuronal transport pathway involves the transport of molecules from the nasal cavity to the brain parenchyma and the pons along the olfactory and trigeminal nerves, respectively. The movement of molecules from the nasal cavity to the olfactory bulb is facilitated through intracellular or extracellular pathways. A very slow axonal transport from the olfactory bulb and other brain regions is performed by passive diffusion or receptor-mediated endocytosis, both facilitating intracellular trafficking in olfactory neurons [22]. By contrast, the extracellular transport of molecules from the nasal cavity to the brain is a much more rapid process. Rapid delivery, almost immediately or up to one hour after intranasal administration [23–26], has been reported for many molecules, hence an extracellular pathway is the most likely mode of transport in those instances. Extracellular transport may play a role in the movement of peptide-loaded nanoparticles within the brain [27]. Lochhead et al. showed the presence of the tracer dextrans 20 min after nasal administration in the perivascular space of the nasal lamina propria and in different brain regions [28]. Similarly, fluorescently labelled insulin was found throughout the brain only 20 min after nasal administration [29]. These findings support the idea of rapid transport of substances from the olfactory bulb throughout the brain by the perivascular pathway. The perivascular transport hypothesis is also supported for the delivery of NPs loaded with a plasmid encoding for hGDNF, where the resulting transfected cells appear to be situated in the perivascular spaces surrounding capillary endothelial cells and are most likely pericytes [30].

While others have reported delivery to multiple brain regions [15,31] upon nasal administration, we aimed to achieve targeted delivery to the cortex in order to exploit the clinical potential for developing effective gene therapies against Alzheimer's disease, posterior cortical atrophy and frontal lobe glioblastomas. Additionally, assuming an extracellular pathway, we sought to examine the effect of the HYD coating of the polyplexes to facilitate brain delivery via the nasal route of administration. HYD has been used as a spreading agent for the subcutaneous route for over 50 years, enabling volumes in excess of the normal 2 mL [32] to be administered due to a loosening of the connective tissue by enzymatic cleavage of ECM biopolymer components. Specifically, hyaluronidase—whether of bacterial or vertebral origin—catalyses the hydrolysis of HA at the 1,4-glycosidic linkages [33]. Vertebrate HYD, as has been used in the current study (endo-β-acetyl-hexosaminidase), also catalyses the degradation of chondroitin and chondroitin-6-sulphate at the 1,4-glycosidic linkage, albeit at a slower rate than for hyaluronic acid. Furthermore, subcutaneous formulations containing HYD that allow rapid injection of increased dose volumes of 5 mL of trastuzumab have recently been approved for human use and more recently a 10 mL volume of subcutaneous rituximab has been administered using HYD [34]. We have previously shown that HYD coating on nanoparticles has a beneficial effect on drug bioavailability when HYD nanoparticles are administered via the subcutaneous route; increasing plasma exposure by two-fold and increasing tumoricidal activity when compared to formulations devoid of HYD [35]. To the best of our knowledge, we have not seen reports of HYD coated nanoparticles being used for nose to brain delivery.

2. Materials and Methods

CellTiter 90® AQ one solution cell proliferation assay, pSV-40 β-Galactosidase control vector, Beta-Glo® and pGL4.13[luc2/SV40] vector, were supplied by Promega (Southampton, UK). Ninety-six well Corning cell culture plates, hydrochloric acid (purity $\geq$ 98%) were supplied by VWR (Fontenay-sous-Bois, France) and Luciferin was supplied by Perkin Elmer (Waltham, MA, USA). T-PER™ tissue protein extraction reagent, EDTA free halt protease inhibitor cocktail, Lipofectamine 2000 and acetonitrile HPLC grade (purity $\geq$ 99.5%) were supplied by Thermo Scientific (Loughborough, UK). Visking dialysis tubing was supplied by Medicell Membranes Ltd. (London, UK). Glycol chitosan Mw = 113 kDa, Mn = 98 kDa was supplied by Wako (Osaka, Japan). Deuterium oxide, sodium acetate anhydrous (purity $\geq$ 99%), glacial acetic acid, hyaluronidase Type I S-400–1000 units mg^{-1}, trifluoracetic acid (purity $\geq$ 99%), hyaluronic acid (Mw 70–90 kDa), bovine serum albumin, Triton™ X-100, magnesium chloride hexahydrate (purity $\geq$ 96%), trypsin (0.02% EDTA, Gibco™ GlutaMAX, penicillin/streptomycin, minimal essential medium eagle (MEME), OptiMEM and foetal bovine serum were all supplied by Sigma Aldrich (Gillingham, UK).

2.1. Acid Degradation of Glycol Chitosan (GC)

Glycol chitosan (10 g) was dissolved in HCl (4 M, 375 mL) as described previously [36]. The flask was incubated for 2 h in a preheated water bath at 50 °C. Dialysis against water was performed over 24 h with 5–6 water changes (3.5 kDa MWCO). The dialyzed solution was freeze-dried on a Christ 1–4 LD plus freeze dryer (Martin Christ, Osterode am Harz, Germany).

2.2. Characterization of Glycol Chitosan (GC)

The samples for NMR analysis were prepared at 20 mg mL^{-1} in deuterium oxide and analysed on either an AMX 400 MHz or an AMX 500 MHz spectrometer (Bruker, Rheinstetten, Germany). Molecular weight (Mw) measurements were performed on a GPC-MALLS dRI with a MALLS 120 mW solid-state laser (wavelength, λ658 nm) DAWN® HELEOS™ and Optilab rEX Interferometric Refractometer, respectively (Wyatt Technology Corporation, Santa Barbara, CA, USA). Size exclusion chromatography (SEC) was performed using PolySep™—GFC-P 4000 column (300 × 7.8 mm) protected by a PolySep™ (Phenomenex, Macclesfield, UK) with a GFG-P guard column (35 × 7.8 mm).

2.3. Preparation of Glycol Chitosan Polyplexes and Lipoplexes with Lipofectamine (GCP 1 and LX 1)

Nanocomplexes for in vitro studies were prepared at a 6 μg mL^{-1} concentration of β-Gal DNA in phosphate buffer (20 mM, pH = 6.8) or in OptiMEM for Lipofectamine in a total volume of 500 μL. Equal volumes of plasmid DNA (250 μL) and polymer or Lipofectamine in phosphate buffer (250 μL) at a polymer, β-Gal DNA mass ratio of 60:1 (GCP1) or a Lipofectamine, β-Gal DNA mass ratio of 2:1 (LX 1) were prepared. The β-Gal DNA solution was always added to the polymer dispersion followed by mixing with a pipette for 10 s. Lipofectamine formulations were prepared by following the manufacturer's instructions. Complexation was performed over 24 h and at 4 °C for GCP 1 and 30 min at room temperature for LX 1.

The polyplexes and lipoplexes for the in vivo experiments were prepared as described above but at a β-Gal DNA concentration of 250 μg mL^{-1} in a total volume of 16 μL (a dose of 0.2 mg kg^{-1} for GCP 3 and LX 3) and at a β-Gal concentration of 84 μg mL^{-1} in a total volume of 16 μL (a dose of 0.067 mg kg^{-1} for GCP 2 and LX 2).

2.4. Preparation of Hyaluronidase Coated Nanocomplexes (GCPH)

Polyplexes with a polymer to DNA weight ratio of 60:1 were prepared containing 6 µg mL^{-1} DNA in phosphate buffer (20 mM, pH = 6.8) in a total volume of 250 µL and stored for 24 h at 4 °C. Working solutions of hyaluronidase in NaCl (20 mM, pH adjusted to 12 with 0.1 M NaOH) were prepared. The hyaluronidase solutions (250 µL) were added to the polyplex dispersion described above (250 µL), dropwise under magnetic stirring for 30 min. Subsequently, the now formed ternary complexes (hyaluronidase, glycol chitosan and DNA) were stored for another 24 h at 4 °C. For the scaled-up formulations for in vivo experiments, the mass ratios of plasmid, polymer and enzyme were kept at 1:60:84.

GCPH 7 for in vivo administration was prepared at a luciferase DNA concentration of 84 µg mL^{-1} (16 µL). Equal volumes of polyplex (8 µL) and hyaluronidase (8 µL 14.2 mg mL^{-1}) were mixed, as described above, followed by incubation at 4 °C for 24 h.

The name codes for the ternary complexes (GCPH) include numbers that represent the amount of hyaluronidase added in mg mL^{-1}. As such, GCPH 7 indicates that the formulation contained hyaluronidase at a concentration of 7 mg mL^{-1}. The ratio of GC to DNA was always at a weight ratio of 60:1.

2.5. Dynamic Light Scattering (DLS)

Size and zeta potential measurements were both performed in a reusable zeta cell on a Malvern Zetasizer Nano ZS machine (Malvern Panalytical, Malvern, UK). Size measurements were performed first, followed by a zeta potential measurement. Prior to the measurements, the instrument was checked with size and zeta potential standards.

2.6. Reversed-Phase High Performance Liquid Chromatography (RP-HPLC)

Hyaluronidase analysis was performed using a reverse-phase PRLP-S column (4.6 × 50 mm in length, pore size = 3 µm) and an RP-HPLC system (Agilent Technologies, Santa Clara, CA, USA). The system was fitted with a guard column and analysis was carried out at a flow rate of 0.7 mL min^{-1}. The column temperature was set to 80 °C, the injection volume set at 10 µL and the wavelength at 280 nm. 0.1% Trifluoroacetic acid (TFA)/Acetonitrile (ACN) was used as the mobile phase and run at a gradient (0.50 min 10% ACN, 0.51 min 90% ACN, 4.00 min 90% ACN, 4.01 min 10% ACN). Samples were prepared in 0.1% TFA and analysed using a standard curve (y = 708.13x − 5.6753, r^2 = 0.991).

2.7. Cell Culture

U-87 MG cells (ATCC® HTB-14™) were maintained in 75 cm^2 blue vent cap culture flasks in 10–12 mL of minimal essential medium eagle (MEME) supplemented with Sodium Pyruvate (1% v/v), GlutaMAX°TM (1% v/v), Penicillin/Streptomycin (1% v/v) and foetal bovine serum (10% v/v).

2.8. In Vitro Transfection Experiments

U-87 cells were seeded in lysine-coated 6 well plates at a density of 5 × 10^5 cells per well in 1 mL of MEME. The cells were left for 72 h to reach the exponential growth phase and were then treated with the nanocomplexes or naked DNA. After 72 h the full MEME from each well of the plate was replaced by FBS free MEME (1.5 mL). An aliquot of the nanocomplexes (0.5 mL) was then added to each well containing FBS free medium MEME (1.5 mL) to make up the total volume to 2 mL per well. The plates were then left for 17 h in an incubator at 37 °C in the presence of 5% CO$_2$. At the end of the incubation period, the FBS-free medium with the treatments was aspirated and replaced with 2 mL per well of full MEME containing FBS (10% v/v). The plates were then left in the incubator at 37 °C for another 24 h before performing the β-Galactosidase assay.

2.9. β-Galactosidase Assay

The β-Galactosidase enzyme assay was purchased from Promega (Southampton, UK) and was performed according to the manufacturer's instructions.

2.10. MTS Assay

U-87 cells were seeded in 96 well plates at a density of 10^3 cells per well in a total volume of 100 µL and left for 72 h to reach the exponential phase. Two-fold serial dilutions across the plate were performed for Lipofectamine at a starting concentration of 0.5 mg mL^{-1} Lipofectamine. Individual solutions were prepared for GC37 at the following concentrations (5 mg mL^{-1}, 4.6 mg mL^{-1}, 4.4 mg mL^{-1}, 4.0 mg mL^{-1}, 3.6 mg mL^{-1}, 3.0 mg mL^{-1}, 2.6 mg mL^{-1}, 2.2 mg mL^{-1} and 1.8 mg mL^{-1}). Cells were treated for 17 h in FBS free medium, then recovered for 24 h in complete medium. Five wells containing cells without any treatment were left as a negative control and 5 wells treated with Triton X 100 (0.05% w/v) were used as a positive control. The MTS reagent (20 µL) was added to all the wells and the absorbance at 490 nm was measured using a SpectraMax M series spectrophotometer (Molecular Devices, San Jose, CA, USA) after 2 h.

IC50 values were calculated from equations generated by fitting data plots to a linear regression model in GraphPad Prism.

2.11. Hyaluronic Acid Digestion Assay

Hyaluronic acid (70–90 kDa, 10 mg) was dissolved in phosphate buffer (0.3 M sodium phosphate, pH = 5.35). The solution was then heated to 90 °C with stirring until all the hyaluronic acid was dissolved, followed by cooling down to 37 °C in a water bath. The assay was performed according to the manufacturer's instructions available at Enzymatic Assay of Hyaluronidase (3.2.1.35) (sigmaaldrich.com) [37].

2.12. Intranasal Dosing

All animal experiments were performed under a UK Home Office licence and in accordance with the UK Animal Scientific Procedures Act 1986 (ASPA). A local ethics committee approved the experimental procedures. The experiments were carried out in the biological safety unit at the UCL School of Pharmacy. Female, BALB/c mice weighing ~20 g (Charles River, Harlow, UK) were initially kept for a week to acclimatise prior to the start of the experimental work in the animal unit, maintained at an ambient temperature, relative humidity of 60% and equal day and night cycles. The animals (n = 4 per group) were anaesthetized in an isoflurane chamber with 3–4% isoflurane connected to an oxygen pump for 3–4 min. Intranasal dosing was performed using methods previously described [38]. The mice were left in a separate cage to recover fully after the anaesthesia. Once nanocomplexes were administered, imaging was performed 24 h post-administration, 15 min and 1 h after intranasal dosing with 16 µL of the LuGal substrate (15 mg mL^{-1}).

The in vivo imaging system (IVIS; IVIS®-Spectrum systems, Xeno-gen-Caliper Life Sciences, Hopkinton, MA, USA) machine with a cabinet and a CCD camera (2048 × 2048 pixels) was used to image the animals. All anaesthetic procedures were performed with 3–4% isoflurane in the chamber and a maintaining dose of 2% isoflurane during the imaging process in the IVIS cabinet. The system was connected to a computer with a Living Image® 3.0 software (Xeno-gen-Caliper Life Sciences, Hopkinton, MA, USA). An image sequence of four exposure times was generated (30 s, 60 s, 120 s and 240 s). Comparisons between images were performed for the same exposure time of 240 s. The average radiance or the sum of the radiance (photons/second) of each pixel in the region of interest (cm^2) was identified with a circular selection divided by the number of pixels (p/s/cm^2/sr), where p = photons, s = seconds, and sr = steradian is compared between treatments.

2.13. Brain Dissection and Homogenisation

Mice (n = 4 per group) were killed by a CO_2 overdose followed by decapitation. For downstream analyses, ~1 mg of tissue was manually homogenised in 20 µL of T-PER reagent, according to the manufacturer's recommendation. T-PER reagent was supplemented with EDTA-free Halt Protease Inhibitor Cocktail (1 mL in 100 mL of T-PER reagent). After preparing the tissue homogenates, the tubes were centrifuged at 10,000× g for 5 min and the supernatants were collected. An aliquot of the supernatant (100 µL) was pipetted onto a white 96-well plate and the LuGal substrate (100 µL) was added to each well. Luminescence was measured on a SpectraMax series M plate reader (Molecular Devices, San Jose, CA, USA). The signal from a control animal was subtracted from all the samples. To normalise the data, the relative luminescent units (RLU) per well were divided by the weight of the samples and converted to RLU mg^{-1} of tissue.

2.14. Statistical Analysis

IC 50 values of Lipofectamine and GC37 were compared using an unpaired t-test. Statistical analysis of datasets involving multiple comparisons was performed using an ordinary one-way ANOVA with a Bonferroni correction in GraphPad Prism 7. p-values less than 0.05 are given one asterisk (* p), p-values less than 0.01 are given two asterisks (** p), p-values less than 0.001 are indicated with three asterisks (*** p), while p-values of less than 0.0001 are marked with four asterisks (**** p).

3. Results

3.1. Acid Degradation of Glycol Chitosan

A relationship between degradation time and molecular weight (Mw) of glycol chitosan has been established previously [36]. Based on this, the time point for degradation was chosen to be 2 h to obtain a glycol chitosan (GC) polymer with a Mw range between 20,000–40,000 kDa. The Mw of the degraded GC batch was measured to be 37,440 Da (GC37) (Mw = 37,440, Mn = 37 200, Mw/Mn = 1.006), while the non-degraded GC had a Mw of approximately 100 kDa (GC100) as reported by the manufacturer, (Figure 1a), after 2 h and 0 h degradation, respectively. Dialysis was used to remove the excess hydrochloric acid from the degradation mixture. NMR analysis provided information on the structure of GC (Figure S1, see Supplementary Information). The structure of GC is presented in Figure 1a.

3.2. Toxicity of the Gene Carrier

As a naturally derived polymer, chitosan is often considered biocompatible by default. Indeed, it is biodegradable in vivo by endogenous enzymes in the body, such as lysozyme, which degrades chitosan to N-acetylglucosamine [39], the latter being a building block of biomacromolecules, such as glycoproteins, proteoglycans, glycosaminoglycans (GAGs) and other components of the connective tissues [40]. However, biocompatibility must be considered in relation to the structural parameters of the polymer, dosage form, the route of administration and the intended use.

The present study was focused on investigating the effect of GC37 and LX as gene carriers rather than on the toxicity of these formulations in the U87 cell line. Although it is proven that cytotoxicity is cell type-dependent [41], experiments in one cell line can provide early evidence of the cytotoxicity profile of the carriers. GC37 as a polymer carrier was almost 10 times less toxic than Lipofectamine; the latter used as a positive control in all transfection experiments (IC50 GC37 = 3.41 mg mL^{-1} vs. IC50 Lipofectamine = 0.36 mg mL^{-1}, * $p < 0.05$), (Figure 1b).

3.3. Polyplex Formation

Polyplex formation is confirmed by DLS where naked β-Gal shows the presence of multiple peaks in the size intensity plot (Figure 2a), while glycol chitosan addition at a 60:1 g g^{-1} mass ratio to DNA results in the formation of a monodisperse population of polyplexes as shown by the intensity size distribution plots (Figure 2b). The scaled-up nanocomplexes for in vivo applications showed an increase in particle size with an increase in the amount of DNA used, an observation which has also been reported by others [42–45] (Figure 2b and Table 1). A possible explanation of the phenomenon has been provided by Mann et al., who investigated the DNA condensation potential of poly-L-ornithine by atomic force microscopy. The authors concluded that with the increase in DNA concentration, multimolecular condensation is observed as opposed to monomolecular

DNA condensation, which is believed to be operational when lower amounts of DNA are used [45]. Uncoated polyplexes presented with a positive charge of +7 mV to +10 mV (Table 1).

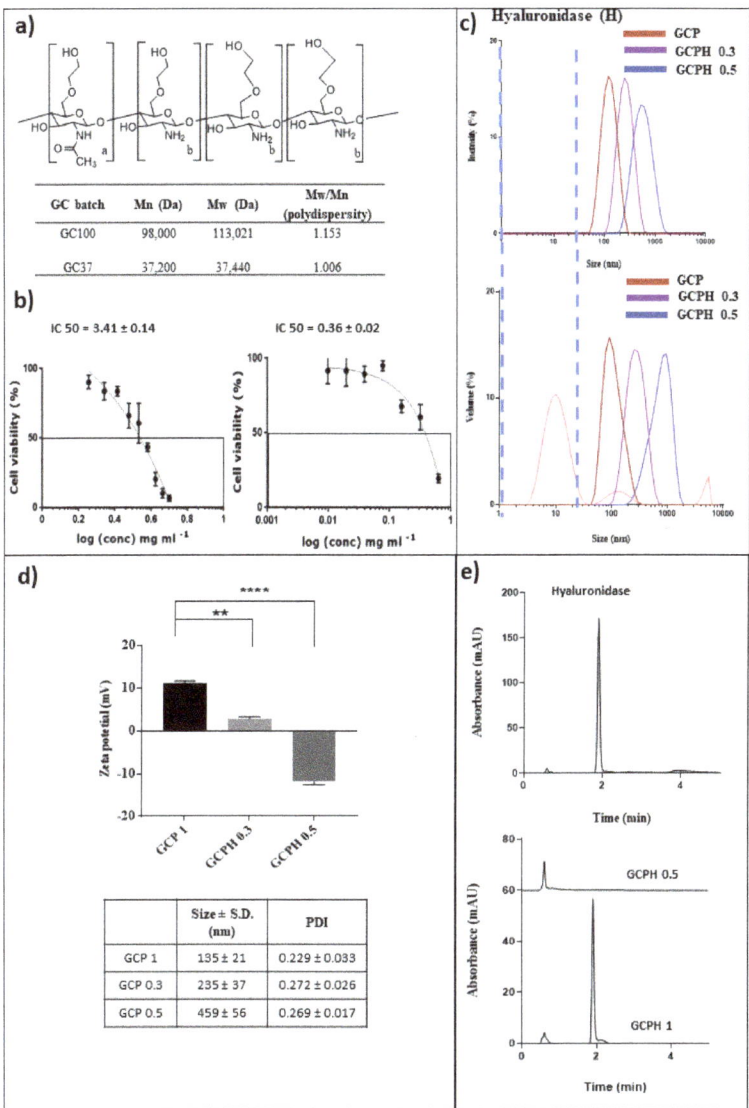

Figure 1. Structure of glycol chitosan (GC), molecular weight and PDI for degraded and non-degraded GC (**a**). IC 50 values for GC37 and Lipofectamine in U87 cells (**b**). Intensity and volume size distribution plots of GCP 1, GCPH 0.3, GCPH 0.5 and hyaluronidase (**c**). Zeta potential values, size and PDI of GCP, GCPH 0.3 and GCPH 0.5 (**d**). The zeta potential of polyplexes without HYD (GCP) is significantly different when compared to polyplexes coated with HYD (GCPH 0.2, ** $p \leq 0.01$) and (GCPH 0.3, **** $p \leq 0.0001$) (**d**). HPLC chromatograms of free hyaluronidase (top) and ternary complexes with 1 mg mL^{-1} hyaluronidase-GCPH 1 and with 0.5 mg mL^{-1} hyaluronidase-GCPH 0.5 (bottom) (**e**).

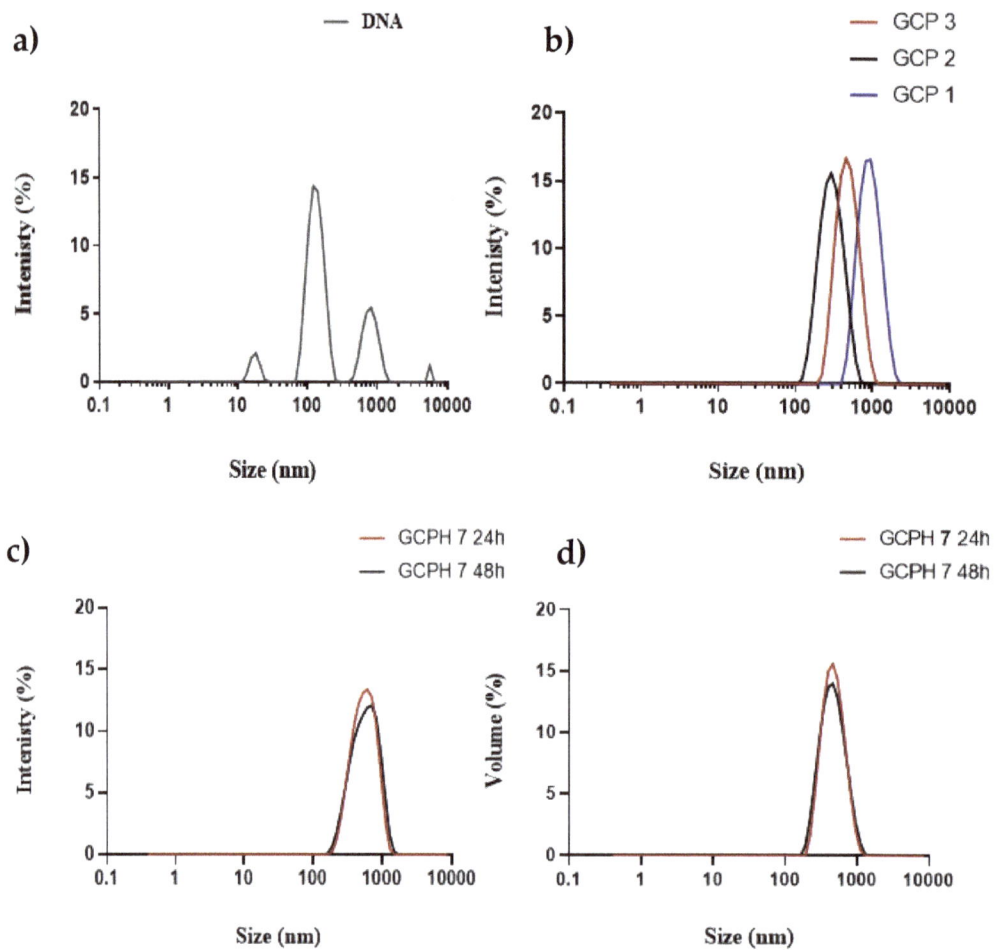

Figure 2. Representative intensity size plots of naked β-Gal DNA (**a**), GCP (GCP 1 contains 6 µg mL^{-1} β-Gal DNA, GCP 2 contains 84 µg mL^{-1} β-Gal DNA, GCP 3 contains 250 µg mL^{-1} β-Gal DNA, all GC, DNA ratios are 60, 1 g g^{-1} (**b**), GCPH 7 (84 µg mL^{-1} β-Gal DNA), with 7.2 mg mL^{-1} of hyaluronidase size distribution by intensity (**c**) and volume (**d**) at 24 and 48 h.

Table 1. Size, PDI and zeta potential of GCP, GCPH and DNA. The data is representative of three independent measurements (=3, mean ± SD).

Polyplex	Size (nm)	PDI	Zeta Potential (mV)
GCP 1	135 ± 21	0.229 ± 0.033	+7 ± 3
GCP 2	482 ± 36	0.113 ± 0.023	+9 ± 4
GCP 3	863 ± 28	0.161 ± 0.021	+10 ± 3
GCPH 7	526 ± 14	0.578 ± 0.053	−10 ± 2
DNA	140 ± 31 (65%) 950 ± 61 (23%) 20 ± 9 (7%)	0.589 ± 0.077	−26 ± 5

3.4. HYD Coated Polyplexes

GCPH 0.3 and GCPH 0.5 showed no free hyaluronidase for both intensity and volume size distribution plots (Figure 1c) and a significant drop in charge from +10 mV for non-coated polyplexes (GCP) to about −12 mV for the coated polyplexes (GCPH 0.5, **** $p < 0.0001$) (Figure 1d).

The isoelectric point (pI) of crude HYD isolated from bovine testes is reported to be 5.4 [33]. Theoretically, pH values above the pI of an enzyme will result in a net negative charge for the protein, which is desired for the interaction between the positively charged polyplex and the negatively charged enzyme. Dissolving HYD in 20 mM NaCl at a pH of 12 resulted in a pronounced negative charge for the enzyme, because of the extreme pH when compared to 20 mM PBS at a pH of 6.8 (−26 mV and −4.5 mV, respectively, Figure S2, see Supplementary Information). The presence of particles of about 11 nm with 82% abundance is visible from the intensity size distribution of HYD in 20 mM NaCl. Volume and number size distribution plots showed particles of 6 nm with 100% abundance (Figure S2A–C, see Supplementary Information).

Intensity and volume size distribution plots of 0.3 and 0.5 mg mL^{-1} HYD coated GC37 polyplexes (GCPH 0.3 and GCPH 0.5) showed no free enzyme, unimodal size distribution (Figure 1c) and a decrease in zeta potential from approximately +10 mV (GCP) to about −12 mV (GCPH 0.5), **** $p < 0.0001$, (Figure 1d). A size increase is visible for GCPH ternary complexes with an increase in enzyme concentration. Similarly, to the size data, PDI also increased for both GCPH 0.3 and GCPH 0.5 when compared to GCP (0.272 vs. 0.189, ** $p < 0.01$ and 0.282 vs. 0.189, ** $p < 0.01$, (Figure 1d)). This observation is made by others; Dai et al. showed a zeta potential drop and an increase in size for their multi-component nanoparticles comprised of a polymeric shell, an anti-cancer drug, gelatine-RGD and HYD all assembled in one electrostatic complex [46].

The DLS measurements for GCPH 0.3 and GCPH 0.5 ternary complexes showed that using 0.3 and 0.5 mg mL^{-1} of HYD for both polyplexes resulted in enzyme-coated particles of increased size and a negative charge. A step further in the characterisation of the ternary complexes was to use a quantitative method to estimate the amount of free enzyme, i.e., based on the calibration curve using the HPLC method described in the experimental part ($r^2 = 0.9907$). The retention time (RT) of HYD was 1.921 min (Figure 1e). Since the size of GCPH 0.5 ternary complexes was ≥200 nm (Figure 1d), a 0.22 μm filter was used to separate coated particles and free enzyme (size of free enzyme ~6 nm) for analytical purposes. A ternary complex with an increased amount of hyaluronidase (GCPH 1) was also used. The filtrate of free hyaluronidase showed an 87% ± 3% recovery after HPLC analysis with the remaining 13% of enzyme putatively left in the dead volume of the filter. The filtrates of GCPH 0.5 and GCPH 1 were analysed and GCPH 1, but not GCPH 0.5, showed a peak with a RT 1.921 in the chromatogram (Figure 1e). By using the area under the curve, it was quantified that 34% ± 5% or 0.34 mg mL^{-1} of free hyaluronidase was present in GCPH 1 filtrate. Due to the filter dead volume, it is uncertain whether all the remaining enzyme is complexed. However, the absence of an HYD peak in the chromatogram of GCPH 0.5 ternary complexes along with the size and zeta potential data provide strong evidence that at a concentration of 0.5 mg mL^{-1} HYD, GCP polyplexes (0.36 mg mL^{-1} GC) are surface coated with the enzyme. Uncoated polyplexes presented with a positive charge of +7 mV to + 10 mV, while GCPH 0.3 and GCPH 0.3 showed a negative charge of about −12 mV, Figure 1d). HYD coated (GCPH 7) polyplexes are stable for 48 h in aqueous media, proven by both intensity and volume size distribution plots (Figure 2c,d).

3.5. In Vitro Hyaluronic Acid Digestion Potential of Polyplexes Coated with Hyaluronidase

We have previously developed enzyme-bound particles, using polymeric vesicles prepared from N-palmitoyl-N-monomethyl-N,N-dimethyl-N,N,N-trimethyl-6-O-glycolchitosan and N-biotinylated dipalmitoylphosphatidlyethanolamine, which were subsequently bound to beta-galactosidase streptavidin [47] and found that enzyme activity was preserved in this system. However, immobilisation strategies of enzymes on nanoparticles have been proven to affect the function of the enzyme because of structural changes during the immobilisation process [48,49]. Although an assembly based on electrostatic interactions does not involve chemical modifications to the structure of the enzyme, a pH alteration could hinder important amino acid residues, which can negatively influence the enzyme function [50]. Therefore, to check the potential of the ternary complexes to digest HA in vitro when compared to the free enzyme, an HA digestion assay was used. All ternary complexes retained approximately 50% of their enzymatic activity when compared to the free enzyme regardless of the concentration used (Figure 3a).

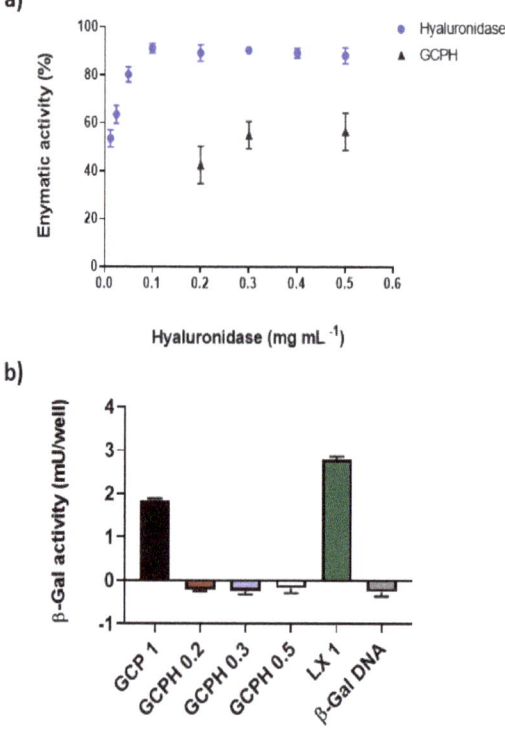

Figure 3. Hyaluronic acid digestion potential of the ternary complexes and free enzyme (**a**). Transfection efficiency of GCP 1 (black bar), GCPH 0.2 (brown bar), GCPH 0.3 (blue bar), GCPH 0.5 (white bar), LX 1 (green bar) and naked β-Gal DNA (grey bar) (**b**). The data is representative of three independent experiments ($n = 3$, mean $\pm$ SD).

3.6. Transfection Efficiency of Polyplexes in U87 Glioma Cell Line

GCP 1 polyplexes containing 6 µg mL^{-1} DNA were transfection competent but were found to be significantly less effective at delivering the reporter plasmid to U87 cells when compared to lipoplexes, LX 1 (1.8 mU/well vs. 2.8 mU/well, **** $p < 0.0001$ (Figure 3b)). GCPH 0.3 and GCPH 0.5 completely lost their in vitro transfection efficiency (delivery of β-Gal DNA to U87 cells). Even a further reduction in the concentration of HYD—GCPH 0.2, showed no active β-Gal enzyme expression in U87 cells, when compared to hyaluronidase-free polyplexes (GCP 1, Figure 3b).

3.7. In Vivo Studies

IVIS imaging of animals 24 h post nanocomplex administration at a dose of 0.067 mg kg^{-1} and 15 min after substrate administration showed an intense luminescent signal in the nasal cavity. Interestingly, the animal treated with naked β-Gal DNA showed the highest signal (5.6×10^8 p/scm^3/sr) with distribution close to the administration site (Figure S3, see Supplementary Materials). However, GCP 2 and especially GCPH 7 showed a different distribution pattern of the signal when compared to naked DNA, where the luminescent signal of the animal treated with GCPH 7 appeared to spread to more caudal parts of the brain. (Figure S3, see Supplementary Materials). Repeated imaging of the same animals an hour post substrate administration showed that the administration of GCP results in a stronger signal when compared to the animal, which received the LX treatment (1.27×10^5 p/s/cm^3/sr and 2.4×10^5 p/s/cm^3/sr, respectively, Figure 4a). The signal from the animal administered with naked DNA was almost at the background level (6.7×10^4 p/s/cm^3/sr) and clearly localised at the tip of the nasal cavity, close to the administration site (Figure 4a). It was then hypothesized that an increase in the dose would allow for the quantification of gene expression. The experiment was repeated with a β-Gal DNA dose increase to 0.2 mg kg^{-1} (250 µg mL^{-1}). Downstream analysis of the homogenised olfactory bulbs, cortex and cerebellum revealed that 24 h post-administration there is no active β-Galactosidase (β-Gal) enzyme in the olfactory bulbs of the animals with any of the treatments (Figure 4b). By contrast, the animals treated with GCP 3 showed significantly higher levels of active β-Gal enzyme in the cortex when compared to animals treated with both LX 3 and naked β-Gal DNA (*** $p \leq 0.001$), (Figure 4c).

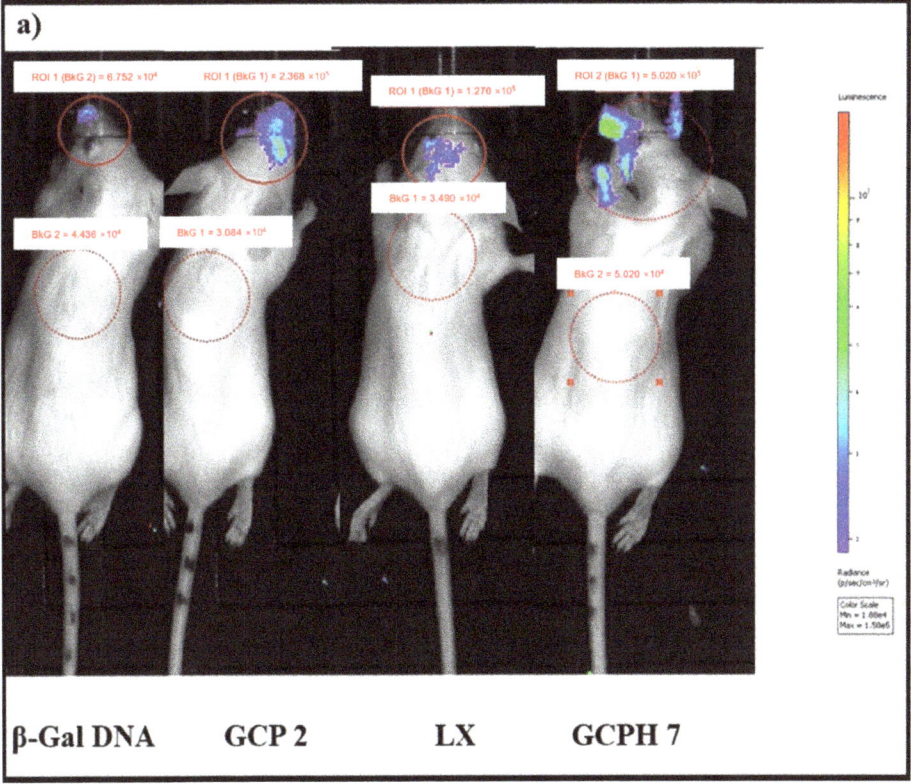

Figure 4. *Cont.*

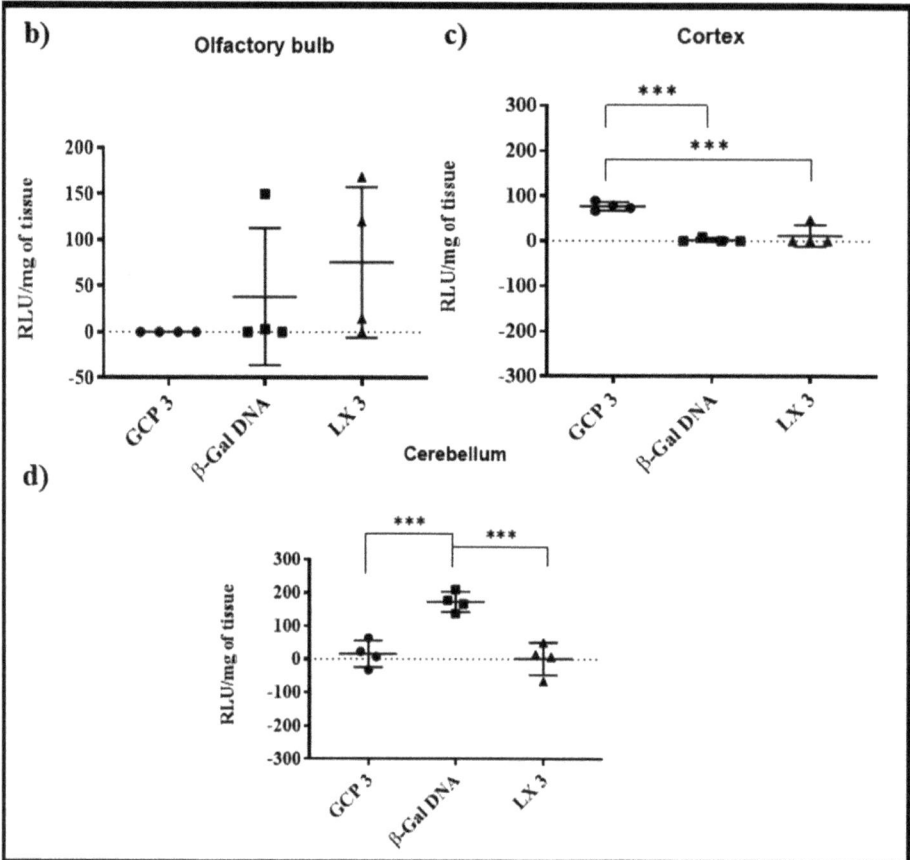

Figure 4. Representative IVIS images from an in vivo intranasal study with nanocomplexes prepared with 84 μg mL^{-1} DNA or a dose of 0.067 mg kg^{-1} DNA (**a**). Imaging was taken 24 h post intranasal administration of the treatments and 1 h after intranasal administration of the substrate and with a 240 s exposure time. Downstream analysis of brain homogenates (mean ± s.d., n = 4) for active β-Gal expression 24 h post nanocomplex administration at a dose of 250 μg mL^{-1} DNA or a dose of 0.2 mg kg^{-1} DNA in olfactory bulbs (**b**), cortex (GCP 3 polyplexes show significantly higher levels of active β-Gal enzyme when compared to naked β-Gal DNA and LX 3 (*** $p \leq 0.001$), (**c**) and cerebellum (naked β-Gal DNA shows a significantly higher level of β-Gal enzyme expression when compared to both GCP 3 and LX 3, *** $p \leq 0.001$). (**d**) The signal from tissue homogenates of olfactory bulbs, cortex and cerebellum of control animals was subtracted from the treatments.

Interestingly, naked β-Gal DNA resulted in significantly higher levels of β-Gal expression in the cerebellum when compared to both LX 3 and GCP 3 (*** $p < 0.001$).

4. Discussion

Neurological disorders are the second leading cause of death and disabilities worldwide [51]. Delivery of drugs to the CNS is a cumbersome task due to the presence of the protective BBB. The BBB blocks the transport of nearly 100% of large molecules to the brain and about 98% of the small molecules [52]. Polymer-mediated gene delivery has still a long way to go before the clinical application becomes widespread. To date, there are no approved polymer-based gene therapeutics on the market and despite seven active clinical trials, none are being developed to target CNS disorders [53]. Although viral vectors are much ahead of the competition, taking over more than 70% of all the active gene therapy clinical trials with thirteen approved therapies, the vast majority of the reports are describing invasive and local administration routes. Exploring intranasal delivery as a non-invasive administration route targeting the CNS and bypassing the BBB has sparked research interest in the area [54]. As stated above, the BBB is a major obstacle to the delivery of therapeutics following systemic application (e.g., intravenous delivery). A growing amount of evidence points unequivocally to an extracellular transport of molecules from the nasal cavity to the olfactory bulb and then throughout the cerebrum via the perivascular pathway [28,30,55]. Therefore, a hyaluronidase coating of the nanoparticle was hypothesized to facilitate the transport of the nanoparticles from the nasal cavity enroute to the brain.

We are motivated to do this work as targeted delivery to the forebrain can offer a significant therapeutic advantage for neurological disorders affecting the cortex including Alzheimer's disease and frontal glioblastoma. It has also been reported that glioblastoma location correlates with specific genetic mutations in patients with frontal glioblastoma associated with isocitrate dehydrogenase 1 (IDH-1) mutations [56], which cause changes in DNA methylation. Additionally, glioblastoma is characterized by the presence of a stiffened and rigid ECM. The stiffened network of overexpressed hyaluronan and other ECM proteins in solid tumours blocks the transport of macromolecules contributing to yet another barrier to the efficient delivery of drugs [57], antibodies [58], immunotoxins [59] and oncolytic adenoviruses [60]. Therefore, the ECM-digestion potential of GCPHs may possibly confer therapeutic benefit to the polyplexes when used via the nose to brain route for gene therapy in glioblastoma.

A 2 h time point for the acid degradation of glycol chitosan was chosen to obtain a polymer with a molecular weight between 20 kDa and 40 kDa, based on previously established molecular weight dependence of GC on degradation time [36]. Figure 1a shows the structure of glycol chitosan as well as the starting molecular weight of the non-degraded material (GC100). The molecular weight of the glycol chitosan obtained after 2 h of acid degradation (GC37) was 37 kDa, as measured by GPC. Peak assignments of corresponding protons in the structure of glycol chitosan are shown in Figure S1 (see Supplementary Information).

Elevated levels of cytotoxicity are often associated with an increased charge density along with a decreased degree of deacetylation for chitosan carriers [61]. The present study showed that glycol chitosan as a gene delivery carrier is 10 times less toxic than Lipofectamine (IC50 in the U87MG cell line = 3.41 mg mL^{-1} vs. 0.36 mg mL^{-1}, respectively, * $p < 0.05$), Figure 1b.

Polyplexes with three different concentrations of β-Gal DNA were prepared (GCP 1, GCP 2 and GCP 3 containing 6 µg mL^{-1}, 84 µg mL^{-1} and 250 µg mL^{-1} DNA) with a resulting size of the nanocomplexes of 135 ± 21, 482 ± 36 and 863 ± 28, respectively (Figure 2b and Table 1). GCP 2 and GCP 3 showed a monodisperse population of particles as determined by DLS with PDI values of <0.2 while GCP 1 showed a PDI value of 0.229. (Table 1). By contrast, unformulated β-Gal DNA presented with a high PDI (>0.5) and three distinct peaks as visible from the intensity size plot (Figure 2a and Table 1).

DLS measurements revealed that GCPH 7 ternary complexes presented with unimodal size distribution and a z-average mean size of 532 ± 71, but also with high PDI ≥ 0.5, which remained unchanged after 48 h. This provides evidence of the short-term stability of the system (Figure 2c,d). Furthermore, no peak indicating free hyaluronidase is present for both intensity and volume size distribution plots (Figure 2c,d). A positive charge was measured for all GCP nanocomplexes ranging from +7 mV to +10 mV and a negative charge of −10 mV for the ternary complexes with hyaluronidase (Table 1). Nanoparticle surface charge is important for stability and prevents the formation of large aggregates. Although glycol chitosan polyplexes and hyaluronidase coated particles possess a slight positive and negative charge respectively, they were stable as confirmed by the unimodal intensity size distribution plots.

Although HYD coated polyplexes GCPH 0.3 and GCPH 0.5 lost their transfection potential in vitro, they retained half of their potential to digest hyaluronic acid when compared to free hyaluronidase Figure 3a,b. LX 1 lipoplexes appeared to be significantly better transfection agents when compared to GCP 1 polyplexes in U87 cells (**** $p < 0.0001$), Figure 3b. The coated polyplexes differ in their size and charge from the non-coated polyplexes, however, even a further reduction of the amount of HYD (GCPH 0.2) did not restore their in vitro transfection potential. While there is more evidence for a positive relationship between increased cationic charge and transfection efficiency, the effect of polyplex size on transfection potential is not clear. Perhaps a 3D spheroid model would be more appropriate to compare the diffusion of the coated nanoparticles in a mimic of the tumour microenvironment. Improved diffusion in tumour spheroids for the multi-component system, when compared to the control nanoparticles, is reported by Dai et al. Additionally the multi-component electrostatic complex with hyaluronidase retained half of its hyaluronic acid digestion potential when compared to the free enzyme [46]. Using electrostatic interactions for complex assembly affects the enzyme function by potentially hindering important amino acids in the active site of the enzyme but does not result in a complete loss of enzyme activity.

Chitosan's mucoadhesive properties make it a suitable candidate over other polymeric gene delivery vectors for intranasal delivery [62]. Intranasal administration of siRNA (via chitosan-based siNS1 nanoparticles) which acts by silencing the viral NS1 gene before or after infection with a respiratory syncytial virus (RSV) showed significantly decreased virus titres in the lungs and decreased inflammation compared to controls [63]. In addition to the significant attenuation of the infection, siNS1 delivered by the low molecular weight oligomeric chitosan induces 4-day protection from RSV infection emphasizing both the prophylactic and therapeutic potential of the nanoparticles. We have previously shown successful delivery of siRNA in the olfactory bulb neurons following nasal administration using ethyl-amino glycol chitosan polyplexes [64]. The nasal route, rather than the conventional delivery to the upper respiratory tract or the lungs, has also been used for the administration of chitosan-mediated gene therapy for brain delivery as described by Ramos et al. [65]. The authors report on the intranasal delivery of Mn2+ incorporating chitosan nanoparticles (MNPs) carrying a dsDNA coding for a red fluorescent protein (RFP). MNPs of 122 nm in size were shown to deliver the highest amount of RFP, which was detected in the cortex, striatum and hippocampus, with the highest protein expression in the striatum 48 h post intranasal administration.

The perivascular hypothesis for the transport of molecules through the olfactory neuroepithelium, unprotected by the BBB is gaining popularity as the leading mechanism of transport from the nasal cavity to the brain. The proof-of-concept studies of intranasally administered peptides, proteins, and polysaccharides discussed earlier show rapid delivery to brain regions, which do not correlate with the intracellular transport option. However, for gene expression or silencing, more time is needed for an effect to take place. IVIS imaging 24 h post nasal administration and 15 min after substrate delivery show the strongest luminescent signal residing predominantly in the nasal cavity for naked β-Gal DNA (Figure S3, see Supplementary Information). GCP 2 and especially GCPH 7 show the presence of transfected cells in more caudal parts of the brain with the signal spreading further from the administration site (Figure S3). These observations are also confirmed by the later imaging time point of 1 h. GCPH 7 appeared as the most effective gene carrier in vivo with the highest luminescent signal measured at 4.7×10^5 p/s/cm^3/sr, Figure 4a. GCP polyplexes showed higher signal levels when compared to LXs (2.4×10^5 vs. 1.27×10^5 p/s/com^3/sr), while naked DNA was at baseline levels (6.7×10^4 p/s/cm^3/sr) and appeared only at the very tip of the nasal cavity, suggesting minimal transport to the brain. By contrast, GCP 2, LX 2 and GCPH 7 showed signal localization further away from the administration site, Figure 4a. Similar findings are reported by others, where complexed DNA results in longer-lasting gene expression when compared to naked DNA [66]. Tissue homogenization and downstream analysis of the olfactory bulbs, cortex and cerebellum of four animals per group for the four treatments (GCP 2, LX 2, naked β-Gal DNA and GCPH 7, all at 84 μg mL^{-1} or 0.067 mg kg^{-1}) resulted in inconclusive data, potentially because of the low dose administered (data not shown). Dose precision in intranasal administration is technically difficult and limiting, as a result of mucociliary clearance and the different anatomies of individual nasal cavities [67]. An increase in the dose of β-Gal DNA at 250 μg mL^{-1} (0.2 mg kg^{-1}) and downstream analysis of tissue homogenates of three brain regions (olfactory bulbs, cortex and cerebellum) at 24 h post intranasal dosing showed no active β-Gal enzyme in the olfactory bulbs of the animals (Figure 4b). Significantly higher levels of active β-Gal enzyme (Figure 4c) were detected in the cortex of animals treated with GCP 3 polyplexes when compared both to the naked plasmid (*** $p \leq 0.001$) and to LX 3 (*** $p \leq 0.001$). Interestingly, animals treated with naked β-Gal DNA showed the highest protein expression in the cerebellum (Figure 4d) when compared to both lipoplexes and polyplexes (GCP 3 and LX 3, *** $p < 0.001$). A possible explanation for the observed differences is transport through the trigeminal pathway. Olfactory neurons connect the olfactory region of the nasal cavity to the brain—olfactory bulb and frontal cortex. By contrast, the trigeminal neurons connect the respiratory region to more caudal parts of the brain—pons, medulla and spinal cord [68]. However, it is hard to differentiate if carriers/delivery vehicles/substances/materials are using the olfactory or the trigeminal pathway, since the olfactory region is also innervated by branches of the trigeminal nerve, and so it is generally believed that both are involved. Moreover, trigeminal nerve branches passing through the cribriform plate (a horizontal segment forming the roof of the nasal cavity) were shown to be involved in the delivery of substances from the nose to the forebrain [69].

The delivery of the glycol chitosan polyplexes (GCP) to the cortex using a non-invasive route of administration such as the nose to brain route offers great potential for targeting neurological disorders in the cerebral cortex. A recent study by Ramos et al., showed effective silencing of the gene responsible for the synthesis of mutant huntingtin protein (HTT) where HTT mRNA was reduced by over 50% in the olfactory bulbs, hippocampus, striatum, and cerebral cortex at a dose of 5.8 nmol after 48 h [70]. GCP nanoparticles do not need manganese for their preparation and manganese could contribute to the toxicity of the carrier system as the authors suggest [65].

5. Conclusions

In summary, we have shown that glycol chitosan polyplexes upon intranasal administration are able to deliver β-Gal DNA plasmid predominantly to the brain cortex and that glycol chitosan is significantly less toxic when compared to the commercial transfection reagent, Lipofectamine. This important finding may be studied further to create gene therapy interventions for neurodegenerative and brain cancer conditions specifically requiring cortex targeting. Naked DNA is preferentially delivered to the cerebellum following intranasal administration and we hypothesize that this is because it utilizes the trigeminal pathway to transport to the deeper brain. Coating polyplexes with hyaluronidase results in gene expression spreading to wider parts of the brain upon intranasal administration, when compared to uncoated polyplexes. However, further studies are needed to prove the role of hyaluronidase coating to facilitate the extracellular transport of molecules from the nasal cavity to the brain.

Supplementary Materials: The following supporting information can be downloaded at: https://www.mdpi.com/article/10.3390/pharmaceutics14061136/s1. Figure S1: Degraded GC37 ^{1}H-NMR (D$_2$O), Figure S2: Size distribution plots of hyaluronidase by intensity, volume and number, Figure S3: Representative IVIS images 24 h post intranasal administration of polyplexes and 15 mins post intranasal administration of the substrate at β-Gal DNA concentration of 84 μg mL^{-1} and a dose of 0.067 mg kg^{-1}.

Author Contributions: I.F.U., A.I.P. and A.G.S.: Conceptualization, data curation and writing—review and editing. A.I.P.: conduct of all experiments, methodology, formal analysis, investigation, data curation, writing—original draft preparation. I.K.: investigation, methodology, review and editing. A.V.: methodology and review and editing. All authors have read and agreed to the published version of the manuscript.

Funding: This research was funded by the EPSRC (EP/L01646X/1, award # 1638294) and the Centre for Doctoral Training in Targeted Therapeutics and Nanomedicines at the UCL School of Pharmacy.

Institutional Review Board Statement: The study was conducted in accordance with the UK Home Office licence and in accordance with the UK Animal Scientific Procedures Act 1986 (ASPA). The experiments were carried out in the biological safety unit at the UCL School of Pharmacy. The animal study protocol was approved by the Named Veterinary Surgeon and Named Animal Care and Welfare Officer in the UCL School of Pharmacy Biological Safety Unit.

Informed Consent Statement: Not applicable.

Data Availability Statement: The data supporting the findings of the study are available from the corresponding author, upon a reasonable request.

Acknowledgments: We would like to thank the CDT for Targeted Therapeutics and Advanced Nanomedicines in UCL School of Pharmacy, London, UK. Additionally, we would like to thank Ryan Mellor for his guidance and technical assistance with the HPLC method for the detection of hyaluronidase.

Conflicts of Interest: The authors declare no conflict of interest. The company had no role in the design of the study; in the collection, analyses, or inter-pretation of data; in the writing of the manuscript; or in the decision to publish the results.

References

1. Zhang, W.; Mehta, A.; Tong, Z.; Esser, L.; Voelcker, N.H. Development of Polymeric Nanoparticles for Blood–Brain Barrier Transfer—Strategies and Challenges. *Adv. Sci.* **2021**, *8*, 2003937. [CrossRef] [PubMed]
2. Owensiii, D.; Peppas, N. Opsonization, biodistribution, and pharmacokinetics of polymeric nanoparticles. *Int. J. Pharm.* **2006**, *307*, 93–102. [CrossRef] [PubMed]
3. Pozzoli, M.; Rogueda, P.; Zhu, B.; Smith, T.; Young, P.M.; Traini, D.; Sonvico, F. Dry powder nasal drug delivery: Challenges, opportunities and a study of the commercial Teijin Puvlizer Rhinocort device and formulation. *Drug Dev. Ind. Pharm.* **2016**, *42*, 1660–1668. [CrossRef] [PubMed]
4. Pardeshi, C.V.; Belgamwar, V.S. Direct nose to brain drug delivery *via* integrated nerve pathways bypassing the blood–brain barrier: An excellent platform for brain targeting. *Expert Opin. Drug Deliv.* **2013**, *10*, 957–972. [CrossRef]
5. Bahadur, S.; Pardhi, D.M.; Rautio, J.; Rosenholm, J.M.; Pathak, K. Intranasal nanoemulsions for direct nose-to-brain delivery of actives for cns disorders. *Pharmaceutics* **2020**, *12*, 1230. [CrossRef]
6. Kim, I.D.; Shin, J.H.; Kim, S.W.; Choi, S.; Ahn, J.; Han, P.L.; Park, J.S.; Lee, J.K. Intranasal delivery of HMGB1 siRNA confers target gene knockdown and robust neuroprotection in the postischemic brain. *Mol. Ther.* **2012**, *20*, 829–839. [CrossRef]
7. Aly, A.E.E.; Waszczak, B.L. Intranasal gene delivery for treating Parkinsons disease: Overcoming the blood-brain barrier. *Expert Opin. Drug Deliv.* **2015**, *12*, 1923–1941. [CrossRef]
8. Claxton, A.; Baker, L.D.; Hanson, A.; Trittschuh, E.H.; Cholerton, B.; Morgan, A.; Callaghan, M.; Arbuckle, M.; Behl, C.; Craft, S. Long-acting intranasal insulin detemir improves cognition for adults with mild cognitive impairment or early-stage Alzheimer's Disease dementia. *J. Alzheimer's Dis.* **2015**, *44*, 897–906. [CrossRef]
9. Craft, S.; Claxton, A.; Baker, L.D.; Hanson, A.J.; Cholerton, B.; Trittschuh, E.H.; Dahl, D.; Caulder, E.; Neth, B.; Montine, T.J.; et al. Effects of Regular and Long-Acting Insulin on Cognition and Alzheimer's Disease Biomarkers: A Pilot Clinical Trial. *J. Alzheimer's Dis.* **2017**, *57*, 1325–1334. [CrossRef]
10. Craft, S.; Raman, R.; Chow, T.W.; Rafii, M.S.; Sun, C.K.; Rissman, R.A.; Donohue, M.C.; Brewer, J.B.; Jenkins, C.; Harless, K.; et al. Safety, Efficacy, and Feasibility of Intranasal Insulin for the Treatment of Mild Cognitive Impairment and Alzheimer Disease Dementia: A Randomized Clinical Trial. *JAMA Neurol.* **2020**, *77*, 1099–1109. [CrossRef]
11. Brambilla, M.; Manenti, R.; de Girolamo, G.; Adenzato, M.; Bocchio-Chiavetto, L.; Cotelli, M. Effects of Intranasal Oxytocin on Long-Term Memory in Healthy Humans: A Systematic Review. *Drug Dev. Res.* **2016**, *77*, 479–488. [CrossRef] [PubMed]
12. Fliedner, S.; Schulz, C.; Lehnert, H. Brain uptake of intranasally applied radioiodinated leptin in Wistar rats. *Endocrinology* **2006**, *147*, 2088–2094. [CrossRef] [PubMed]
13. Lee, M.R.; Shnitko, T.A.; Blue, S.W.; Kaucher, A.V.; Winchell, A.J.; Erikson, D.W.; Grant, K.A.; Leggio, L. Labeled oxytocin administered via the intranasal route reaches the brain in rhesus macaques. *Nat. Commun.* **2020**, *11*, 2783. [CrossRef]
14. Berger, S.; Pho, H.; Fleury-Curado, T.; Bevans-Fonti, S.; Younas, H.; Shin, M.K.; Jun, J.C.; Anokye-Danso, F.; Ahima, R.S.; Enquist, L.W.; et al. Intranasal leptin relieves sleep-disordered breathing in mice with diet-induced obesity. *Am. J. Respir. Crit. Care Med.* **2019**, *199*, 773–783. [CrossRef] [PubMed]

15. Harmon, B.T.; Aly, A.E.; Padegimas, L.; Sesenoglu-Laird, O.; Cooper, M.J.; Waszczak, B.L. Intranasal administration of plasmid DNA nanoparticles yields successful transfection and expression of a reporter protein in rat brain. *Gene Ther.* **2014**, *21*, 514–521. [CrossRef] [PubMed]
16. Aly, A.E.E.; Harmon, B.T.; Padegimas, L.; Sesenoglu-Laird, O.; Cooper, M.J.; Waszczak, B.L. Intranasal Delivery of pGDNF DNA Nanoparticles Provides Neuroprotection in the Rat 6-Hydroxydopamine Model of Parkinson's Disease. *Mol. Neurobiol.* **2019**, *56*, 688–701. [CrossRef]
17. Ha, J.; Kim, M.; Lee, Y.; Lee, M. Intranasal delivery of self-assembled nanoparticles of therapeutic peptides and antagomirs elicits anti-tumor effects in an intracranial glioblastoma model. *Nanoscale* **2021**, *13*, 14745–14759. [CrossRef]
18. Chapman, C.D.; Frey, W.H.; Craft, S.; Danielyan, L.; Hallschmid, M.; Schiöth, H.B.; Benedict, C. Intranasal treatment of central nervous system dysfunction in humans. *Pharm. Res.* **2013**, *30*, 2475–2484. [CrossRef]
19. Wang, Z.; Xiong, G.; Tsang, W.C.; Schätzlein, A.G.; Uchegbu, I.F. Nose-to-brain delivery. *J. Pharmacol. Exp. Ther.* **2019**, *370*, 593–601. [CrossRef]
20. Alexander, A.; Saraf, S. Nose-to-brain drug delivery approach: A key to easily accessing the brain for the treatment of Alzheimer's disease. *Neural Regen. Res.* **2018**, *13*, 2102. [CrossRef]
21. Crowe, T.P.; Greenlee, M.H.W.; Kanthasamy, A.G.; Hsu, W.H. Mechanism of intranasal drug delivery directly to the brain. *Life Sci.* **2018**, *195*, 44–52. [CrossRef] [PubMed]
22. Dhuria, S.V.; Hanson, L.R.; Frey, W.H. Intranasal delivery to the central nervous system: Mechanisms and experimental considerations. *J. Pharm. Sci.* **2010**, *99*, 1654–1673. [CrossRef] [PubMed]
23. Hashizume, R.; Ozawa, T.; Gryaznov, S.M.; Bollen, A.W.; Lamborn, K.R.; Frey, W.H.; Deen, D.F. New therapeutic approach for brain tumors: Intranasal delivery of telomerase inhibitor GRN163. *Neuro. Oncol.* **2008**, *10*, 112–120. [CrossRef] [PubMed]
24. Nonaka, N.; Farr, S.A.; Kageyama, H.; Shioda, S.; Banks, W.A. Delivery of Galanin-Like Peptide to the Brain: Targeting with Intranasal Delivery and Cyclodextrins. *J. Pharmacol. Exp. Ther.* **2008**, *325*, 513–519. [CrossRef] [PubMed]
25. Charlton, S.T.; Whetstone, J.; Fayinka, S.T.; Read, K.D.; Illum, L.; Davis, S.S. Evaluation of Direct Transport Pathways of Glycine Receptor Antagonists and an Angiotensin Antagonist from the Nasal Cavity to the Central Nervous System in the Rat Model. *Pharm. Res.* **2008**, *25*, 1531–1543. [CrossRef]
26. Hada, N.; Netzer, W.J.; Belhassan, F.; Wennogle, L.P.; Gizurarson, S. Nose-to-brain transport of imatinib mesylate: A pharmacokinetic evaluation. *Eur. J. Pharm. Sci.* **2017**, *102*, 46–54. [CrossRef]
27. Godfrey, L.; Iannitelli, A.; Garrett, N.L.; Moger, J.; Imbert, I.; King, T.; Porreca, F.; Soundararajan, R.; Lalatsa, A.; Schätzlein, A.G.; et al. Nanoparticulate peptide delivery exclusively to the brain produces tolerance free analgesia. *J. Control. Release* **2018**, *270*, 135–144. [CrossRef]
28. Lochhead, J.J.; Wolak, D.J.; Pizzo, M.E.; Thorne, R.G. Rapid transport within cerebral perivascular spaces underlies widespread tracer distribution in the brain after intranasal administration. *J. Perinatol.* **2015**, *35*, 371–381. [CrossRef]
29. Thorne, R.G.; Pronk, G.J.; Padmanabhan, V.; Frey, W.H. Delivery of insulin-like growth factor-I to the rat brain and spinal cord along olfactory and trigeminal pathways following intranasal administration. *Neuroscience* **2004**, *127*, 481–496. [CrossRef]
30. Aly, A.E.E.; Harmon, B.; Padegimas, L.; Sesenoglu-Laird, O.; Cooper, M.J.; Yurek, D.M.; Waszczak, B.L. Intranasal delivery of hGDNF plasmid DNA nanoparticles results in long-term and widespread transfection of perivascular cells in rat brain. *Nanomed. Nanotechnol. Biol. Med.* **2019**, *16*, 20–33. [CrossRef]
31. Das, M.; Wang, C.; Bedi, R.; Mohapatra, S.S.; Mohapatra, S. Magnetic micelles for DNA delivery to rat brains after mild traumatic brain injury. *Nanomed. Nanotechnol. Biol. Med.* **2014**, *10*, 1539–1548. [CrossRef] [PubMed]
32. Scodeller, P.; Catalano, P.N.; Salguero, N.; Duran, H.; Wolosiuk, A.; Soler-Illia, G.J.A.A. Hyaluronan degrading silica nanoparticles for skin cancer therapy. *Nanoscale* **2013**, *5*, 9690–9698. [CrossRef] [PubMed]
33. Monroe Freeman, R.E.; Anderson, P.; Wezster, M.E.; Dorfman, A. Ethanolic fractionation of bovine testicular hyaluronidase. *J. Biol. Chem.* **1950**, *186*, 201–206. [CrossRef]
34. Wang, S.S.; Yan, Y.; Ho, K. US FDA-approved therapeutic antibodies with high-concentration formulation: Summaries and perspectives. *Antib. Ther.* **2021**, *4*, 262–272. [CrossRef]
35. Soundararajan, R.; Wang, G.; Petkova, A.; Uchegbu, I.F.; Schä, A.G. Hyaluronidase Coated Molecular Envelope Technology Nanoparticles Enhance Drug Absorption via the Subcutaneous Route. *Mol. Pharm.* **2020**, *17*, 2599–2611. [CrossRef]
36. Wang, W.; Mcconaghy, A.M.; Tetley, L.; Uchegbu, I.F. Controls on Polymer Molecular Weight May Be Used To Control the Size of Palmitoyl Glycol Chitosan Polymeric Vesicles. *Langmuir* **2001**, *17*, 631–636. [CrossRef]
37. Enzymatic Assay of Hyaluronidase. Available online: https://www.sigmaaldrich.com/BG/en/technical-documents/protocol/protein-biology/enzyme-activity-assays/enzymatic-assay-of-hyaluronidase (accessed on 5 May 2022).
38. Hanson, L.R.; Fine, J.M.; Svitak, A.L.; Faltesek, K.A. Intranasal administration of CNS therapeutics to awake mice. *J. Vis. Exp.* **2013**, *74*, e4440. [CrossRef]
39. Lončarević, A.; Ivanković, M.; Rogina, A. Lysozyme-Induced Degradation of Chitosan: The Characterisation of Degraded Chitosan Scaffolds. *J. Tissue Repair Regen.* **2017**, *1*, 12–22. [CrossRef]
40. Chen, J.-K.; Shen, C.-R.; Liu, C.-L. N-acetylglucosamine: Production and applications. *Mar. Drugs* **2010**, *8*, 2493–2516. [CrossRef]
41. Sohaebuddin, S.K.; Thevenot, P.T.; Baker, D.; Eaton, J.W.; Tang, L. Nanomaterial cytotoxicity is composition, size, and cell type dependent. *Part. Fibre Toxicol.* **2010**, *7*, 22. [CrossRef]

42. Mann, A.; Richa, R.; Ganguli, M. DNA condensation by poly-l-lysine at the single molecule level: Role of DNA concentration and polymer length. *J. Control. Release* **2008**, *125*, 252–262. [CrossRef] [PubMed]
43. Cherng, J.Y.; Talsma, H.; Verrijk, R.; Crommelin, D.J.; Hennink, W.E. The effect of formulation parameters on the size of poly-((2-dimethylamino)ethyl methacrylate)-plasmid complexes. *Eur. J. Pharm. Biopharm.* **1999**, *47*, 215–224. [CrossRef]
44. Ogris, M.; Steinlein, P.; Kursa, M.; Mechtler, K.; Kircheis, R.; Wagner, E. The size of DNA/transferrin-PEI complexes is an important factor for gene expression in cultured cells. *Gene Ther.* **1998**, *5*, 1425–1433. [CrossRef] [PubMed]
45. Mann, A.; Khan, M.A.; Shukla, V.; Ganguli, M. Atomic force microscopy reveals the assembly of potential DNA "nanocarriers" by poly-l-ornithine. *Biophys. Chem.* **2007**, *129*, 126–136. [CrossRef]
46. Dai, J.; Han, S.; Ju, F.; Han, M.; Xu, L.; Zhang, R.; Sun, Y. Preparation and evaluation of tumour microenvironment response multistage nanoparticles for epirubicin delivery and deep tumour penetration. *Artif. Cells Nanomed. Biotechnol.* **2018**, *46*, 860–873. [CrossRef]
47. Uchegbu, I.F. Pharmaceutical nanotechnology: Polymeric vesicles for drug and gene delivery. *Expert Opin. Drug Deliv.* **2006**, *3*, 629–640. [CrossRef]
48. Hanefeld, U.; Cao, L.; Magner, E. Enzyme immobilisation: Fundamentals and application. *Chem. Soc. Rev.* **2013**, *42*, 6211. [CrossRef]
49. Fernandez-Lafuente, R. Editorial Special Issue: Enzyme Immobilization. *Molecules* **2014**, *19*, 20671–20674. [CrossRef]
50. Karmakar, S. Enzyme Activity—An overview | ScienceDirect Topics. In *Handbook of Nanomaterials for Industrial Applications*; Elsevier: Amsterdam, The Netherlands, 2018.
51. Feigin, V.L.; Nichols, E.; Alam, T.; Bannick, M.S.; Beghi, E.; Blake, N.; Culpepper, W.J.; Dorsey, E.R.; Elbaz, A.; Ellenbogen, R.G.; et al. Global, regional, and national burden of neurological disorders, 1990–2016: A systematic analysis for the Global Burden of Disease Study 2016. *Lancet Neurol.* **2019**, *18*, 459–480. [CrossRef]
52. Pardridge, W.M. The blood-brain barrier: Bottleneck in brain drug development. *NeuroRx* **2005**, *2*, 3–14. [CrossRef]
53. Nyamay'antu, A.; Dumont, M.; Kedinger, V.; Erbacher, P. Non-Viral Vector Mediated Gene Delivery: The Outsider to Watch out for in Gene Therapy. *Cell Gene Ther. Insights* **2019**, *5*, 51–57. [CrossRef]
54. Villate-Beitia, I.; Puras, G.; Zarate, J.; Agirre, M.; Ojeda, E.; Pedraz, J.L. First Insights into Non-invasive Administration Routes for Non-viral Gene Therapy. In *Gene Therapy—Principles and Challenges*; InTech: Vienna, Austria, 2015.
55. Hadaczek, P.; Yamashita, Y.; Mirek, H.; Tamas, L.; Bohn, M.C.; Noble, C.; Park, J.W.; Bankiewicz, K. The 'Perivascular Pump' Driven by Arterial Pulsation Is a Powerful Mechanism for the Distribution of Therapeutic Molecules within the Brain. *Mol. Ther.* **2006**, *14*, 69–78. [CrossRef] [PubMed]
56. Paldor, I.; Pearce, F.C.; Drummond, K.J.; Kaye, A.H. Frontal glioblastoma multiforme may be biologically distinct from non-frontal and multilobar tumors. *J. Clin. Neurosci.* **2016**, *34*, 128–132. [CrossRef] [PubMed]
57. Frantz, C.; Stewart, K.M.; Weaver, V.M. The extracellular matrix at a glance. *J. Cell Sci.* **2010**, *123*, 4195–4200. [CrossRef]
58. Pluen, A.; Boucher, Y.; Ramanujan, S.; McKee, T.D.; Gohongi, T.; di Tomaso, E.; Brown, E.B.; Izumi, Y.; Campbell, R.B.; Berk, D.A.; et al. Role of tumor-host interactions in interstitial diffusion of macromolecules: Cranial vs. subcutaneous tumors. *Proc. Natl. Acad. Sci. USA* **2001**, *98*, 4628–4633. [CrossRef]
59. Wenning, L.A.; Murphy, R.M. Coupled cellular trafficking and diffusional limitations in delivery of immunotoxins to multicell tumor spheroids. *Biotechnol. Bioeng.* **1999**, *62*, 562–575. [CrossRef]
60. Li, Z.-Y.; Ni, S.; Yang, X.; Kiviat, N.; Lieber, A. Xenograft models for liver metastasis: Relationship between tumor morphology and adenovirus vector transduction. *Mol. Ther.* **2004**, *9*, 650–657. [CrossRef]
61. Huang, M.; Khor, E.; Lim, L.-Y. Uptake and Cytotoxicity of Chitosan Molecules and Nanoparticles: Effects of Molecular Weight and Degree of Deacetylation. *Pharm Res.* **2004**, *21*, 344–353. [CrossRef]
62. Yilmaz, E. Chitosan: A Versatile Biomaterial. In *Advances in Experimental Medicine and Biology*; Springer: Boston, MA, USA, 2004; pp. 59–68.
63. Zhang, W.; Yang, H.; Kong, X.; Mohapatra, S.; Juan-Vergara, H.S.; Hellermann, G.; Behera, S.; Singam, R.; Lockey, R.F.; Mohapatra, S.S. Inhibition of respiratory syncytial virus infection with intranasal siRNA nanoparticles targeting the viral NS1 gene. *Nat. Med.* **2005**, *11*, 56–62. [CrossRef]
64. Simão Carlos, M.I.; Zheng, K.; Garrett, N.; Arifin, N.; Workman, D.G.; Kubajewska, I.; Halwani, A.A.; Moger, J.; Zhang, Q.; Schätzlein, A.G.; et al. Limiting the level of tertiary amines on polyamines leads to biocompatible nucleic acid vectors. *Int. J. Pharm.* **2017**, *526*, 106–124. [CrossRef]
65. Sanchez-Ramos, J.; Song, S.; Kong, X.; Foroutan, P.; Martinez, G.; Dominguez-Viqueira, W.; Mohapatra, S.; Mohapatra, S.; Haraszti, R.A.; Khvorova, A.; et al. Chitosan-Mangafodipir nanoparticles designed for intranasal delivery of siRNA and DNA to brain. *J. Drug Deliv. Sci. Technol.* **2018**, *43*, 453–460. [CrossRef] [PubMed]
66. Yurek, D.M.; Fletcher, A.M.; McShane, M.; Kowalczyk, T.H.; Padegimas, L.; Weatherspoon, M.R.; Kaytor, M.D.; Cooper, M.J.; Ziady, A.G. DNA nanoparticles: Detection of long-term transgene activity in brain using bioluminescence imaging. *Mol. Imaging* **2011**, *10*. [CrossRef] [PubMed]
67. Gänger, S.; Schindowski, K. Tailoring Formulations for Intranasal Nose-to-Brain Delivery: A Review on Architecture, Physico-Chemical Characteristics and Mucociliary Clearance of the Nasal Olfactory Mucosa. *Pharmaceutics* **2018**, *10*, 116. [CrossRef] [PubMed]
68. Selvaraj, K.; Gowthamarajan, K.; Karri, V.V.S.R. Nose to brain transport pathways an overview: Potential of nanostructured lipid carriers in nose to brain targeting. *Artif. Cells Nanomed. Biotechnol.* **2018**, *46*, 2088–2095. [CrossRef]

69. Liu, X.-F.; Fawcett, J.R.; Hanson, L.R.; Frey, W.H. The window of opportunity for treatment of focal cerebral ischemic damage with noninvasive intranasal insulin-like growth factor-I in rats. *J. Stroke Cerebrovasc. Dis.* **2004**, *13*, 16–23. [CrossRef]
70. Sava, V.; Fihurka, O.; Khvorova, A.; Sanchez-Ramos, J. Enriched chitosan nanoparticles loaded with siRNA are effective in lowering Huntington's disease gene expression following intranasal administration. *Nanomed. Nanotechnol. Biol. Med.* **2020**, *24*, 102119. [CrossRef]

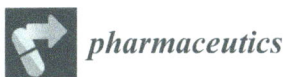

Article

Thymoquinone-Enriched Naringenin-Loaded Nanostructured Lipid Carrier for Brain Delivery via Nasal Route: In Vitro Prospect and In Vivo Therapeutic Efficacy for the Treatment of Depression

Farheen Fatima Qizilbash [1], Muhammad Usama Ashhar [1], Ameeduzzafar Zafar [2], Zufika Qamar [1], Annu [1], Javed Ali [1], Sanjula Baboota [1], Mohammed M. Ghoneim [3], Sultan Alshehri [4] and Asgar Ali [1,*]

[1] Department of Pharmaceutics, School of Pharmaceutical Education and Research, Jamia Hamdard University, New Delhi 110062, India; farheenfqizilbash_sch@jamiahamdard.ac.in (F.F.Q.); usamas132@gmail.com (M.U.A.); zufikakaqamar_sch@jamiahamdard.ac.in (Z.Q.); atriannu407@gmail.com (A.); jali@jamiahamdard.ac.in (J.A.); sbaboota@jamiahamdard.ac.in (S.B.)

[2] Department of Pharmaceutics, College of Pharmacy, Jouf University, Sakaka 72341, Al-Jouf, Saudi Arabia; zzafarpharmacian@gmail.com or azafar@ju.edu.sa

[3] Department of Pharmacy Practice, College of Pharmacy, AlMaarefa University, Ad Diriyah 13713, Ad Diriyah, Saudi Arabia; mghoneim@mcst.edu.sa

[4] Department of Pharmaceutics, College of Pharmacy, King Saud University, Riyadh 11451, Riyadh, Saudi Arabia; salshehri1@ksu.edu.sa

* Correspondence: aali@jamiahamdard.ac.in or alipharm786@gmail.com; Tel.: +91-9899571926

Abstract: In the current research, a thymoquinone-enriched naringenin (NGN)-loaded nanostructured lipid carrier (NLC) was developed and delivered via the nasal route for depression. Thymoquinone (TQ) oil was used as the liquid lipid and provided synergistic effects. A TQ- and NGN-enriched NLC was developed via the ultrasonication technique and optimized using a central composite rotatable design (CCRD). The optimized NLC exhibited the following properties: droplet size, 84.17 to 86.71 nm; PDI, 0.258 to 0.271; zeta potential, −8.15 to −8.21 mV; and % EE, 87.58 to 88.21%. The in vitro drug release profile showed the supremacy of the TQ-NGN-NLC in comparison to the NGN suspension, with a cumulative drug release of 82.42 ± 1.88% from the NLC and 38.20 ± 0.82% from the drug suspension. Ex vivo permeation study displayed a 2.21-fold increase in nasal permeation of NGN from the NLC compared to the NGN suspension. DPPH study showed the better antioxidant potential of the TQ-NGN-NLC in comparison to NGN alone due to the synergistic effect of NGN and TQ oil. CLSM images revealed deeper permeation of the NGN-NLC (39.9 µm) through the nasal mucosa in comparison to the NGN suspension (20 µm). Pharmacodynamic studies, such as the forced swim test and the locomotor activity test, were assessed in the depressed rat model, which revealed the remarkable antidepressant effect of the TQ-NGN-NLC in comparison to the NGN suspension and the marketed formulation. The results signify the potential of the TQ-enriched NGN-NLC in enhancing brain delivery and the therapeutic effect of NGN for depression treatment.

Keywords: naringenin; nanostructured lipid carrier; intranasal delivery; central composite rotatable design; depression

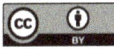

1. Introduction

Depression is a major public health issue that affects all age groups globally. As per the World Health Organization (WHO), depression affects around 280 million people across the globe and is known to be the main factor contributing to global disability [1]. An imbalance in the levels of neurotransmitters (NTs) such as norepinephrine, dopamine, and serotonin, which have a major function that plays a significant role in conducting information through the presynaptic to the postsynaptic neuron, is commonly attributed to the cause of depression [2]. Issues such as oxidative stress, mitochondrial dysfunction, and inflammation are the most explored aspects that occur in patients with depression [3]. Conventionally available treatment for depression is associated with several adverse effects, such as cognitive impairment, tachycardia, etc., most of which have bioavailability issues and thus low therapeutic efficacy. Natural drugs have been widely used in treating depression and anxiety in recent years due to better therapeutic windows and fewer adverse effects. Naringenin (NGN) is a natural flavonoid that is used for treating numerous neurological ailments. It works by hindering monoamine oxidase-A (MAO-A), which results in the restoration of serotonin, epinephrine, and dopamine levels [4]. It also raises the levels of brain-derived neurotrophic factor (BDNF) in the hippocampus, demonstrating its effectiveness in treating depression [5,6]. NGN, when administered by conventional routes, leads to extensive first-pass metabolism with reduced bioavailability of 5.81% in the brain because of its inability to pass via the blood/brain barrier (BBB) [7]. Therefore, TQ-enriched NLC has been used to achieve a synergistic effect and enhance the BA of NGN in the brain.

Nanostructured lipid carriers (NLCs) were developed because they offer several benefits, including drug protection, low toxicity, no organic solvents during manufacture, and controlled release [8,9]. NLCs also protect the loaded medication from degradation and efflux ions, leading to increased drug bioavailability in the blood and brain [10]. NLCs can also be administered via the intranasal route to achieve brain-targeted action. Since the target site for depression is the brain, the administration of an NLC via the nasal route can result in direct delivery of the medication into the brain by avoiding drug delivery to nontarget sites. The intranasal route is known to circumvent the hepatic metabolism and intestinal metabolism, as well as the BBB. It is a non-delivery-invasive and safer route to achieve improved bioavailability and therapeutic effectiveness of a drug with minimal side effects [11,12].

As one of the components of NLCs is a liquid lipid, thymoquinone (TQ) has been employed as an oil phase or a liquid lipid for the development of NLCs. Thymoquinone (TQ) is known to be the chief component of *Nigella sativa* seeds and has several pharmacological actions, such as anti-inflammatory and antioxidant effects [13]. It also offers peroxidation to the lipid membrane, hindering neuroinflammation by blocking the development of inflammatory mediators, known to be a causative factor for the progression of depression [14,15]. TQ also helps in modulating γ-aminobutyric acid (GABA) and nitric oxide levels and upregulates the levels of 5-hydroxytryptamine in the brain, showing its antidepressant activity [16,17]. Thus, using TQ as a liquid lipid in the formulation provides an added advantage in the treatment of depression [18].

Natural products have been demonstrated to have considerable pharmacological effects that affect many important cell signaling pathways and induce mitogenic, cytotoxic, and genotoxic reactions needed for disease treatment and prophylaxis [19,20]. These herbs, including various flavonoids, triterpenoids, and saponins, have been explored by 75% of the world for various ailments. Some work by hindering the monoamine oxidase, serotonin, dopamine, and norepinephrine transporters, while others work by enhancing hippocampal dopamine levels. Some traditional Chinese medicinal plants, such as flavonoids extracted from *Tilia Americana*, have been found to be effective in treating sleep disorders, while some plants, such as *Polygala tenuifolia, Panax ginseng, Fructus aurantii*, and Shen Yuan, are medication extensively used to stimulate BDNF in depressive models of rodents [21]. Herbal extracts are known to target various biological pathways and several receptors [22]. However, the basic mechanisms of these herbs have been repeatedly described without a fundamental pathway. Thus, these herbs and their extracts need to be further explored in terms of clinical studies to understand their underlying pathways and therapeutic efficacy in humans [23,24].

In recent years, scientists have discovered the use of chemicals, such as statins, chemically known as 3-hydroxy-3-methyl-glutaryl-CoA (HMG-CoA) inhibitors, derived from plants, which have gained attention due to their therapeutic effects that occur by targeting several molecular pathways. These statins, including fluvastatin, simvastatin, atorvastatin, and pravastatin, are known to have significant effects in lowering cholesterol levels, while lovastatin, derived from *Aspergillus terreus*, was approved by the Food and Drug Administration in 1987 to stimulate autophagy, which further suppresses the growth of cancer cells [25,26].

As a matter of fact, some anticancer drugs, such as vinca alkaloids and paclitaxel, have been made from plant sources and used as first-line treatment for ovarian cancer [27]. Another compound, known as apigenin, has gained attention due to its pharmacological effects, such as anti-inflammation and neuroprotective effects. It helps in targeting several signaling pathways, such as phosphatidylinositol 3-kinase/protein kinase B (PI3K/AKT), nuclear factor kappa B (NF-kB), etc., and thus helps in the treatment of cancer by diminishing the proliferation of tumors [28]. Celastrol is another compound also known to possess an anticancer effect by stimulating various cellular pathways, which further works by triggering the mitochondrial apoptotic pathway and hindering NF-kB, resulting in cell cycle arrest. It is also known to tackle bioavailability issues when loaded into a nanocarrier and has proved to be a safer compound. These phytochemicals have expanded their use due to their safer toxicity windows and multifactorial effects [29].

From previous studies, the neurodegenerative effects of NGN and TQ have been established separately against Alzheimer's disease, Parkinson's diseases, depression, anxiety, etc. However, there are various limitations associated with NGN, such as low aqueous solubility, poor absorption across the gastrointestinal tract, and extensive gut flora metabolism, leading to the deterioration of NGN [30]. Similarly, TQ also suffers from low bioavailability due to its chemical properties and poor penetration ability across the membrane [31]. Thus, to mask these associated limitations of NGN and TQ, this combination was loaded into an NLC for the treatment of depression and was administered through the intranasal route for uninterrupted delivery to the brain.

Previously, Gaba et al. reported an NGN nanoemulsion encapsulated with vitamin E for treating Parkinson's disease [32]. The nanoemulsion approach requires the incorporation of large quantities of surfactants and cosurfactants that can be reduced by formulating them into an NLC. Similarly, Ahmad et al. reported a poloxamer/chitosan-loaded NGN nanoemulsion for the treatment of cerebral ischemia [33]. However, both studies lacked a discussion of the stability issues of the prepared nanoemulsion. According to a study, nanoemulsions exhibit major stability issues such as coalescence, Ostwald ripening, creaming, phase separation, burst release [34], and sedimentation upon storage or during the preparation of the formulation [35]. However, these issues can be circumvented by incorporating the drug into an NLC-based formulation. Alam et al. prepared a TQ-loaded solid lipid carrier to attain an antidepressant effect in Wistar rats [36]. This study did not include in vitro and ex vivo assessment of the prepared formulation, which is a major pharmaceutical consideration for assessing the drug release pattern of a formulation. However, the drug loading efficiency in a solid lipid nanocarrier is comparatively lower than that of NLCs. Single lipids are incorporated into solid lipid nanocarriers due to their limited drug loading ability. Additionally, solid lipid nanocarriers undergo gelation and polymorphic transitions due to their highly ordered crystal lattice structure; therefore, NLCs may be a better approach compared to other nanolipid carriers [37].

The purpose of this research work was to formulate and evaluate a naringenin-encapsulated nanostructured lipid carrier (NGN-NLC) with TQ oil as a liquid lipid to provide synergistic efficacy for treating depression. This study also focuses on enhancing the central nervous system (CNS) bioavailability of NGN by avoiding the BBB via the intranasal route. The antidepressant potential of the NGN-NLC was further investigated by performing pharmacodynamic studies.

2. Materials and Methods
2.1. Materials

Naringenin and TQ oil were purchased as gift samples from Sigma-Aldrich Co. (Spruce St Saint Louis, MO, USA). Gelucire 39/01, glyceryl monostearate, Compritol, Precirol ATO-

5, Labrafil M 2130 CS, and Cremophor-EL were purchased from Gattefosse India Pvt. Ltd (Mumbai, India). Ascorbic acid and Rhodamine B were purchased from Sigma-Aldrich (Mumbai, India). Methanol and ethanol were obtained from Merck (Mumbai, India). 1,1-Diphenyl-2-picrylhydrazyl and 5,5'-dithiobis-2-nitrobenzoic acid were purchased from Sigma-Aldrich Chemicals Pvt. Ltd. (Bangalore, Karnataka, India). Sefsol® 218 was purchased from S D Fine Chem Limited (Mumbai, India). All other purchased solvents and chemicals were of analytical grade.

2.2. Methods

2.2.1. Solid Lipid and Liquid Lipid Screening

The selection of the solid lipid was made on the basis of the solubility of a drug in the lipid. A 1 g amount of several solid lipids was added to separate vials and heated on a magnetic stirrer at 5 ± 1 °C, taken a few degrees beyond the melting point of the solid lipid. Then, the addition of NGN in an incremental order was performed until saturation was reached, which was assessed visibly. The solubility of NGN in the liquid lipid, which was taken as TQ oil, was assessed by the addition of an excessive quantity of NGN to 2 mL of TQ oil and Sefsol® 218 (S-218) in the ratio of 1:1 in a stoppered vial with a 5 mL capacity [38]. Thereafter, for 5 min, the mixture was vortexed and placed in an isothermal shaker for 48 h at a temperature of 25 ± 0.5 °C. The supernatant obtained was later collected, diluted by methanol, and examined by UV spectrophotometry (UV-1601, Shimadzu, Japan) at 287 nm that was done after performing the centrifugation which was carried out for 13 min at 3000 rpm [39].

2.2.2. Assessment of Binary Mixture

The binary mixture of liquid lipid (TQ oil:S-218) and solid lipid was taken in several ratios (90:10, 85:15, 80:20, 70:30, 75:25, and 60:40) to assess the miscibility between the two lipids. The lipid mixture contained Precirol ATO-5 as the solid lipid, and TQ oil along with S-218 (1:1) as liquid lipids were taken in the above-mentioned ratios and stirred at 200 rpm on a magnetic stirrer for 1 h maintained at 85 ± 1 °C. A cooled sample of the solid combination was smeared on filter paper to evaluate the miscibility, followed by a visual inspection of the filter paper for the occurrence of any liquid oil droplets. The ratio that did not show any appearance of droplets of the lipids on the filter paper was preferred for the development of the NGN-NLC [40,41].

2.2.3. Screening of Surfactants

The surfactant was preferred based on its emulsification capability to emulsify the lipidic mixture. Different surfactants were chosen based on the literature review and their capacity to liquefy lipids. Methylene chloride (3 mL) was employed to liquefy the 100 mg lipidic mixture (Precirol ATO-5 and TQ oil/S-218 in a 1:1 ratio), which was added in the ratio of 70:30 to 10 mL of 5% solution of various surfactants. The organic phase was heated at 40 ± 1 °C for 30 min to obtain a mixture free from methylene chloride. The diluted sample's percentage transmittance was evaluated using a UV spectrophotometer at 510 nm [42].

2.3. Optimization and Formulation of Nanostructured Lipid Carrier (NLC)

2.3.1. NLC Optimization

The prepared NLC was optimized using Design Expert® (version 12.0.1.0, State-Ease Inc. Minneapolis, MN, USA). The binary lipid phase and surfactant were taken as independent variables in the central composite rotatable design (CCRD), and droplet size, entrapment efficiency (% EE), and polydispersity index (PDI) were taken as dependent variables (Table 1).

Table 1. Independent and dependent variables that have been considered in CCRD.

Factors	Levels Used				
Independent Variable	Axial (−α)	Low (−1)	Medium (0)	High (+1)	Axial (+α)
A: Binary lipid concentration (w/w%)	0.292	0.5	1	1.5	1.707
B: Surfactant concentration (w/w%)	1.171	2	4	6	6.828
Dependent variable	Constraints used				
R1: Droplet size (nm)	Minimum				
R2: PDI	Minimum				
R3: Entrapment efficiency (%)	Maximum				

2.3.2. Formulation of NLC

The solvent diffusion method was used to formulate the NGN-NLC, followed by the ultrasonication method. The preparation of the organic phase was done by prepending the lipidic mixture (70:30) and half the quantity of the surfactant (Cremophor-EL), along with NGN (0.72 mg/mL). Whereas, the preparation of aqueous phase was carried out by adding the left over quantity of the surfactant to 10 mL of distilled water. Both phases were maintained at the same temperature (70 °C), with continuous stirring at 500 rpm on a magnetic stirrer. Dropwise addition of the aqueous phase to the organic phase on a magnetic stirrer was performed with uninterrupted stirring at 800 rpm for 30 min, keeping both phases at 70 ± 5 °C. The resultant was then sonicated for 5 min using a probe sonicator (Hielscher, Germany) in an ice bath, that was subsequently cooled to room temperature [42].

2.4. Characterization of Optimized NGN-NLC Formulation

2.4.1. Zeta Potential, Droplet Size, and Polydispersity Index (PDI)

Zeta potential, droplet size, and PDI were assessed using the technique of dynamic light scattering (Malvern Zetasizer, Nano ZS, UK). The optimized NGN-NLC was diluted approximately 50 times before the analysis of the above-mentioned parameters. The scattering angle was maintained at 90°, whereas the temperature was maintained around 25 ± 2 °C. For the formulations that were not diluted, distilled water was used as a blank before experimenting. Experiments were performed in triplicate [43,44].

2.4.2. Entrapment Efficiency (% EE)

The quantity of free drug in the NLC that was entrapped was calculated by estimating the % EE. A 1 mL volume of the NGN-NLC was centrifuged at 4 ± 1 °C for 1 h at 15,120 g force (Sigma-3K30, Osterode am Harz, Germany). After diluting with methanol, the supernatant was collected, and the free drug was analyzed using UV spectroscopy at 287 nm. The calculation of the % EE was performed using the following equation [45].

$$Entrapment\ Efficiency = \frac{(W_t - W_s)}{(W_t)} \times 100 \quad (1)$$

where, W_t is the quantity of NGN added to the system, and W_s is the quantity of NGN in the supernatant upon centrifugation.

2.4.3. Determination of Surface Morphology

TEM (CM 200, Philips Briarcliff Manor, NY, USA)) was implemented to determine the surface morphology of the optimized NGN-NLC (CM 200, Philips Briarcliff Manor, NY, USA)). The optimized NGN-NLC formulation was subjected to dilution following the addition of a drop of the NGN-NLC on a copper grid coated with carbon, which was then dried and negatively stained with 1% phosphotungstic acid. The grid was then placed in the instrument and examined by TEM [46].

2.4.4. Stability Studies

Stability studies of the NGN-NLC were carried out for 3 months at room temperature ($25 \pm 2\ °C/60 \pm 5\%$ RH). The samples of these studies were taken at 0, 1, and 3 months and later examined for variation in physical appearance, droplet size, PDI, and % EE [47].

2.4.5. Drug Release Studies Using Dialysis Membrane

The release study of the drug from the NGN-NLC and NGN suspension were performed on a magnetic stirrer with the aid of a dialysis membrane with assembly placed at $37 \pm 2\ °C$. In the dialysis bag (12–14 KD), 2 mL of the optimized NGN-NLC formulation and NGN suspension containing 0.72 mg/mL of NGN was placed, which was kept in phosphate-buffered solution (PBS, pH = 6.4) (100 mL). A 1 mL volume of the sample was taken at 0.25, 0.5, 1, 2, 4, and 12 h and substituted with the same quantity of fresh media (PBS, pH = 6.4). The samples were examined three times ($n = 3$) by UV spectroscopy at 287 nm [48]. Then, drug release by the dialysis membrane was calculated using the following equation:

$$\% \text{ Drug Release} = \frac{\text{Concentration } (\mu g/mL) \times \text{Dilution Factor} \times \text{Volume of Release Medium } (mL)}{\text{Initial Dose } (\mu g)} \times 100 \quad (2)$$

2.4.6. Ex Vivo Nasal Permeation Study

The depth permeation of the NGN-NLC and NGN-suspension across goat nasal mucosa was evaluated using the CLSM technique, in which the nasal mucosa was positioned on a Franz diffusion cell filled with PBS (pH = 6.4). The NGN-NLC and NGN suspension treated with Rhodamine B (0.03% w/v) were added to the donor compartment of the Franz diffusion cell. The whole setup was placed on a magnetic stirrer, which was stirred at 100 rpm and maintained at 36 °C for 2 h. The experiment was carried out using isolated goat nasal mucosa and not an artificial membrane, as it was not easily available from a nearby slaughterhouse. Moreover, it was derived from the literature review that goat nasal mucosa is readily and cheaply available, and its morphology is relatively similar to that of humans. A 1 mL volume of the optimized NGN-NLC and NGN suspension both containing 0.72 mg/mL of NGN was placed in the donor section, the volume of which was 10 mL. A 1 mL volume of the sample was taken at 0.25, 0.5, 1, 2, 4, and 12 h and replaced with the same quantity of fresh media (PBS, pH = 6.4). The samples were analyzed in triplicate ($n = 3$) employing UV spectroscopy at 287 nm. The amount of NGN permeated was estimated using the following equation [49]:

$$\text{Permeability Coefficient } (P_{app}) = \frac{Flux}{\text{Initial Drug Concentration}} \quad (3)$$

2.4.7. Antioxidant Activity: DPPH Assay

Dithiobis-2-nitrobenzoic acid (DPPH) that is known to be a stable radical that produces a deep violet color upon the delocalization of its spare electron or hydrogen radical. The antioxidant potential of the NGN-NLC was compared to a standard of ascorbic acid, as well as pure NGN suspension. The evaluation was based on the ability of DPPH to scavenge free radicals at room temperature. Various concentrations (1–80 µg/mL) of all three samples were prepared in methanol, and each sample (1 mL) was diluted by the methanolic solution of DPPH (1 mL). After 30 min, the mixture was scanned, maintaining methanol (95%) as a blank at 515 nm [50]. The percentage inhibition of DPPH was determined using the following equation:

$$\% \text{ Inhibition of DPPH Radical} = \frac{A_0 - A_1}{A_0} \times 100 \quad (4)$$

where A_0 and A_1 are the absorbance of the control (blank) and sample, respectively. The 50% inhibitory dose, i.e., IC_{50} value, was evaluated using GraphPad Prism 8.0 (GraphPad Software, San Diego, CA, USA).

2.4.8. Estimation of Depth of Permeation by Confocal Laser Scanning Microscopy (CLSM)

The depth of permeation of the formulation and suspension across goat nasal mucosa was evaluated using the CLSM technique, in which the nasal mucosa was employed on a Franz diffusion cell filled with PBS (pH = 6.4). Then, the nasal mucosa was removed after 2 h, washed using distilled water, and isolated at a temperature of $-20\ ^\circ C$, followed by cutting off approximately 20 µm of thin slices of isolated nasal mucosa kept on coverslips made of glass. The formulation and suspension were treated with Rhodamine B (0.03% w/v), which was added to the donor compartment of the Franz diffusion cell. The whole setup was placed on a magnetic stirrer, which was stirred at 100 rpm and maintained at 36 $^\circ C$ for 2 h. These sections were later assessed on an LSM 710 scanning confocal microscope (TCS SP5II, Leica Microsystem Ltd., Wetzlar, Germany) at 580 nm, where the extent of depth of penetration between the NGN-NLC and NGN suspension was compared [51,52].

2.5. Pharmacodynamic Studies

The therapeutic effectiveness of the antidepressant drugs was investigated by performing behavior studies. NTs present in the brain are responsible for the normal functioning of the brain. Thus, the current research work was performed to examine the effect of the NGN-NLC (i.n) when compared to that of the NGN suspension (i.n) and oral administration of the duloxetine suspension (marketed formulation) by performing a forced swim test and locomotor activity test. The formulations were evaluated for inducing their antidepressant effect on rats to downregulate the symptoms linked with depression.

Wistar rats weighing between 200 and 250 g (11–12 weeks old) of either sex were chosen for performing pharmacodynamic tests. The animal study protocol was permitted by the Institutional Animal Ethical Committee (IAEC) (Jamia Hamdard, New Delhi, India), with the approved animal study protocol 173/Go/Re/ S/2000/CPCSEA (Approval No. 1647, 2019). The current study was performed following the guidelines of the Declaration of Helsinki. The experiment was conducted in a manner to reduce suffering. The Wistar rats were categorized into five groups, with three rats in each group. Normal and control groups consisted of non-depressed and depressed rats, respectively. The DLX suspension (oral) (duloxetine suspension) group consisted of depressed rats that were treated with a marketed antidepressant, i.e., DLX suspension with a dosage of 2.06 mg kg^{-1}. The doses of the different formulations were administered before determining the pharmacodynamic parameters.

Depressed rats of the last two groups were NGN suspension (i.n) and NGN-NLC (i.n) (0.72 mg kg^{-1}). Forced swim tests and locomotor activity tests (behavioral studies) were performed on the above-mentioned groups.

To induce depression, Wistar rats weighing between 200 and 250 g were chosen for the experiment. The rats were positioned in a cylindrical glass tank individually containing water up to a depth of approximately 30 cm at 28 $\pm$ 2 $^\circ C$ for 15 min. The animals were then taken out of the water and dried gently by patting them with a clean and dry towel. This procedure was performed for 15 days, and on the same day (15th day), pharmacodynamic parameters were determined after performing the forced swim test and the locomotor activity test [53].

2.5.1. Forced Swim Test

The forced swim test relies on the phenomenon of causing immobility in rats, which is subsequently tested for reversal by antidepressant drug delivery. Swimming time, immobility time, and climbing time are the three components used in the forced swim test. This test is based on the stimulation of immobility. It is a fast, easy, common, and cost-effective test, where immobility represents depressive behavior in rats. The rats were laid in a cylinder-shaped tank with a depth of 30 cm consisting of water at an optimal temperature of 28 ± 2 °C. The 6 min test was performed 30 min after administration of each formulation in the respective groups for a period of 15 days. Animals were re-exposed to a similar environment to swim for 6 min after each dose was administered on the 15th day, and forced swimming, immobility, and climbing times were recorded for 300 s [54].

2.5.2. Locomotor Activity Test

The locomotor activity test is also employed to investigate the efficacy of antidepressant drugs. The locomotor test was conducted to calculate the movements of rats using a digital photoactometer (Hicon, Chandigarh, India) consisting of photocells of infrared light. Rats were positioned in the photoactometer for 15 days before the experiment. The number of times the animal moved was counted using beam light, which was considered the locomotor activity performed by the rats. Different group comparisons were performed after the administration of the NGN-NLC and suspensions [55].

2.6. Statistical Analysis

The outcomes of the studies were analyzed by GraphPad Prism 8.0 (GraphPad Software, San Diego, CA, USA). The studies were carried out three times, and the results were expressed as the mean ± standard deviation (SD) using one-way ANOVA analysis. Data were considered statistically significant at $p < 0.05$.

3. Results and Discussion

3.1. Selection of Liquid Lipid and Solid Lipid

TQ oil was chosen as the liquid lipid for the formulation of the NLC due to its therapeutic effect as a potent antidepressant. In depression, an imbalance of brain NTs such as dopamine and serotonin occurs. TQ oil has been reported to restore these brain chemicals, thus indicating its antidepressant property. TQ oil also exhibits enhanced resistance to oxidative stress by diminishing the elevated levels of superoxide dismutase, lipid peroxidase, malondialdehyde, and glutathione in the brain and has been shown to reduce the pro-inflammatory mediators responsible for depression [56,57]. Thus, TQ oil was chosen as the lipidic phase. The drug solubility (NGN) in TQ oil was found to be 11.43 ± 0.09 mg/mL. This concentration of the selected liquid lipid led to the deposition of the drug at the bottom. Therefore, to enhance the solubility of NGN in TQ oil, S-218 was added as a solubilizing agent. The result was obtained after the incorporation of TQ oil with S-218 in the ratio of 1:1, indicating increased solubility of the drug in the selected liquid lipid. The solubility thus obtained was found to be 16.32 ± 0.21 mg/mL. Hence TQ: S-218 in the ratio of 1:1 was selected [58].

Among the various solid lipids, Gelucire 39/01, glyceryl monostearate (GMS), Compritol, Precirol ATO-5, and Labrafil M 2130 CS were screened. The highest solubility of NGN was in Precirol ATO-5, which was 15.91 ± 0.47 mg/g, as shown in Figure 1. On mixing with liquid lipid, Precirol ATO-5 has been reported to offer drug release in a sustained manner, improve solubility, and lessen the adverse effects associated with the drug [58,59].

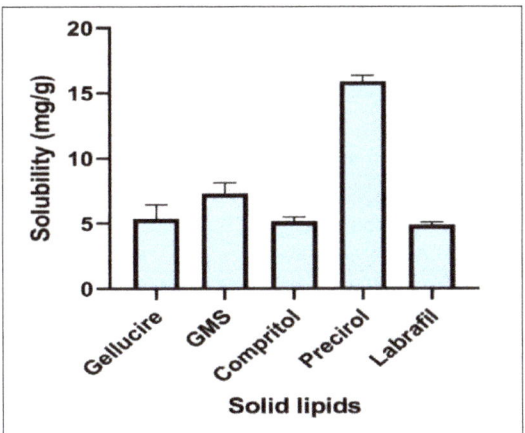

Figure 1. Solubility of NGN in various solid lipids: Precirol ATO-5 exhibited maximum solubility = 16.32 ± 0.21 mg/mL. Data expressed using mean ± SD ($n = 3$).

3.2. Assessment of Binary Mixture

The optimized ratio of binary lipid was chosen based on the stability of the binary lipid. On performing the test on the filter paper, it was perceived that no oil spots were detected on it after the application of a smear of the binary lipids consisting of a ratio of 70:30, signifying the miscibility of both lipids (i.e., solid and liquid lipids) compared to the other ratios. Hence, Precirol ATO-5 and TQ oil/S-218 (1:1) in the ratio of 70:30 were chosen for the formulation [56].

3.3. Screening of Surfactants

Various surfactants were employed to emulsify the selected binary mixture. The percentage transmittance of dispersion of the selected ratio was determined with different surfactants (Table 2). It was found that the drug demonstrated maximum miscibility in Cremophor-EL, including the utmost percent transmittance with the binary mixture; thus, it was considered a surfactant for the development of the NLC. Cremophor-EL is a surfactant used for poorly water-soluble drugs and also provides stability to the NGN-NLC by linking the long-chain fatty acids into the core of the lipidic phase [56].

Table 2. Transmittance in various surfactants ($n = 3$).

Surfactants	Transmittance (%) ± S.D
Tween 80	40.61 ± 0.53
Tween 20	70.18 ± 0.09
Cremophor-EL	91.11 ± 0.67
Labrasol	0.40 ± 0.35
Poloxamer	41.20 ± 0.77
Tween 60	25.36 ± 0.55
Span 20	0.40 ± 0.73
Solutol	0.73

3.4. Optimization and Formulation of Nanostructured Lipid Carrier (NLC)

A total of 13 runs were generated by the CCRD based on the selected independent variables. According to the suggested runs (Table 3), preparation of various formulations was performed and considered to predict the outcome of the dependent variables on the independent variables (R1, R2, and R3). Adjusted R^2 and predicted R^2 values of all dependents are mentioned in Table 4.

Table 3. CCRD experimental design and observed responses.

Runs	Independent Variable		Dependent Variable		
	Factor 1 A: Binary Mixture Concentration (Solid/Liquid Lipid Concentration) (w/w)	Factor 2 B: Surfactant Concentration (w/w)	R1: Droplet Size (nm)	R2: PDI	R3: (% EE)
1	0.29	4.0	49.32	0.326	59.54
2	0.50	6.0	59.43	0.316	69.88
3	0.50	2.0	63.43	0.309	62.34
4	1.00	1.1	97.44	0.259	66.78
5	1.00	4.0	82.33	0.261	88.99
6	1.00	6.8	50.32	0.332	80.98
7	1.00	4.0	81.88	0.277	91.23
8	1.00	4.0	84.34	0.267	89.45
9	1.00	4.0	82.65	0.274	88.43
10	1.00	4.0	85.32	0.266	90.34
11	1.50	6.0	64.66	0.239	73.42
12	1.50	2.0	99.39	0.188	77.78
13	1.70	4.0	79.33	0.162	76.87

Table 4. Overall ANOVA analysis results for CCRD.

Response	Statistics of Model Summary				Suggested Model
	Std. Dev.	R2	Adjusted R2	Predicted R2	
R1: Droplet Size	4.14	0.9628	0.9362	0.7500	Quadratic
R2: PDI	0.0087	0.9824	0.9698	0.8818	Quadratic
R3: EE%	2.52	0.9702	0.9490	0.8067	Quadratic

3.4.1. Outcome of the Independent Variables on Dependent Variables

Outcome of binary mixture concentration and surfactant concentration on the dependent variable (droplet size).

The concentration of surfactant had a significant effect on the size of the droplet ($p < 0.0001$), followed by the concentration of the binary lipidic phase ($p < 0.0002$). The size of the droplet of the respective batch was found to be in the range of 49.32–99.39 nm. The binary lipid phase had a positive effect on droplet size, while surfactant concentration had a negative effect, according to the quadratic equation. This also suggested that the binary phase concentration increased as the droplet size of the formulation increased. The effect of the concentration of surfactant on droplet size was such that increasing surfactant concentration decreased droplet size. This was attributed to a decline in the interfacial tension between the oil and aqueous phases, which resulted in a smaller droplet size [57]. The combination of independent variables such as binary lipid and surfactant concentration (AB) had a negative effect on droplet size (Figure 2a).

$$R1 = 83.37 + 10.45A - 13.17B - 7.68AB - 8.83A^2 - 4.06B^2 \qquad (5)$$

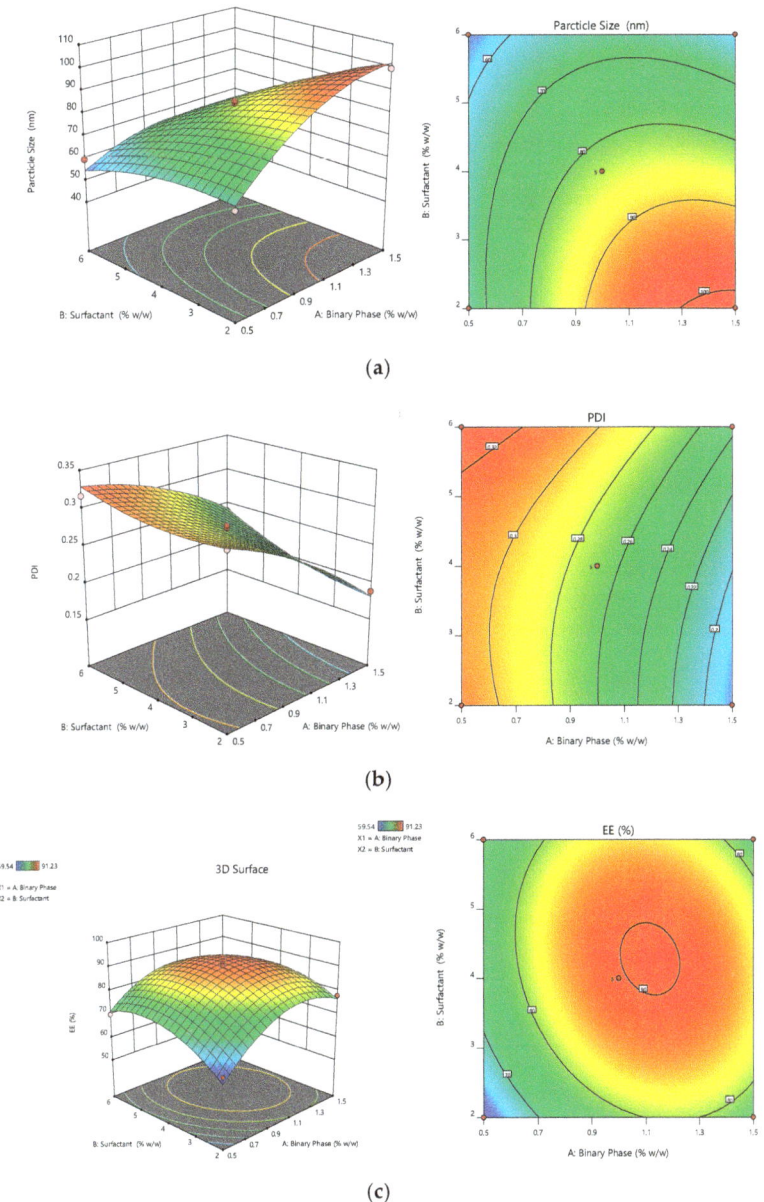

Figure 2. Response surface graphs showing effect of binary mixture concentration and surfactant concentration. (**a**) Droplet size: concentration of binary mixture increased with an increase in droplet size, while concentration of surfactant increased with an increase in droplet size. (**b**) PDI: concentration of binary mixture decreased with an increase in PDI, while with an increase in concentration of surfactant, PDI increased. (**c**) % EE: concentration of binary mixture increased with an increase in % EE, while the concentration of surfactant also increased with an increase in % EE.

The outcome of binary mixture concentration and surfactant concentration on the dependent variable (PDI).

The PDI is one of the most crucial factors in developing the NGN-NLC. The concentration of surfactant had a significant effect on the size of the droplet ($p < 0.0001$), succeeded by the concentration of the binary lipidic phase ($p < 0.0001$). On applying analysis, the experimental data were analyzed and fitted in the quadratic model. The PDI of the respective batch was in the range of 0.162–0.326. The quadratic equation showed that the concentration of surfactant had a positive effect, whereas the concentration of the binary lipid phase had a negative effect on the PDI. However, the effect was not that significant. The effect of the various factors on the PDI is shown in Figure 2b.

$$R2 = + 0.26190 - 0.0537A + 0.0202B + 0.0110AB - 0.0142A^2 + 0.0116B^2 \qquad (6)$$

The outcome of binary mixture concentration and surfactant concentration on the dependent variable (% EE).

% EE had a main role in the formulation of the NGN-NLC. It was witnessed that the concentration of the binary lipid phase ($p < 0.0005$) and surfactant ($p < 0.0138$) showed a significant effect on the entrapment efficiency. The prepared NGN-NLC showed % EE in the range of 59.54–91.23%. The quadratic equation showed that the binary lipid and the surfactant concentration had a positive effect. This suggested that the entrapment efficiency of the formulation increased with an increase in the concentration of the binary lipid, as well as the concentration of surfactant. Combining the two lipids may result in an improved amalgamation of the drug into the binary lipid, followed by the solubility of the drug and assimilation into voids of the imperfect binary lipid matrix. The multilayered presence of the molecules around the droplets enabled more space for NGN to be incorporated, causing increased entrapment efficiency [58]. On the other hand, the combination of the independent variables such as the binary lipid and surfactant concentration (AB) displayed a negative effect on the entrapment efficiency. The effect of different factors on entrapment efficiency is shown in Figure 2c.

$$R3 = +89.69 + 5.44 + 2.91B - 2.97AB - 10.79A^2 - 7.95B^2 \qquad (7)$$

3.4.2. Validation of Experimental Design

A comparison was made between the validation of the experimental design for the optimized formulation, and the obtained responses revealed an optimal formula consisting of 1% binary lipid mixture concentration and 4% concentration of surfactant. The experimental results were found to be analogous with each other denoting the validation and reliability for the optimized formulation.

3.5. Evaluation of Optimized NGN-NLC

3.5.1. Zeta Potential, Droplet Size, and Polydispersity Index (PDI)

The value of zeta potential of the optimized NGN-NLC was in the range of −8.15 to −8.21 mV (Figure 3a). Here, the negative charge could be credited to the lipids and nonionic surfactant used in the formulation, leading to a lower magnitude of nano-based particles without the presence of aggregation, thus indicating the stability of the NGN-NLC [59].

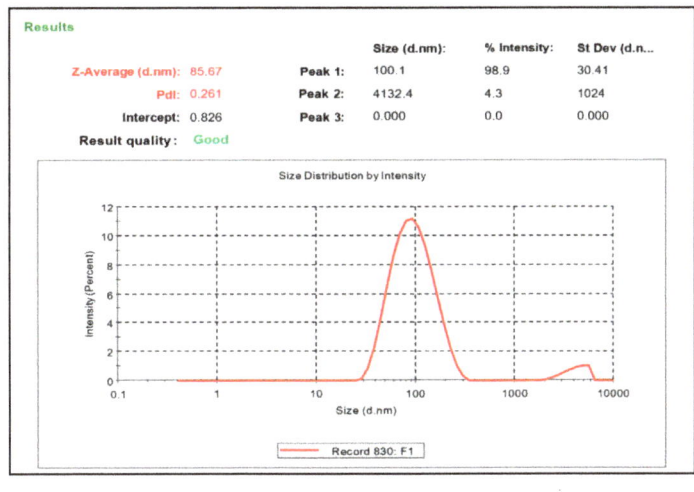

(a)

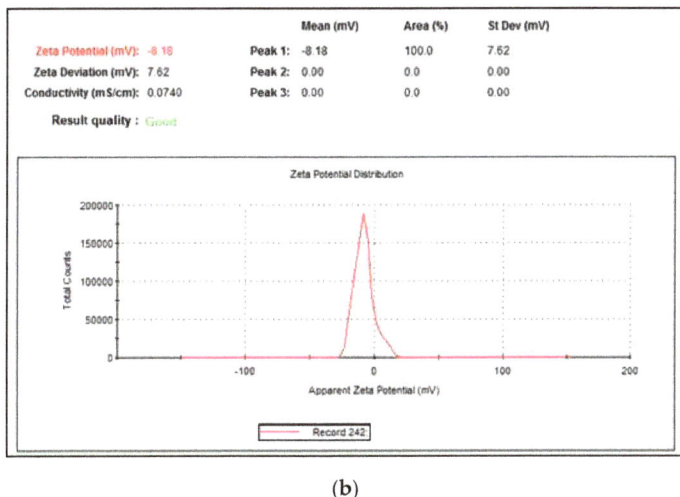

(b)

Figure 3. (**a**) Zeta potential of optimized NGN-NLC was found to be in the range of −8.15 to −8.21 mV. (**b**) Droplet size and PDI of optimized NGN-NLC were found to be in the range of 84.17 to 86.71 nm and 0.258 to 0.271, respectively.

The droplet size and PDI of the optimized NGN-NLC were found to be in the range of 84.17 to 86.71 nm and 0.258 to 0.271, respectively (Figure 3b). The droplet size of the formulations has a significant role in the absorption of drugs via the i.n route because of the opening and closing of the tight junctions located in the epithelium cells of the nasal membrane. Smaller droplet size and larger surface area would help in the rapid absorption of the drug. Furthermore, a decreased size of the droplet would result in improved drug carriage via the olfactory route to the brain. The PDI signifies the distribution of the size of the nanocarriers in the formulation. PDI values less than 0.5 signify that the formulation is monodispersed (homogeneity), whereas a PDI value more than 0.5 signifies the polydispersity of the formulation [60].

3.5.2. Entrapment Efficiency (% EE)

The optimized formulation exhibited a range of 87.58 to 88.21% for % EE, which signified that the drug was entrapped into the nanocarrier-mediated system. The lipophilicity of NGN could be the reason for the high entrapment efficiency that allowed it to solubilize in the lipid matrix. NLCs have irregularities in the crystal lattice that enable adequate space for drug molecules to be accommodated, further resulting in enhanced drug entrapment efficiency. The main goal of the greater % EE is to attain a maximal drug concentration in the lipidic matrix that results in a greater amount of drug release at a lower dose [61].

3.5.3. Determination of Surface Morphology

TEM was employed to determine the morphology of the surface of the optimized formulation. The droplets of the NGN-NLC seemed to be dark and spherical with uniform droplet size distribution with a diameter of 60–90 nm (0.06–0.09 µm) (Figure 4a). No aggregation of particles was observed in the formulation.

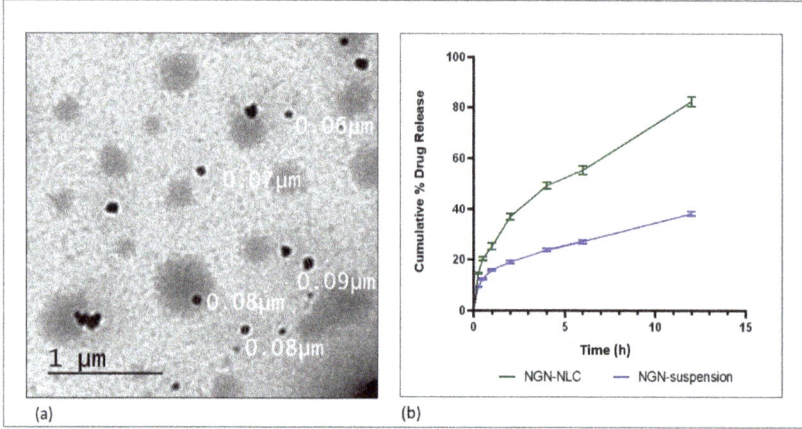

Figure 4. (**a**) Surface morphology determination using TEM, showing the uniform distribution of droplets in optimized NGN-NLC. (**b**) The drug release profile of NGN from NGN-NLC and NGN suspension in phosphate buffer (pH = 6.4) using the dialysis membrane, showed a 2.15-fold increase in drug release from NGN-NLC in comparison to that of NGN suspension. The result was found to be statistically significant, whereas data were expressed using mean ± SD (n = 3).

3.6. Stability Studies

The 3-month stability studies confirmed the stability of the NGN-NLC at room temperature (25 ± 2 °C/60 ± 5% RH). The NGN-NLC was assessed for changes in physical appearance, occurrence of phase separation, caking, changes in droplet size, PDI, and entrapment efficiency. The NGN-NLC did not show any changes in physical appearance phase separation and caking. An insignificant change (p > 0.05) was observed in the droplet size, PDI, and % EE of the formulation. The formulation did not show any precipitate formation (Table 5). The high stability of the formulation could be due to the high zeta potential and small droplet size [62].

Table 5. Stability studies of NGN-NLC at room temperature (25 ± 2 °C/60 ± 5% RH) (n = 3).

Time (Months)	Change in Appearance	Phase Separation	Caking	Droplet Size (nm) (Mean ± SD) (n = 3)	PDI (Mean ± SD) (n = 3)	% EE (Mean ± SD) (n = 3)
0	No	No	No	85.43 ± 1.21	0.263 ± 0.012	87.58 ± 4.69
1	No	No	No	85.96 ± 1.59	0.271 ± 0.015	87.21 ± 3.46
3	No	No	No	86.21 ± 3.90	0.281 ± 0.017	86.57 ± 3.55

3.7. Drug Release Studies by Dialysis Membrane

The drug release study was performed using a dialysis membrane to investigate the release of NGN from the NGN-NLC and NGN suspension in phosphate buffer (pH = 6.4), respectively. The percentage cumulative release of NGN from the formulation was found to be 82.42 ± 1.88% in 12 h; however, in the case of the NGN suspension, the release of the drug was way too slow, with only 38.20 ± 0.82% drug release after 12 h along with drug precipitation in the dialysis bag. Initially, the drug was seen to escape quickly from the lipidic surface of the NGN-NLC, followed by a slower release pattern due to drug release from the lipid matrix. The results were found to be statistically significant ($p > 0.001$). The optimized NGN-NLC displayed the biphasic type of release from the NGN-NLC and NGN suspension. The NGN-NLC had a 12 h release time (Figure 4b), which could be due to the lower droplet size of the generated NLC.

The results signified that the drug release of the NGN-NLC followed the Korsmeyer–Peppas release model because of the maximum value of the coefficient of correlation ($R2$), i.e., 0.9958, and followed the Fickian diffusion with a biphasic drug release pattern, thus proving the encapsulation of the drug in the core of the lipid. The NGN-NLC showed a 2.15-fold increase in drug release compared to that of the NGN suspension, thereby proving its effectiveness in drug release studies.

3.8. Ex Vivo Nasal Permeation Study

The ex vivo permeation study was used to compare the permeation of the drug (NGN) from the NLC and suspension by means of goat nasal mucosa as a diffusion barrier on the Franz diffusion cell. The NGN-NLC revealed 85.91 ± 9.23% permeation in 12 h in contrast to the NGN suspension, which revealed 38.76 ± 5.00% permeation (Figure 5). The steady-state flux for the NGN-NLC and NGN suspension was found to be 17.7 $\mu gcm^{-2} h^{-1}$ and 1.56 10^{-1} $\mu gcm^{-2} h^{-1}$, respectively, while the permeability coefficient was found to be 8.54 $\mu gcm^{-2} h^{-1}$ and 0.74 10^{-1} $\mu gcm^{-2} h^{-1}$ for the NGN-NLC and NGN suspension, respectively. The flux and permeability coefficient of the NGN-NLC was comparatively higher than that of the NGN suspension. The results were found to be statistically significant ($p > 0.001$). The pattern of drug release from the ex vivo permeation studies was seen to be in correspondence with that of the in vitro studies. The NGN-NLC displayed a 2.21-fold increase in drug permeation compared to that of the NGN suspension. This could be due to the higher retention time of the NGN-NLC, which further led to an enhanced permeation rate and also to the desired sustained release of the drugs across the nasal mucosa that acted as a reservoir for drugs, thereby proving its effectiveness in drug permeation studies [63].

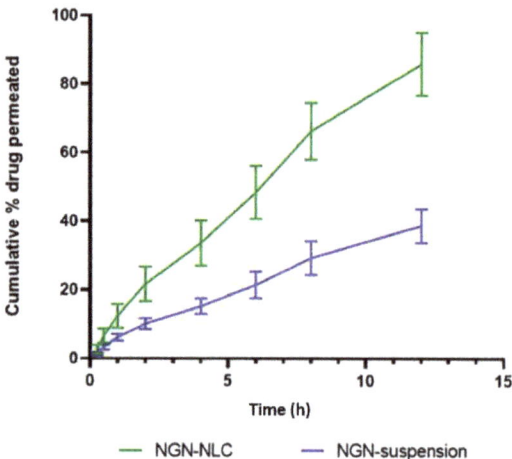

Figure 5. Ex vivo permeation of NGN from the NGN-NLC and NGN-suspension on isolated goat nasal mucosa, showing 2.21-fold increase in NGN from NGN-NLC in comparison to NGN suspension. Data expressed using mean ± SD (n = 3).

3.9. Antioxidant Activity: DPPH Assay

The reducing potential of DPPH was assessed by observing the change in color from purple to yellow which was evaluated at absorbance 515 nm. The data displayed that free radical scavenging was strongly influenced by the NGN-NLC. The increase in the antioxidant property of nanoformulations is usually preferred for improving their potential in neurological brain disorders [50]. The antioxidant activity of the NGN-NLC was found to be higher because of the combined effect of NGN and TQ, thus proving their efficacy as strong antioxidants (Figure 6). It is predicted that the reason for effective antioxidant potential in the NGN-NLC could be due to the synergistic effect of NGN along with TQ oil possessing powerful antioxidant activity. The IC_{50} value for the NGN solution, NGN-NLC, and ascorbic acid was found to be 41.79 µg/mL, 23 µg/mL, and 14 µg/mL, respectively [63].

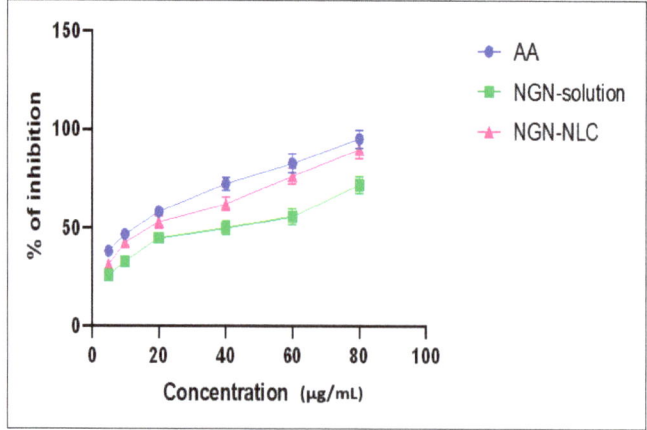

Figure 6. Antioxidant potential of AA, NGN solution, and NGN-NLC, showing % inhibition increase of 1.2-fold from NGN-NLC in comparison with NGN solution due to synergistic effect of NGN and TQ. Data expressed using mean ± SD (n = 3).

3.10. Estimation of Depth of Permeation by Confocal Laser Scanning Microscopy (CLSM)

CLSM investigation was conducted to assess the permeability of the NGN-NLC and NGN suspension across the goat's nasal mucosa. It was observed that the maximum intensity of fluorescence for the NGN suspension was up to a depth of 20.0 μm, which diminished at 25.0 μm (Figure 7a). However, for the NGN-NLC, it was spotted up to a depth of 39.9 μm, that diminished at 44.9 μm (Figure 7b), indicating the uniform distribution of NGN in the NGN-NLC compared to that of the NGN suspension. Thus, the NGN-NLC displayed about 1.99-fold deeper permeation in the nasal mucosa in comparison with the NGN suspension. These results were found to be in accordance with the ex vivo permeation study.

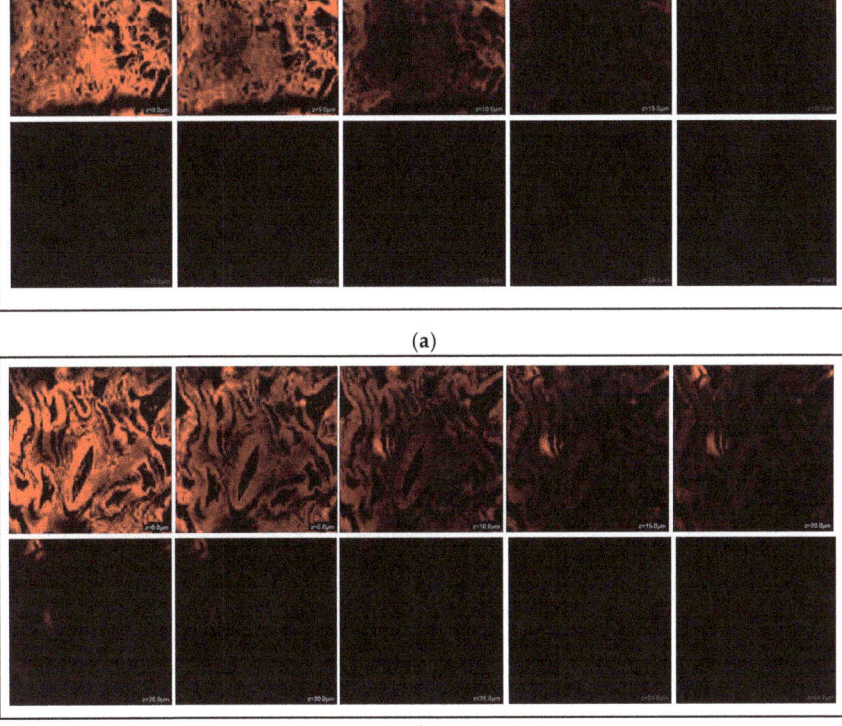

Figure 7. (a) CLSM images after administration of NGN suspension across isolated goat nasal mucosa. (b) CLSM images after administration of NGN-NLC across isolated goat nasal mucosa, showing 1.99-fold enhanced permeation in comparison to NGN suspension.

3.11. Pharmacodynamic Studies

3.11.1. Forced Swim Test (FST)

The forced swim test is the generally used animal model for evaluating the effectiveness of antidepressants. The FST revealed that the control group showed a mean swimming time of 82.33 ± 1.42 s. Additionally, on the administration of the NGN suspension via the i.n route, a significant increase ($p < 0.001$) in the mean swimming time (162.66 ± 2.22 s) was observed compared to the DLX suspension after following the oral administration, which showed a mean swimming time of 131.33 ± 1.56 s.

However, after the administration of the NGN-NLC via the i.n route, a significant increase ($p < 0.001$ versus control) with a mean swimming time of 213 ± 2.51 s indicated the therapeutic effectiveness of the formulation (Figure 8a).

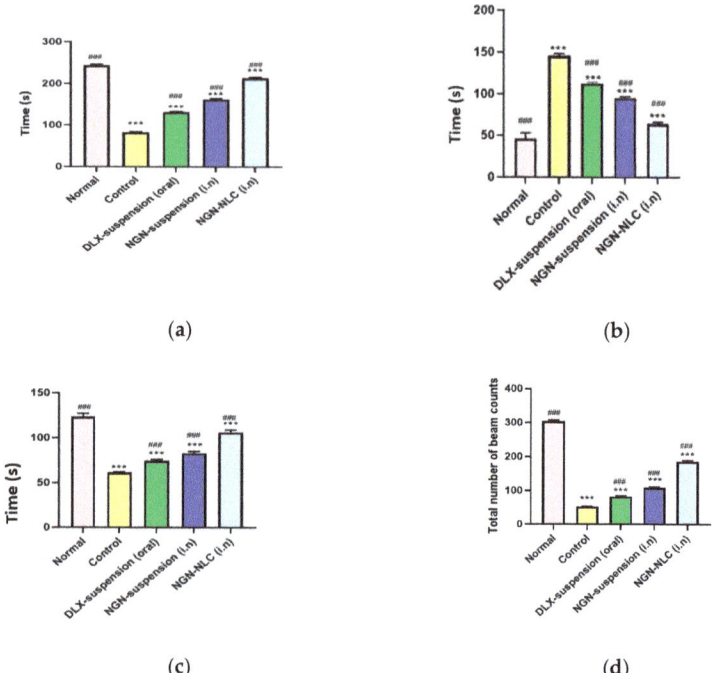

Figure 8. Pharmacodynamic investigation of different groups after performing behavioral studies such as (**a**) forced swim test, (**b**) immobility test, (**c**) climbing time, and (**d**) locomotor activity test. (*** indicates that the comparison was made between normal vs. other groups; whereas ### indicates that the comparison was made between control and other groups). Data expressed using mean ± SD (n = 3).

The immobility time refers to the motionless behavior of rats when they were placed in a cylinder consisting of water. The mean immobility time of the control group showed a significant increase ($p < 0.001$) compared to that of the DLX suspension (oral) group. After the administration of the NGN suspension through the i.n route, a significant decrease ($p < 0.001$) was observed in contrast to the control group. On the other hand, the administration of the NGN-NLC (i.n) displayed a significant decrease ($p < 0.001$) in the immobility time (64 ± 1.52 s) against that of the control group (Figure 8b).

The climbing time for the normal and control groups was found to be 123.33 ± 3.78 and 61.33 ± 3.87 s, respectively. The depressed group treated with the DLX suspension orally and the NGN suspension intranasally showed a climbing time of 74.66 ± 1.21 and 83.01 ± 1.89 s, respectively. The depressed group treated with the NGN-NLC via the i.n route showed a climbing time of about 106 ± 3.03 s (Figure 8c). It was observed that the rats exhibited a fall in the time spent trying to escape from the cylindrical glass tank filled with water, but this time duration was significantly extended after the administration of the NGN-NLC ($p < 0.001$) via the i.n route against the control group, the DLX suspension (oral) group and the group treated with the NGN suspension (i.n). The significant increase in the climbing time of rats treated with the NGN-NLC (i.n) could be credited to the occurrence of NGN and TQ oil in the hippocampus of the brain, leading to the synergistic effect of the drugs, and thus allowing the inhibition of the reuptake of serotonin, thus causing an enhanced amount of serotonin in the brain [64].

3.11.2. Locomotor Activity Test

The locomotor activity test was conducted with the help of a digital photoactometer for 5 min. It was observed that the normal and control groups showed a beam count of 304 ± 3.51 and 52.66 ± 1.12 s, respectively, while the DLX suspension (oral) and NGN suspension (i.n) groups were seen to exhibit a total beam count of 83.33 ± 1.52 and 109.01 ± 2.64 s ($p < 0.001$). However, after the administration of the NGN-NLC (i.n), a significant increase of $p < 0.001$ with a total beam count of 186.33 ± 2.82 s against that of the control group was witnessed (Figure 8d). The results proved the efficacy of the NGN-NLC when administered via the i.n route in comparison to that of the NGN suspension and DLX suspension, which were administered intranasally and orally, respectively [65].

Successful outcomes were obtained from the pharmacodynamic studies consisting of the FST and the locomotor activity test, which further proved the therapeutic efficacy and synergistic effect after the i.n administration of the NGN-NLC. The administration of the NGN-NLC not only enhanced the uptake of drugs through the i.n route against suspensions but also led to the desired antidepressant effect. The therapeutic effectiveness of the NGN-NLC (i.n) could be attributed to the lipid nanocarriers that helped in the direct targeting of the brain through the olfactory route, whereas the orally administered formulation showed poor results because of the extensive hepatic first-pass metabolism and its inability to cross via tight junctions present at the BBB. Nonetheless, the mechanisms exhibited by the NTs led to behavioral changes exhibited by the rats. The increase in the concentration of serotonin in the hypothalamus and frontal cortex of rats was attributed to the i.n administration of the NGN-NLC, which further increased the availability of serotonin in the presynaptic neurons and caused a remarkable increase in the mean swimming and climbing times of the rats [64,65].

4. Conclusions

The NGN-NLC was successfully prepared and optimized utilizing a CCRD. The optimized NLC exhibited the following properties: droplet size, 84.17 to 86.71 nm; polydispersity index, 0.258 to 0.271; zeta potential, -8.15 to -8.21 mV; and entrapment efficiency, 87.58 to 88.21%. The NGN-NLC showed controlled release for 12 h that revealed 2.15-fold enhancement of NGN release from the NLC compared to the NGN suspension. Ex vivo results showed enhanced permeation (2.21-fold) of the NLC through the nasal mucosa compared to the NGN suspension. DPPH study revealed the improved antioxidant potential of NGN. The results of the CLSM study showed a higher amount of penetration by the NGN-NLC than the NGN suspension, while the stability study showed good stability of the NLC over 3 months. Furthermore, pharmacodynamic data revealed an increase in the antidepressant potential of the NGN-NLC. The present study concluded the successful optimization of the NGN-NLC and its potential in augmenting brain bioavailability and the therapeutic effectiveness of NGN for the effective treatment of depression after nasal administration. The research findings indicated that transporting the drug via the olfactory pathway can help in targeting the drug directly to the brain. Nevertheless, the current research work still lacks clinical study data, which can help in assessing its therapeutic effectiveness, as well as the risk/benefit ratio in humans.

Author Contributions: Conceptualization, F.F.Q., S.B., J.A., M.M.G. and S.A.; software, M.U.A. and A.; formal analysis, M.U.A., A. and J.A.; data curation, J.A.; writing—original draft preparation, F.F.Q.; writing—review and editing, Z.Q., S.B., A.A., A.Z., M.M.G. and S.A.; supervision, A.A.; project administration, A.A. All authors have read and agreed to the published version of the manuscript.

Funding: This research received no external funding.

Institutional Review Board Statement: The animal study protocol was permitted by the Institutional Animal Ethical Committee (IAEC) (Jamia Hamdard, New Delhi, India), with the approved animal study protocol 173/Go/Re/ S/2000/CPCSEA (Approval No. 1647, 2019). The current study was performed following the guidelines of the Declaration of Helsinki.

Informed Consent Statement: Not applicable.

Data Availability Statement: This study did not report any data (All the data is included in the current manuscript).

Conflicts of Interest: The authors declare no conflict of interest.

Abbreviations

AA: ascorbic acid, BBB; blood/brain barrier, CCRD; central composite rotatable design, CLSM; confocal laser scanning microscopy, CPCSEA; Committee for the Purpose of Control and Supervision of Experiments on Animals, DLX suspension; duloxetine suspension, DPPH; dithiobis-2-nitrobenzoic acid, % EE; entrapment efficiency, i.n; intranasal, MAO; monoamine oxidase, NLC; nanostructured lipid carrier, NGN-NLC; naringenin-loaded nanostructured lipid carrier, NT; neurotransmitter, PDI; polydispersity index, S-218; Sefsol®, SD; standard deviation, TEM; transmission electron microscope, TQ; thymoquinone.

References

1. Liu, Q.; He, H.; Yang, J.; Feng, X.; Zhao, F.; Lyu, J. Changes in the global burden of depression from 1990 to 2017: Findings from the Global Burden of Disease study. *J. Psychiatr. Res.* **2020**, *126*, 134–140. [CrossRef] [PubMed]
2. Pandey, Y.R.; Kumar, S.; Gupta, B.K.; Ali, J.; Baboota, S. Intranasal delivery of paroxetine nanoemulsion via the olfactory region for the management of depression: Formulation, behavioural and biochemical estimation. *Nanotechnology* **2015**, *27*, 25102. [CrossRef] [PubMed]
3. Michel, T.M.; Pulschen, D.; Thome, J. The Role of Oxidative Stress in Depressive Disorders. *Curr. Pharm. Des.* **2012**, *18*, 5890–5899. [CrossRef] [PubMed]
4. Olsen, H.T.; Stafford, G.I.; van Staden, J.; Christensen, S.B.; Jäger, A.K. Isolation of the MAO-inhibitor naringenin from *Mentha aquatica* L. *J. Ethnopharmacol.* **2008**, *117*, 500–502. [CrossRef] [PubMed]
5. Hritcu, L.; Ionita, R.; Postu, P.A.; Gupta, G.K.; Turkez, H.; Lima, T.C.; Carvalho, C.U.S.; de Sousa, D. Antidepressant Flavonoids and Their Relationship with Oxidative Stress. *Oxidative Med. Cell. Longev.* **2017**, *2017*, 5762172. [CrossRef]
6. Olugbemide, A.S.; Ben-Azu, B.; Bakre, A.G.; Ajayi, A.M.; Femi-Akinlosotu, O.; Umukoro, S. Naringenin improves depressive- and anxiety-like behaviors in mice exposed to repeated hypoxic stress through modulation of oxido-inflammatory mediators and NF-kB/BDNF expressions. *Brain Res. Bull.* **2021**, *169*, 214–227. [CrossRef]
7. Shulman, M.; Cohen, M.; Soto-Gutierrez, A.; Yagi, H.; Wang, H.; Goldwasser, J.; Lee-Parsons, C.W.; Benny-Ratsaby, O.; Yarmush, M.L.; Nahmias, Y. Enhancement of Naringenin Bioavailability by Complexation with Hydroxypropoyl-β-Cyclodextrin. *PLoS ONE* **2011**, *6*, e18033. [CrossRef]
8. Cunha, S.; Costa, C.P.; Loureiro, J.A.; Alves, J.; Peixoto, A.F.; Forbes, B.; Lobo, J.M.S.; Silva, A.C. Double Optimization of Rivastigmine-Loaded Nanostructured Lipid Carriers (NLC) for Nose-to-Brain Delivery Using the Quality by Design (QbD) Approach: Formulation Variables and Instrumental Parameters. *Pharmaceutics* **2020**, *12*, 599. [CrossRef]
9. Emad, N.A.; Ahmed, B.; Alhalmi, A.; Alzobaidi, N.; Al-Kubati, S.S. Recent progress in nanocarriers for direct nose to brain drug delivery. *J. Drug Deliv. Sci. Technol.* **2021**, *64*, 102642. [CrossRef]
10. Erdő, F.; Bors, L.A.; Farkas, D.; Bajza, Á.; Gizurarson, S. Evaluation of intranasal delivery route of drug administration for brain targeting. *Brain Res. Bull.* **2018**, *143*, 155–170. [CrossRef]
11. Costa, C.P.; Moreira, J.; Amaral, M.H.; Lobo, J.M.S.; Silva, A. Nose-to-brain delivery of lipid-based nanosystems for epileptic seizures and anxiety crisis. *J. Control. Release* **2019**, *295*, 187–200. [CrossRef] [PubMed]
12. Alam, M.I.; Baboota, S.; Ahuja, A.; Ali, M.; Ali, J.; Sahni, J.K. Intranasal infusion of nanostructured lipid carriers (NLC) containing CNS acting drug and estimation in brain and blood. *Drug Deliv.* **2013**, *20*, 247–251. [CrossRef] [PubMed]
13. Kadil, Y. The neuropharmacological preclinical effects of Nigella Sativa: A review. *Curr. Bioact. Compd.* **2021**, *17*, 1. [CrossRef]
14. Benkermiche, S.; DjemLi, S.; Haloui, M.; Bena-Bed, M.L.; Tahraoui, A. Preventive Effects of Ginger Extract and Nigella sativa Oil on Anxiety and Depression Behavior in Wistar Rats Exposed to Mercuric Chloride. *Pharmacogn. Res.* **2021**, *14*, 1–4. [CrossRef]
15. Farkhondeh, T.; Samarghandian, S.; Shahri, A.M.P.; Samini, F. The Neuroprotective Effects of Thymoquinone: A Review. *Dose-Response* **2018**, *16*, 1–11. [CrossRef] [PubMed]
16. Jakaria, M.D.Y.; Cho, D.-Y.; Haque, E.; Karthivashan, G.; Kim, I.-S.; Ganesan, P.; Choi, D.-K. Neuropharmacological Potential and Delivery Prospects of Thymoquinone for Neurological Disorders. *Oxidative Med. Cell. Longev.* **2018**, *2018*, 1209801. [CrossRef]
17. Beheshti, F.; Khazaei, M.; Hosseini, M. Neuropharmacological effects of Nigella sativa. *Avicenna J. Phytomed.* **2016**, *6*, 124–141.

18. Kaymak, E.; Akin, A.T.; Öztürk, E.; Karabulut, D.; Kuloğlu, N.; Yakan, B. Thymoquinone has a neuroprotective effect against inflammation, oxidative stress, and endoplasmic reticulum stress in the brain cortex, medulla, and hippocampus due to doxorubicin. *J. Biochem. Mol. Toxicol.* **2021**, *35*, e22888. [CrossRef]
19. Yadav, V.P.; Jaswal, V.; Sharma, A.; Kashyap, D.; Tuli, H.S.; Garg, V.K.; Das, S.K.; Srinivas, R. Celastrol as a pentacyclic triterpenoid with chemopreventive properties. *Pharm. Pat. Anal.* **2018**, *7*, 155–167. [CrossRef]
20. Ramana, K.V.; Singhal, S.S.; Reddy, A.B. Therapeutic Potential of Natural Pharmacological Agents in the Treatment of Human Diseases. *BioMed Res. Int.* **2014**, *2014*, 573452. [CrossRef]
21. Jiang, N.; Wang, H.; Huang, H.; Lv, J.; Zeng, G.; Wang, Q.; Bao, Y.; Chen, Y.; Liu, X. The Antidepressant-Like Effects of Shen Yuan in a Chronic Unpredictable Mild Stress Rat Model. *Front. Psychiatry* **2021**, *12*, 1263. [CrossRef] [PubMed]
22. Moragrega, I.; Ríos, J.L. Medicinal Plants in the Treatment of Depression: Evidence from Preclinical Studies. *Planta Med.* **2021**, *87*, 656–685. [CrossRef] [PubMed]
23. Zhou, N.; Gu, X.; Zhuang, T.; Xu, Y.; Yang, L.; Zhou, M. Gut Microbiota: A Pivotal Hub for Polyphenols as Antidepressants. *J. Agric. Food Chem.* **2020**, *68*, 6007–6020. [CrossRef] [PubMed]
24. Elias, E.; Zhang, A.Y.; Manners, M.T. Novel Pharmacological Approaches to the Treatment of Depression. *Life* **2022**, *12*, 196. [CrossRef]
25. Ashrafizadeh, M.; Ahmadi, Z.; Farkhondeh, T.; Samarghandian, S. Modulatory effects of statins on the autophagy: A therapeutic perspective. *J. Cell. Physiol.* **2020**, *235*, 3157–3168. [CrossRef] [PubMed]
26. Galluzzi, L.; Green, D.R. Autophagy-Independent Functions of the Autophagy Machinery. *Cell* **2019**, *177*, 1682–1699. [CrossRef] [PubMed]
27. Xu, L.; Hu, G.; Xing, P.; Zhou, M.; Wang, D. Paclitaxel alleviates the sepsis-induced acute kidney injury via lnc-MALAT1/miR-370-3p/HMGB1 axis. *Life Sci.* **2020**, *262*, 118505. [CrossRef]
28. Ahmed, S.A.; Parama, D.; Daimari, E.; Girisa, S.; Banik, K.; Harsha, C.; Dutta, U.; Kunnumakkara, A.B. Rationalizing the therapeutic potential of apigenin against cancer. *Life Sci.* **2021**, *267*, 118814. [CrossRef]
29. Lim, H.Y.; Ong, P.S.; Wang, L.; Goel, A.; Ding, L.; Wong, A.L.-A.; Ho, P.C.-L.; Sethi, G.; Xiang, X.; Goh, B.C. Celastrol in cancer therapy: Recent developments, challenges and prospects. *Cancer Lett.* **2021**, *521*, 252–267. [CrossRef]
30. Salehi, B.; Fokou, P.V.T.; Sharifi-Rad, M.; Zucca, P.; Pezzani, R.; Martins, N.; Sharifi-Rad, J. The Therapeutic Potential of Naringenin: A Review of Clinical Trials. *Pharmaceuticals* **2019**, *12*, 11. [CrossRef]
31. Khan, A.; Tania, M.; Fu, S.; Fu, J. Thymoquinone, as an anticancer molecule: From basic research to clinical investigation. *Oncotarget* **2017**, *8*, 51907–51919. [CrossRef] [PubMed]
32. Gaba, B.; Khan, T.; Haider, F.; Alam, T.; Baboota, S.; Parvez, S.; Ali, J. Vitamin E Loaded Naringenin Nanoemulsion via Intranasal Delivery for the Management of Oxidative Stress in a 6-OHDA Parkinson's Disease Model. *BioMed Res. Int.* **2019**, *2019*, 2382563. [CrossRef] [PubMed]
33. Ahmad, N.; Ahmad, R.; Ahmad, F.; Ahmad, W.; Alam, A.; Amir, M.; Ali, A. Poloxamer-chitosan-based Naringenin nanoformulation used in brain targeting for the treatment of cerebral ischemia. *Saudi J. Biol. Sci.* **2020**, *27*, 500–517. [CrossRef] [PubMed]
34. Md, S.; Alhakamy, N.A.; Aldawsari, H.M.; Husain, M.; Kotta, S.; Abdullah, S.T.; Fahmy, U.A.; AlFaleh, M.A.; Asfour, H.Z. Formulation Design, Statistical Optimization, and In Vitro Evaluation of a Naringenin Nanoemulsion to Enhance Apoptotic Activity in A549 Lung Cancer Cells. *Pharmaceutics* **2020**, *13*, 152. [CrossRef] [PubMed]
35. Rai, V.K.; Mishra, N.; Yadav, K.S.; Yadav, N.P. Nanoemulsion as pharmaceutical carrier for dermal and transdermal drug delivery: Formulation development, stability issues, basic considerations and applications. *J. Control. Release* **2018**, *270*, 203–225. [CrossRef] [PubMed]
36. Thymoquinone Loaded Solid Lipid Nanoparticles Demonstrated Antidepressant-Like Activity in Rats via Indoleamine 2, 3-Dioxygenase Pathway. Drug Research. Available online: https://sci-hub.se/10.1055/a-1131-7793 (accessed on 5 January 2022).
37. Elmowafy, M.; Al-Sanea, M.M. Nanostructured lipid carriers (NLCs) as drug delivery platform: Advances in formulation and delivery strategies. *Saudi Pharm. J.* **2021**, *29*, 999–1012. [CrossRef] [PubMed]
38. Shafiq, S.; Shakeel, F.; Talegaonkar, S.; Ahmad, F.J.; Khar, R.K.; Ali, M. Development and bioavailability assessment of ramipril nanoemulsion formulation. *Eur. J. Pharm. Biopharm.* **2007**, *66*, 227–243. [CrossRef]
39. Xi, J.; Chang, Q.; Chan, C.K.; Meng, Z.Y.; Wang, G.N.; Sun, J.B.; Wang, Y.T.; Tong, H.H.Y.; Zheng, Y. Formulation Development and Bioavailability Evaluation of a Self-Nanoemulsified Drug Delivery System of Oleanolic Acid. *AAPS PharmSciTech* **2009**, *10*, 172–182. [CrossRef]
40. Khan, S.; Yar, M.S.; Fazil, M.; Baboota, S.; Ali, J. Tacrolimus-loaded nanostructured lipid carriers for oral delivery—Optimization of production and characterization. *Eur. J. Pharm. Biopharm.* **2016**, *108*, 277–288. [CrossRef] [PubMed]
41. Negi, L.; Jaggi, M.; Talegaonkar, S. Development of protocol for screening the formulation components and the assessment of common quality problems of nano-structured lipid carriers. *Int. J. Pharm.* **2014**, *461*, 403–410. [CrossRef]
42. Iqbal, B.; Ali, J.; Ganguli, M.; Mishra, S.; Baboota, S. Silymarin-loaded nanostructured lipid carrier gel for the treatment of skin cancer. *Nanomedicine* **2019**, *14*, 1077–1093. [CrossRef] [PubMed]
43. Ashhar, M.U.; Kumar, S.; Ali, J.; Baboota, S. CCRD based development of bromocriptine and glutathione nanoemulsion tailored ultrasonically for the combined anti-parkinson effect. *Chem. Phys. Lipids* **2021**, *235*, 105035. [CrossRef] [PubMed]
44. Tsai, M.-J.; Wu, P.-C.; Huang, Y.-B.; Chang, J.-S.; Lin, C.-L.; Tsai, Y.-H.; Fang, J.-Y. Baicalein loaded in tocol nanostructured lipid carriers (tocol NLCs) for enhanced stability and brain targeting. *Int. J. Pharm.* **2012**, *423*, 461–470. [CrossRef] [PubMed]

45. Boche, M.; Pokharkar, V. Quetiapine Nanoemulsion for Intranasal Drug Delivery: Evaluation of Brain-Targeting Efficiency. *AAPS PharmSciTech* **2016**, *18*, 686–696. [CrossRef] [PubMed]
46. Mandpe, L.; Pokharkar, V. Quality by design approach to understand the process of optimization of iloperidone nanostructured lipid carriers for oral bioavailability enhancement. *Pharm. Dev. Technol.* **2013**, *20*, 320–329. [CrossRef]
47. Praveen, A.; Aqil, M.; Imam, S.S.; Ahad, A.; Moolakkadath, T.; Ahmad, F. Lamotrigine encapsulated intra-nasal nanoliposome formulation for epilepsy treatment: Formulation design, characterization and nasal toxicity study. *Colloids Surf. B Biointerfaces* **2019**, *174*, 553–562. [CrossRef] [PubMed]
48. Aboud, H.; Ali, A.; El-Menshawe, S.F.; Elbary, A.A. Nanotransfersomes of carvedilol for intranasal delivery: Formulation, characterization and in vivo evaluation. *Drug Deliv.* **2015**, *23*, 2471–2481. [CrossRef] [PubMed]
49. Haque, S.; Md, S.; Sahni, J.K.; Ali, J.; Baboota, S. Development and evaluation of brain targeted intranasal alginate nanoparticles for treatment of depression. *J. Psychiatr. Res.* **2014**, *48*, 1–12. [CrossRef]
50. Cryan, J.F.; Markou, A.; Lucki, I. Assessing antidepressant activity in rodents: Recent developments and future needs. *Trends Pharmacol. Sci.* **2002**, *23*, 238–245. [CrossRef]
51. Lee, H.; Ohno, M.; Ohta, S.; Mikami, T. Regular Moderate or Intense Exercise Prevents Depression-Like Behavior without Change of Hippocampal Tryptophan Content in Chronically Tryptophan-Deficient and Stressed Mice. *PLoS ONE* **2013**, *8*, e66996. [CrossRef]
52. Ahmada, A.; Husainb, A.; Mujeebc, M.; Khan, S.; Najmi, A.; Siddique, N.A.; Damanhouri, Z.A.; Anwarh, F. A review on therapeutic potential of Nigella sativa: A miracle herb. *Asian Pac. J. Trop. Biomed.* **2013**, *3*, 337–352. [CrossRef]
53. Victor, M.D.S.; Crake, C.; Coussios, C.; Stride, E. Properties, characteristics and applications of microbubbles for sonothrombolysis. *Expert Opin. Drug Deliv.* **2014**, *11*, 187–209. [CrossRef] [PubMed]
54. Almousallam, M.; Moia, C.; Zhu, H. Development of nanostructured lipid carrier for dacarbazine delivery. *Int. Nano Lett.* **2015**, *5*, 241–248. [CrossRef]
55. Tichota, D.M.; Silva, A.C.; Lobo, J.M.S.; Amara, M.H. Design, characterization, and clinical evaluation of argan oil nanostructured lipid carriers to improve skin hydration. *Int. J. Nanomed.* **2014**, *9*, 3855–3864.
56. Shete, H.; Patravale, V. Long chain lipid based tamoxifen NLC. Part I: Preformulation studies, formulation development and physicochemical characterization. *Int. J. Pharm.* **2013**, *454*, 573–583. [CrossRef]
57. Velmurugan, R.; Selvamuthukumar, S. Development and optimization of ifosfamide nanostructured lipid carriers for oral delivery using response surface methodology. *Appl. Nanosci.* **2016**, *6*, 159–173. [CrossRef]
58. Duong, V.-A.; Nguyen, T.-T.-L.; Maeng, H.-J.; Chi, S.-C. Data on optimization and drug release kinetics of nanostructured lipid carriers containing ondansetron hydrochloride prepared by cold high-pressure homogenization method. *Data Brief.* **2019**, *26*, 104475. [CrossRef] [PubMed]
59. Shah, B.; Khunt, D.; Bhatt, H.; Misra, M.; Padh, H. Intranasal delivery of venlafaxine loaded nanostructured lipid carrier: Risk assessment and QbD based optimization. *J. Drug Deliv. Sci. Technol.* **2016**, *33*, 37–50. [CrossRef]
60. Fatima, N.; Rehman, S.; Nabi, B.; Baboota, S.; Ali, J. Harnessing nanotechnology for enhanced topical delivery of clindamycin phosphate. *J. Drug Deliv. Sci. Technol.* **2019**, *54*, 101253. [CrossRef]
61. Khan, S.; Rehman, S.; Nabi, B.; Iqubal, A.; Nehal, N.; Fahmy, U.; Kotta, S.; Baboota, S.; Shadab; Ali, J. Boosting the Brain Delivery of Atazanavir through Nanostructured Lipid Carrier-Based Approach for Mitigating NeuroAIDS. *Pharmaceutics* **2020**, *12*, 1059. [CrossRef]
62. Jazuli, I.; Annu, B.; Nabi, B.; Moolakkadath, T.; Alam, T.; Baboota, S.; Ali, J. Optimization of Nanostructured Lipid Carriers of Lurasidone Hydrochloride Using Box-Behnken Design for Brain Targeting: In Vitro and In Vivo Studies. *J. Pharm. Sci.* **2019**, *108*, 3082–3090. [CrossRef] [PubMed]
63. Costantino, H.R.; Illum, L.; Brandt, G.; Johnson, P.H.; Quay, S.C. Intranasal delivery: Physicochemical and therapeutic aspects. *Int. J. Pharm.* **2007**, *337*, 1–24. [CrossRef] [PubMed]
64. Deshkar, S.S.; Jadhav, M.S.; Shirolkar, S.V. Development of Carbamazepine Nanostructured Lipid Carrier Loaded Thermosensitive Gel for Intranasal Delivery. *Adv. Pharm. Bull.* **2020**, *11*, 150–162. [CrossRef] [PubMed]
65. Liaquat, L.; Batool, Z.; Sadir, S.; Rafiq, S.; Shahzad, S.; Perveen, T.; Haider, S. Naringenin-induced enhanced antioxidant defence system meliorates cholinergic neurotransmission and consolidates memory in male rats. *Life Sci.* **2018**, *194*, 213–223. [CrossRef] [PubMed]

Article

Improved Efficiency of Pomegranate Seed Oil Administrated Nasally

Hiba Natsheh and Elka Touitou *

The Institute for Drug Research, School of Pharmacy, Faculty of Medicine, The Hebrew University of Jerusalem, Jerusalem 9112102, Israel; hiba.natsheh@mail.huji.ac.il
* Correspondence: elka.touitou@mail.huji.ac.il

Abstract: Pomegranate seed oil (PSO) is currently administrated orally as a food supplement for improving memory. However, the efficiency of the oral dosage forms for such purposes is low, mainly due to the blood brain barrier impeding a good delivery to brain. In this work, we designed and characterized a PSO phospholipid oily gel for nasal administration. We tested the performance of the new PSO delivery system in animal models for impaired memory and locomotor activity. The experimental results indicated a statistically significant improvement ($p < 0.05$) of more than 1.5 fold in the behavior of animals treated nasally, in comparison to those treated with orally administrated oil. Furthermore, in multiphoton microscopy and near infrared imaging studies, the nasal administration of fluorescent probes, fluorescein isothiocyanate (FITC), and indocyanine green (ICG) incorporated in the PSO system showed enhanced delivery to the brain. Results of the histopathologic examination of the nasal cavity and mucosa, as carried out by a pathologist, indicated the safety of the PSO phospholipid oily gel. In conclusion, the results of this work encourage further investigation of the phospholipid oily gel composition as a new way of PSO administration.

Keywords: pomegranate seed oil; nasal delivery system; memory impairment; movement impairment; delivery to brain; improved memory; phospholipid oily gel

1. Introduction

The plant *Punica granatum* (*Punicaceae* family) is known for its medical uses since ancient times. Pomegranate seed oil (PSO) contains polyunsaturated fatty acids, monounsaturated fatty acids, and saturated fatty acids. PSO exhibits in vitro antioxidant, anti-inflammatory, and neuroprotective activities [1–3]. This oil is currently administrated orally for memory improvement and prevention of the progression of neurodegenerative diseases [4–6].

Growing evidence suggests that pomegranate seed oil and extract have therapeutic potential for the treatment and prevention of various central nervous system diseases. Sarkaki reported that two weeks of oral administration of pomegranate seed extract improved the memory of rats after ischemic injury and permanent cerebral ischemia [7,8]. Other studies have focused on the neuroprotective effect of long-term oral administration of PSO nanoemulsions for the prevention and treatment of neurodegenerative disease in an animal model of genetic Creutzfeldt–Jacob disease (CJD) [5]. Braidy et al. [9] demonstrated evidence of protection against the loss of synaptic structure proteins and neuro-inflammation in a transgenic mice model of Alzheimer's disease (AD) that consumed a diet containing 4% ground pomegranates for 15 months.

However, the oral administration of PSO results in partial bioavailability due to its high metabolism in the GI [10]. Moreover, the efficiency of the oral dosage forms for the management of brain disorders is low. This is mainly due to the blood brain barrier (BBB) that limits the absorption of molecules into the brain [11].

The nasal pathway is an alternative route of administration of active substances. It has been traditionally used to treat localized ailments such as allergic rhinitis and symptoms of common cold. For more than three decades, this route has been explored for the systemic delivery of drugs [12]. More recently, the possibility of nasal drug delivery to the brain and the central nervous system (CNS) has become an attractive field of research [13–16]. The main advantages of the nasal pathway reside in the possibility to bypass the BBB and to avoid the hepatic first-pass metabolism associated with the oral intake [12,17].

Despite the advantages of this route, nasal administration of pure PSO can be inconvenient due to nasal leakage or aspiration into the lungs [18]. Furthermore, the low permeation across the nasal mucosa prevents good absorption of many molecules [12].

Therefore, there is a need for new approaches to overcome the present obstacles for the nasal administration of PSO. Many strategies were investigated to enhance the nasal delivery to brain of various molecules. These include nanoparticles and surfactants. Nanovesicular carriers have been shown to be very efficient for the treatment of multiple sclerosis [13], hot flushes [14], pain [15,16,19–21], Parkinson's disease [19], inflammation, migraine, and insomnia [22,23].

In this work, we investigated the efficiency of the nasal delivery of a PSO phospholipid oily gel in animal models for impaired memory and movement. To test the treatment efficiency of the nasal administration of PSO systems, we used mouse models of memory and movement impairment and compared the effect to that of oral administration of the pure oil. The ability to deliver to the mouse brain was tested using fluorescent probes in multiphoton microscopy and near infrared (NIR) imaging studies. The potential irritation of the nasal PSO system on the nasal cavity was examined following sub-chronic administration of the composition to rats.

2. Materials and Methods

2.1. Materials

PSO, containing (w/v) 90% polyunsaturated fatty acids, 5% monounsaturated fatty acids and 5% saturated fatty acids (based on the certificate of analysis provided by N.S. Oils Ltd., Kibbutz Saad, Israel) was used in this study. The phospholipids (PL) Phospholipon 90G, Lipoid, Germany, and Lecithin soya, Fagron, Spain, were used in this work. Reserpine, Fluorescein isothiocyanate (FITC), Indocyanine green (ICG), Sesame oil, and Tween 80 were purchased from Sigma Aldrich, Israel. Dimethyl sulfoxide (DMSO) was purchased from Bio Lab Ltd., Jerusalem, Israel. Propylene glycol (PG) and vitamin E were bought from Tamar, Israel. *Olivae Oleum* (Oleic acid) from Henry Lamotte Oils GMBH, Bremen, Germany was used. All other chemicals were of pharmaceutical grade.

2.2. Animals

All procedures carried out on animals were according to the National Institute of Health's regulations and were approved by the Committee for Animal Care and Experimental Use of the Hebrew University of Jerusalem (MD-11-12821-3; MD-19-15895-3; MD-21-16402-3; MD-21-16474-4).

Mice (male CD-1 ICR) 24–33 g and rats (male HSD) 220–250 g were housed under standard conditions of light and temperature in plastic cages in the specific-pathogen unit (SPF) of the School of Pharmacy at the Hebrew University of Jerusalem. Animals were kept in separated cages with smooth flat floors and provided with unlimited access to water and food.

Nasal administration of the PSO delivery systems was performed under short (2–3 min) anesthesia with isoflurane to prevent loss of the formulation by sneezing. The animals were held in an upright position to mimic human position. The compositions were applied to both nostrils of the animal by a positive displacement pipette coupled with CP25 capillaries and pistons (Microman®, precision microliter pipette, Gilson, France).

2.3. Methods

2.3.1. Preparation of PSO Phospholipid Nasal Oily Gel Systems

The systems comprised of PSO and PL at a weight ratio of 2:1–4:1. The two components were mixed using a mortar and pestle at room temperature until a homogenous gel was obtained. Then, vitamin E (0.5% w/w) was added as an antioxidant. Then, to the obtained gel, other additives such as vegetable oils (oleic acid and sesame oil) up to 40% w/w, and/or propylene glycol (20–75% w/w) could be added. The additives were gradually mixed with the gel using an overhead stirrer (Heidolph, Hei Torque 200, Schwabach, Germany) at 500 rpm for 5 min.

Four PSO delivery systems containing 2:1, 2.3:1, 3:1, or 4:1 PSO:PL ratios were prepared.

2.3.2. Characterization of PSO Phospholipid Nasal Oily Gel Systems

Nasal systems containing 2:1, 2.3:1, 3:1, or 4:1 PSO:PL ratios were characterized for their appearance, spreadability, viscosity, and pH.

The spreadability of the PSO systems were measured by a modified method published by Sherafudeen and Vasantha [24]. This parameter was determined using a 7.6 × 2.6 cm^2 glass slide (Marienfield, Lauda-Konigshofen, Germany). The basal side of porcine skin (Kibutz Lahav, Negev, Israel) was tied to the surface of the slide with a thread. The slide was kept in a mini-incubator (Labnet International, Edison, NJ, USA) at 37 °C. One hundred microliters of the PSO delivery systems were placed on the tissue at an angle of 120°. The spreadability of the system was considered to be the distance that it traveled in 10 s. The average of three readings was recorded for each system.

Viscosity measurement for PSO phospholipid nasal oily systems was carried out using a Brookfield DV III Rheometer LV (Brookfield Engineering Labs., Stoughton, MA, USA) coupled with spindle S4 at 10 rpm and room temperature.

It was interesting to know which pH is generated following the application of the formulation into the nasal cavity. For this purpose, the oily gel system was dispersed in normal saline. The pH of the dispersed system, at a volume ratio of 1:10 [24], was assessed with a Seven Easy pH meter and an InLab Expert Pro electrode (Mettler Toledo, Changzhou, China). All measurements were duplicated.

2.3.3. Visualization of Nasal Delivery to Brain

Nasal Delivery of Fluorescein Isothiocyanate (FITC) to Mice Brain: A Multiphoton Imaging Study

In this experiment, we tested the formulation containing a ratio of PSO:PL. The ability of the PSO phospholipid nasal oily system to deliver FITC to mice brain was assessed by multiphoton imaging. A PSO system containing 0.5% FITC and 20% PSO was investigated. Mice received either 10 µL of nasal PSO system or 10 µL of a control composition containing 0.5% FITC and 20% PSO in paraffin oil. Ten minutes after treatment, the animals were sacrificed and the brains were removed and washed with normal saline. The olfactory region in the brain was observed under a multiphoton microscope A1-MP (NIKON, Tokyo, Japan). The field of image was 818 × 818 × 200 nm (width × height × depth), the scanning was performed using × 20 objective lens with an excitation wavelength of 740 nm, a laser intensity of 6%, and a scan speed of 0.125. The FITC fluorescence intensity (Arbitrary units, A.U.) in the scanned brain region was further analyzed using ImageJ software. The brain of an untreated mouse was examined to rule out the auto-fluorescence of the brain olfactory region.

Visualization of Nasal Delivery of Indocyanine Green (ICG) to Mice Brain: A Near Infrared (NIR) Imaging Study

The delivery of ICG to the mice brain from the nasal PSO delivery system containing PSO: PL ratio of 4:1 was examined by the Odyssey® Infrared Imaging System (LI-COR, Lincoln, NE, USA).

Mice were treated with 10 µL of PSO phospholipid nasal gel comprising 0.5% ICG and 5% PSO or with a control nasal composition containing the same concentration of ICG dissolved in 99.5% PG and compared to untreated mice. Thirty minutes after treatment, the animals were sacrificed and brains were removed, washed with normal saline, and observed under the imaging system. The scanning was performed using offset 2, resolution 339.6 µm, channel 800 nm, and intensity 1. The fluorescence intensity of the probe (A.U.) in the brain was further analyzed using ImageJ software.

2.3.4. Measurement of the Effect of PSO Phospholipid Nasal System in Animal Model of Impaired Memory by the Novel Object Recognition Test (NORT)

A PSO system comprised of 25% PSO at a PSO:PL ratio of 3:1 was tested in this experiment and compared to the oral administration of pure PSO. A modified reserpine induced memory impairment mice model was used [25].

The reserpinized mice were divided randomly into three groups: two PSO treated animal groups, PSO administrated nasally in the delivery system, PSO given orally, and one untreated reserpinized control group (n = 6/group). An additional untreated and un-reserpinized group served as a control with normal memory to test the suitability of the animal model. Reserpinized mice in the treatment groups received PSO at a dose of 300 mg/kg twice daily for five days and the last dose was given on the sixth day, one hour before running the behavioral test.

On days three and five of the experiment, the animals of the three reserpinized groups received intraperitoneal injections of reserpine at doses of 0.5 and 0.4 mg/kg from 0.05% and 0.004% reserpine solutions, respectively, at an injection volume of 10 mL/kg. The reserpine injections were prepared by suspending the compound in water for injection containing 0.1% DMSO and 0.3% Tween 80.

A modified NORT test [25,26] was conducted in a transparent individual cage (29 × 28.5 × 30 cm) for each mouse. Briefly, the animals were placed in the cage to explore two objects similar in terms of size, shape, and color for 6 min. Then, they were returned to their home cage and the arena, including the objects, was thoroughly cleaned with 70% alcohol to avoid leaving odorous cues. After one hour, one of the familiar objects was replaced with a novel object (different in size, shape, and color). The mice were returned to the testing arena and their ability to explore each object was recorded for five minutes. Exploration was defined as the orientation of an animal's snout toward the object, sniffing, or touching. The percentage of novel object recognition was calculated as follows: the time spent exploring the new object × 100/time total of exploration (time exploring new object + time exploring familiar object).

2.3.5. Evaluation of Motor Behavior of Reserpinized Mice in Open Field Test: Effect of PSO Phospholipid Delivery System Administrated Nasally vs. Oral Administration of the Oil

The goal of this experiment was to evaluate the effect of PSO administrated nasally in the phospholipid oily gel carrier in comparison to orally administrated PSO. A PSO system comprised of 25% PSO at a PSO:PL ratio of 3:1 was tested. The motor behavior of reserpinized mice modified model of movement impairment was tested using the open field test [27].

The reserpinized mice were divided randomly into three groups: two PSO treated groups, the PSO nasal system and the PSO oral system, and one untreated control group (n = 6/group). Animals in the treatment groups received PSO at a dose of 300 mg/kg twice daily for five days, then the last dose was given on the sixth day 1.5 h before the test. On the fifth day of the experiment, the animals of the three groups received an intraperitoneal injection of 4 mg/kg Reserpine.

The spontaneous locomotor activity of the animals was measured 23 h after the reserpine injection and 1.5 h after the last administration of PSO. Mice were placed in the center of a cage (29 × 28.5 × 30 cm) with a flat floor divided into nine equal squares. The number of squares crossed by the animal was counted for 5 min, without a habituation session.

2.3.6. Assessment of Local Safety of PSO Phospholipid Oily Gel on Rats' Nasal Cavity and Mucosa following Sub-Chronic Administration

In this test, the safety of the PSO nasal system containing 25% PSO at a PSO:PL ratio of 3:1 on the nasal cavity and mucosa was evaluated in rats using a method previously described by Duchi et al. [20]. In brief, nine male HSD rats (220–250 g) were divided equally into two treatment groups and one untreated control group. Rats in the treatment groups received nasally 15 µL PSO phospholipid oily system or normal saline into both nostrils twice a day, for one week. At the end of the experiment, the animals were sacrificed and the nasal cavities were removed and fixed in 3.7% formaldehyde PBS. Sections of the nasal cavity were cut serially at 5 µm thickness and stained with hematoxylin and eosin. The sections were examined by a histopathologist (Authority for Animal Facilities, Hebrew University of Jerusalem, Jerusalem, Israel) using an Olympus light microscope BX43 and an Olympus digital camera DP21 with Olympus cellSens Entry 1.13 software (Olympus, Tokyo, Japan) using a magnification of ×10. Local toxicity was assessed by evaluating the histopathological alterations in different regions of the nasal cavity including cartilage and turbinate bone, lamina propria and submucosa, mucosal epithelium, and lumen.

2.3.7. Statistical Analysis

Data are reported as mean ± SD and analyzed using one-way ANOVA with Bonferroni's multiple comparison test or using a two-tailed Mann–Whitney test using the GraphPad Prism 5 software (GraphPad Software, Inc., San Diego, CA, USA). A $p < 0.05$ is considered significant in all cases.

3. Results

3.1. Properties of PSO Nasal Phospholipid Oily Gel Systems

PSO phospholipid systems composed of PSO:PL at various ratios were characterized by their appearance, viscosity, spreadability, and pH. Their properties are presented in Table 1.

Table 1. Compositions and properties of various PSO phospholipid oily gel systems.

Composition (Weight Ratio)	Appearance	Viscosity (cP)	Spreadability (cm)	pH *
PSO: PL 4:1	Yellow, slightly viscous liquid	72.7 ± 11.45	1.17 ± 0.15	5.71 ± 0.025
PSO: PL 3:1	Yellow flowing gel	240.0 ± 2.0	1.03 ± 0.06	5.87 ± 0.02
PSO: PL 2.3:1	Yellow semisolid gel	377.0 ± 5.7	0.90 ± 0.0	6.16 ± 0.04
PSO: PL 2:1	Yellow semisolid gel	488.5 ± 13.4	0.87 ± 0.06	6.38 ± 0.14

* pH of dispersed systems in saline (1:10).

PSO phospholipid oily gel systems are homogenous low viscosity gels. The viscosity of these PSO systems was found to be higher than that of the pure oil which is liquid at RT with a viscosity value of 21.5 ± 1.06 cP. The viscosity of the nasal delivery systems increased proportionally with the PL ratio, ranging between 72 cP for the system containing 4:1 PSO:PL and 488 cP for the system containing the two components at a ratio of 2:1. It is noteworthy that a higher viscosity is advantageous in nasal administration, avoiding oil leakage and lung aspiration. The range of spreadability of the formulations was 0.87–1.17 cm. The obtained pH range of 5.71–6.38 is considered acceptable for nasal administration.

3.2. Nasal Delivery to Brain from the PSO System: A Multiphoton Microscopy Study

Figure 1 presents multiphoton micrographs for the olfactory region of mouse brains 10 min after nasal treatment with FITC in the PSO phospholipid delivery system versus a control containing the same PSO concentration but without PL.

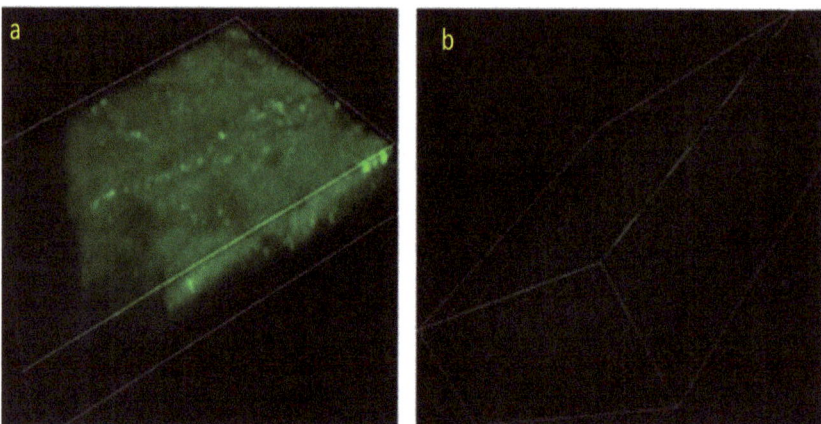

Figure 1. Representative multiphoton micrographs for the olfactory region of mouse brains treated nasally with (**a**) PSO nasal phospholipid system or (**b**) control composition containing PSO but lacking PL, each containing 0.5% w/w FITC. Field of images: Height = 818 μm and width = 818 μm for the both images. Depth = 100 μm for brains of mice which received PSO system and 200 μm for those who received the control composition. Lens × 20 (A1-MP microscope NIKON—Tokyo, Japan).

It can be seen that the nasal administration of PSO phospholipid oily gel containing 0.5% FITC yielded a strong fluorescent signal in the olfactory region of the animal brain as compared to the control FITC composition.

Semi-quantification of the obtained brain images gave a fluorescent intensity of 51.7 A.U. for the PSO Nasal system. On the other hand, nasal administration of FITC from a composition containing an equal amount of PSO not in the gel system yielded a fluorescent intensity of only 9.4 A.U. The multiphoton micrographs and their semi-quantification indicated a more than 500% increased delivery.

3.3. Delivery to the Brain of Molecules from the Nasal Phospholipid Gel System: An NIR Imaging Study

In this experiment, the effect of the PSO phospholipid system on the delivery of ICG to brain was examined in mice by NIR imaging of the brain 30 min following treatment. The obtained NIR images show that the nasal administration of the PSO phospholipid oily gel system yielded a strong fluorescent signal of ICG, as compared to the control composition of the probe (Figure 2).

The semi-quantification of the images and the normalization of the fluorescence intensity (by subtracting the auto-fluorescence of the untreated brain from the fluorescence intensity of each image) showed a fluorescent intensity of 7.5 A.U. for the nasal PSO phospholipid system. On the other hand, nasal administration of the control ICG composition yielded a fluorescent intensity of only 0.4 A.U. This result points towards the role of the PSO phospholipid oily gel nasal system in improving the delivery of this molecule to the brain.

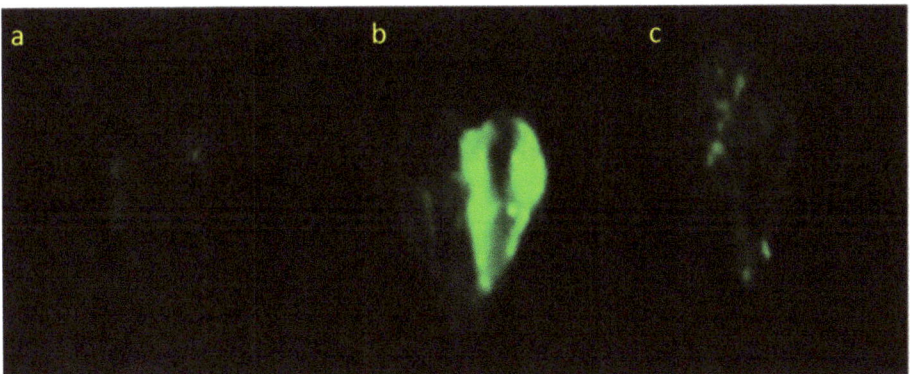

Figure 2. Representative NIR images for (**a**) brain of untreated mice (**b**) brain of mice 30 min following nasal treatment with the PSO delivery system and (**c**) brain of mice treated with a control composition. Each system contained 0.5% w/w ICG. Odyssey® Infrared Imaging System (LI-COR, Lincoln, NE, USA).

3.4. Effect on Memory of an Animal Model

3.4.1. Animal Model of Memory Impairment

The reserpine-induced memory impairment mice model and the novel object recognition test were used to evaluate the effect of PSO phospholipid nasal oily gel on memory. The first step was to validate the reserpine-induced memory impairment animal model by comparing the behavior of untreated reserpinized animals to those of normal memory. The results indicated that animals with normal memory exhibited a recognition percentage of 72.3 ± 2.2%, as compared to 48.3 ± 6.8% for animals with impaired memory ($p < 0.001$) (Figure 3). This 60% reduction in the animal's memory following reserpine sub-chronic administration indicates the suitability and reliability of the impaired memory model.

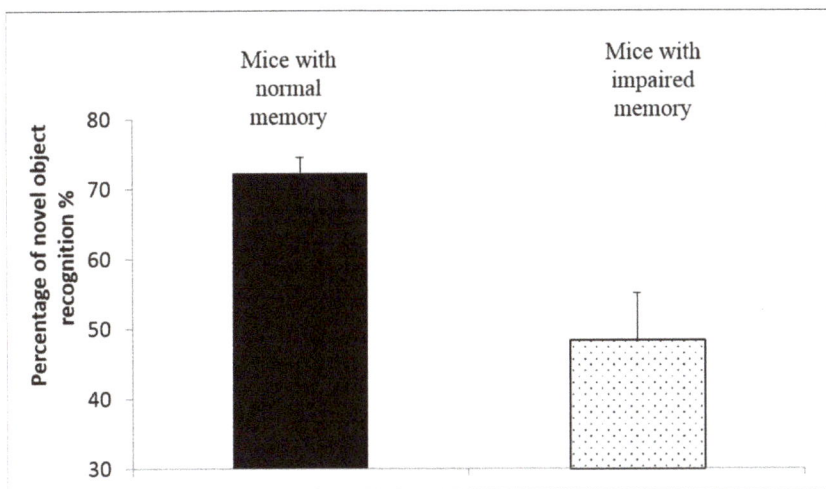

Figure 3. Percentage of novel object recognition for mice with normal memory and for mice with impaired memory ($n = 6$/group), (mean ± SD). $p < 0.001$ for mice with normal memory vs. mice with impaired memory, determined by two-tailed Mann–Whitney Test.

3.4.2. Effect of Nasal Administration of PSO Phospholipid Oily System on Animal Behavior in the Animal Model for Impaired Memory

The effect of the PSO phospholipid nasal system on the behavior of animals with reserpine-induced memory impairment was evaluated in this experiment in comparison to the oral administration of PSO. The data obtained in this part of the experiment showed that pretreatment and treatment with the PSO nasal system for six days led to a significant increase in the recognition percentage in mice with impaired memory.

Figure 4 shows a novel object recognition percentage of 75.9 ± 4.5% in mice pretreated and treated with the PSO phospholipid oily gel. On the other hand, the recognition of animals treated with PSO orally was only 44.4 ± 7.4%, similar to the untreated mice with impaired memory ($p > 0.05$).

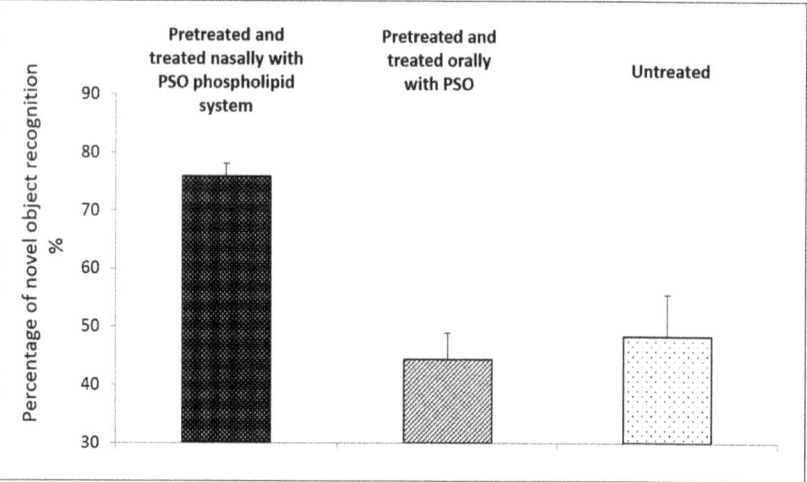

Figure 4. Percentage of novel object recognition by three groups of mice with impaired memory: 1. Pretreated and treated twice daily nasally for six days with the PSO oily phospholipid gel, 2. pretreated and treated twice daily for six days orally with PSO, and 3. untreated animals ($n = 6$/group), (mean ± SD). $p < 0.001$ for nasal PSO nasal system vs. untreated group with impaired memory and $p < 0.001$ for nasal PSO nasal system vs. orally treated, as determined by one-way ANOVA with Bonferroni's multiple comparison test.

This superior effect of the PSO nasal system emphasizes the important role of administrating PSO nasally from the phospholipid oily gel carrier for enhanced efficiency of PSO treatment.

3.5. *Effect of Nasal Administration of the PSO Nasal System Compared to the Oral Administration of PSO on the Motor Behavior of Reserpinized Mice: Results of Open Field Test*

In this experiment, animals with locomotor impairment were treated nasally with PSO phospholipid oily gel or orally with pure oil. Figure 5 presents the number of squares crossed in the open field test by 3 groups of reserpinized mice: 1. treated with PSO phospholipid oily nasal gel system, 2. treated with PSO orally, and 3. untreated animals.

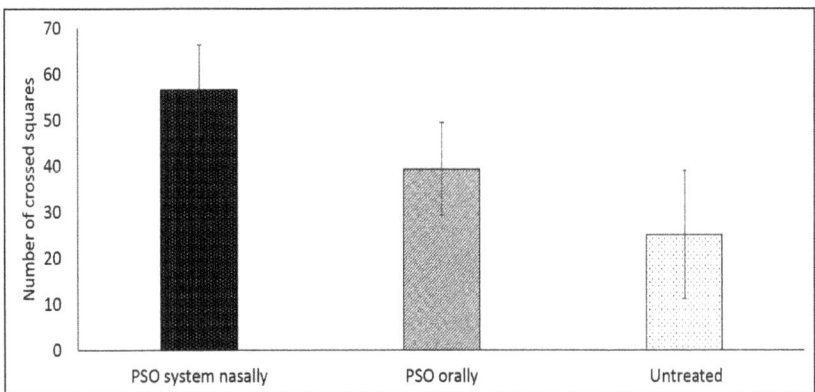

Figure 5. Number of squares crossed in the open field test by reserpinized mice: 1. treated twice daily for five days with PSO system nasally (PSO phospholipid oily gel nasal system), 2. treated twice daily for five days with PSO orally, and 3. untreated animals ($n = 6$/group) (mean ± SD). $p < 0.001$ for PSO nasal system vs. untreated control, $p < 0.05$ for PSO nasal system vs. PSO orally, $p > 0.05$ (considered not significant), for PSO orally vs. untreated control, as determined by one-way ANOVA with Bonferroni's multiple comparison test.

Figure 5 shows that mice treated with the new PSO phospholipid oily gel nasal system expressed increased locomotor activity, crossing 56.6 ± 9.7 squares while the PSO oral group crossed only 39.3 ± 10.0 squares. The untreated animals were able to cross only 25.0 ± 13.9 squares. The results are statistically significant: $p < 0.05$ for the PSO phospholipid oily gel nasal system versus PSO orally and $p < 0.001$ for the PSO phospholipid oily gel nasal system versus the untreated control. This 200% improved movement emphasizes the effect of the new nasal PSO system to reverse the effects of reserpine and enhance locomotor activity in the tested animal model.

3.6. Local Safety of the PSO Phospholipid Nasal Delivery System

The safety of the PSO phospholipid oily gel system on the nasal cavity and mucosa of rats was tested following sub-chronic treatment twice daily for 7 days as compared to normal saline application or to the cavity of untreated animals.

The histopathologic examination, carried out by a pathologist, indicates that the nasal cavity and mucosa of animals treated with the PSO phospholipid oily gel system were similar to those treated with normal saline nasally at the same treatment regimen and were also similar to untreated rats. The bone was symmetrical and the turbinate was intact. No leukocyte infiltration or loss of cilia was noticed in the lamina propria. The submucosal integrity was preserved without any loss of cilia. No evidence was found for leukocyte or non-cellular material infiltration in the lumen (Figure 6).

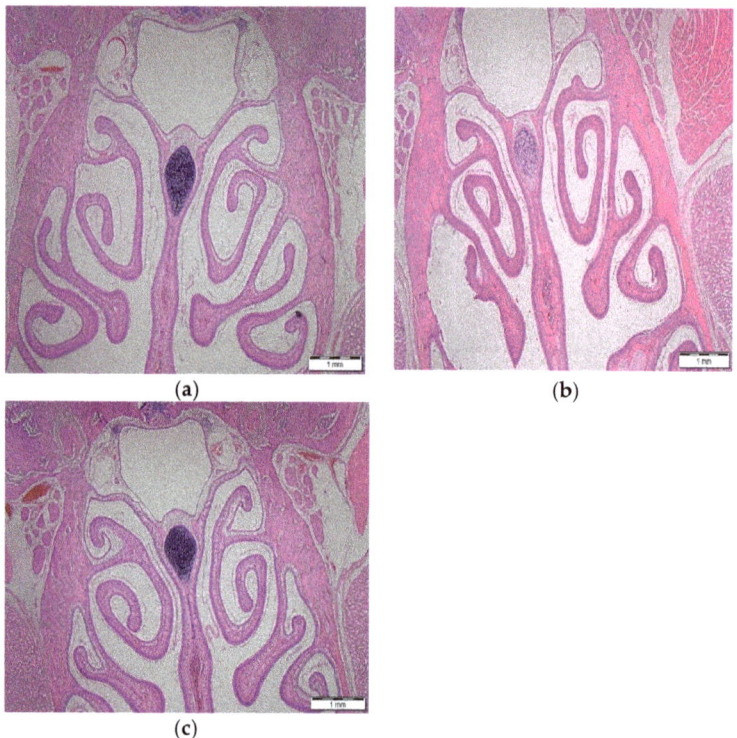

Figure 6. Representative micrographs of nasal cavities excised from rats: (**a**) treated nasally with PSO phospholipid gel system, (**b**) treated nasally with normal saline, and (**c**) untreated rats. Bar = 1 mm.

4. Discussion

This work presents a new PSO phospholipid gel delivery system for nasal administration for the treatment of impaired memory. The viscosity of the gel, as a result of the presence of phospholipid, is an important property to avoid the nasal leakage of PSO and its lung aspiration. The gel system has a relatively low viscosity (72–488 cP). Although we have not tested the residence time, another work on systems with much higher viscosity showed an improved residential time in the nasal mucosa with an increase in viscosity [28]. Another important property of PSO systems is that their pH values upon dispersion in a physiological fluid.

The novel delivery system presented in this work shows an enhanced nasal delivery of molecules to the brain and an improved efficiency of the oil tested in animals. This feature was demonstrated by multiphoton microscopy, where a five-fold increase in the delivery of FITC to the olfactory region of mouse brain ten minutes post nasal administration was evidenced, as compared to control composition. Moreover, in a NIR imaging study, nasal delivery to mice brain of ICG in PSO system, 30 min post-administration, was enhanced by 18-fold, versus a control composition. The enhanced delivery to brain of FITC and ICG, administrated nasally in the PSO phospholipid gel, emphasizes the role of the carrier. The phospholipid has two roles in this delivery carrier: it acts as a permeation enhancer and contributes to the viscosity of the gel.

The next set of experiments in this study focused on the evaluation of the effect of PSO phospholipid oily gel administrated nasally on the memory and movement of animals. Six days of treatment with the new system prevented memory impairment in the reserpinized mouse model. This was not obtained with the PSO administrated orally. Furthermore, a 200% improvement in movement behavior was evidenced in mice model of locomotor impairment, following five days of nasal administration of the PSO phospholipid system. These data point towards a stronger neuroprotective effect of PSO when administered nasally in the phospholipid gel but not following oral administration of PSO.

The neuroprotective mechanism of PSO in the brain remains unclear. It is suggested that PSO acts as a strong antioxidant against oxidative stress and free radical damage. This hypothesis is supported by an in vitro study by Sabahi et al. [29] indicating the ability of PSO to neutralize reactive oxygen species (ROS) and enhance the expression of the antioxidant gene in rat pheochromocytoma (PC12) neuronal cells neuro-intoxicated by 3-nitropropionic acid (3-NP).

Oxidative stress and free radical damage seem to play a key role in neurodegenerative disorders such as Alzheimer's disease and Parkinson's disease. Previous studies indicated that oxidative stress induces neuroinflammation, protein aggregation, and mitochondrial dysfunction leading to neuronal death, depression-like behavior, and memory impairment [30,31].

As mentioned in the introduction, several works have investigated the neuroprotective effect of PSO animal models of CNS diseases [5–9].

Recently, Fathy et al. [32] studied the effect of pomegranate seed extract on a paraquat-induced mouse model of Parkinson's disease. Animals started to receive the extract orally on daily basis for two weeks then continued concomitantly with intraperitoneal injections of paraquat twice daily for three weeks. The reported results indicated that the treatment reduced oxidative stress via a significant reduction of malondialdehyde levels and augmentation of antioxidant enzyme activity in the substantia nigra region of the brain.

Previous publications investigated the potential therapeutic effect of long-term administration of pomegranate seed oil and extract. Treatment regimens in these reports reached more than 6 months [5,9]. One noteworthy finding of our work is the efficiency of PSO delivered nasally from the new system evidenced in just a few days of treatment. To the best of our knowledge, this is the first work investigating the effect of nasal delivery of PSO for the treatment and prevention of CNS diseases in a short period of time.

Nasal drug delivery is a convenient and noninvasive alternative route to the oral way of administration. By using nasal treatment, the disadvantages related to the gastrointestinal tract and hepatic first-pass metabolism can be avoided. Another advantage of nasal administration is the ability to deliver molecules directly to the brain by bypassing the BBB via the olfactory and trigeminal nerves allowing for an improved treatment [11,17].

In our previous work, we have shown that some carriers, such as soft phospholipid nanovesicles, enhanced the direct nose to brain delivery of the incorporated drug, leading to a rapid onset of action and an improved treatment outcome [13–16,18–21]. In this work, we investigated a phospholipid oily gel system of PSO for enhanced delivery of molecules to brain and improved the efficiency of PSO treatment.

The safety of nasally administered delivery systems is a critical parameter. Therefore, we examined the local safety on the nasal cavity and mucosa following sub-chronic nasal administration of the PSO phospholipid system to rats. The histopathologic examination of the nasal cavities indicated the absence of pathological local side effects for the tested period.

Overall, the new PSO nasal system was found to enhance the oil activity without causing nasal toxicity or irritation in the tested period.

To our knowledge, this is the first investigation on nasal delivery of PSO to the brain and CNS and its efficacy for the treatment of impaired memory. It opens the door for future research focusing on a number of directions, including the antioxidant effect of PSO components delivered nasally and the stability of PSO and the nasal system.

5. Conclusions

In this work, a PSO phospholipid oily gel for nasal administration was designed and investigated. The system shows an enhanced nasal delivery of molecules to brain and improved efficiency of PSO to treat memory and movement impairment in animal models. The histopathologic examination of the nasal cavities indicated the absence of pathological local side effects for the tested period.

Author Contributions: Conceptualization, E.T; methodology, E.T. and H.N.; investigation, E.T. and H.N.; experimental, E.T. and H.N.; resources, E.T.; writing—original draft preparation, E.T. and H.N.; writing—review and editing, E.T. and H.N; supervision, E.T. All authors have read and agreed to the published version of the manuscript.

Funding: This research received no external funding.

Institutional Review Board Statement: All procedures carried out on animals were according to the National Institute of Health's regulations and were approved by the Committee for Animal Care and Experimental Use of the Hebrew University of Jerusalem (MD-11-12821-3; MD-19-15895-3; MD-21-16402-3; MD-21-16474-4).

Informed Consent Statement: Not applicable.

Acknowledgments: The authors would like to thank Musa Mujahed and Ana Maria Botero-Anug, from the Authority for Biological and Biomedical Models, Hebrew University of Jerusalem, for the nasal cavity and mucosa sectioning and histopathological examination.

Conflicts of Interest: The authors declare no conflict of interest.

References

1. Costantini, S.; Rusolo, F.; De Vito, V.; Moccia, S.; Picariello, G.; Capone, F.; Guerriero, E.; Castello, G.; Volpe, M.G. Potential Anti-Inflammatory Effects of the Hydrophilic Fraction of Pomegranate (*Punica granatum* L.) Seed Oil on Breast Cancer Cell Lines. *Molecules* **2014**, *19*, 8644–8660. [CrossRef] [PubMed]
2. Rojo-Gutiérrez, E.; Carrasco-Molinar, O.; Tirado-Gallegos, J.M.; Levario-Gómez, A.; Chávez-González, M.L.; Baeza-Jiménez, R.; Buenrostro-Figueroa, J.J. Evaluation of green extraction processes, lipid composition and antioxidant activity of pome-granate seed oil. *J. Food Meas. Charact.* **2021**, *15*, 2098–2107. [CrossRef]
3. Račková, L.; Ergin, V.; Bali, E.B.; Kuniakova, M.; Karasu, C. Pomegranate Seed Oil Modulates Functions and Survival of BV-2 Microglial Cells in vitro. *Int. J. Vitam. Nutr. Res.* **2014**, *84*, 295–309. [CrossRef] [PubMed]
4. Boroushaki, M.T.; Mollazadeh, H.; Afshari, A.R. Pomegranate seed oil: A comprehensive review on its therapeutic effects. *Int. J. Pharm. Sci. Res.* **2016**, *7*, 1000–1013.
5. Mizrahi, M.; Friedman-Levi, Y.; Larush, L.; Frid, K.; Binyamin, O.; Dori, D.; Fainstein, N.; Ovadia, H.; Ben-Hur, T.; Magdassi, S.; et al. Pomegranate seed oil nanoemulsions for the prevention and treatment of neurodegenerative diseases: The case of genetic CJD. *Nanomed. Nanotechnol. Biol. Med.* **2014**, *10*, 1353–1363. [CrossRef]
6. Binyamin, O.; Larush, L.; Frid, K.; Keller, G.; Friedman-Levi, Y.; Ovadia, H.; Abramsky, O.; Magdassi, S.; Gabizon, R. Treatment of a multiple sclerosis animal model by a novel nanodrop formulation of a natural antioxidant. *Int. J. Nanomed.* **2015**, *10*, 7165–7174. [CrossRef]
7. Sarkaki, A.; Hajipour, S.; Mansouri, M.T.; Pilevarian, A.; Rad, M.R. Pomegranate seed hydroalcoholic extract improves memory deficit due to permanent cerebral hypoperfusion/ischemia in male rats. *Health Med.* **2013**, *7*, 863–871.
8. Sarkaki, A.; Rezaiei, M.; Naseri, M.G.; Rafieirad, M. Improving active and passive avoidance memories deficits due to permanent cerebral ischemia by pomegranate seed extract in female rats. *Malays. J. Med. Sci.* **2013**, *20*, 25–34.
9. Braidy, N.; Essa, M.M.; Poljak, A.; Selvaraju, S.; Al-Adawi, S.; Manivasagm, T.; Thenmozhi, A.J.; Ooi, L.; Sachdev, P.; Guil-lemin, G.J. Consumption of pomegranates improves synaptic function in a transgenic mice model of Alzheimer's disease. *Oncotarget* **2016**, *7*, 64589. [CrossRef]
10. Yuan, G.; Sinclair, A.J.; Xu, C.; Li, D. Incorporation and metabolism of punicic acid in healthy young humans. *Mol. Nutr. Food Res.* **2009**, *53*, 1336–1342. [CrossRef]
11. Patel, M.M.; Goyal, B.R.; Bhadada, S.V.; Bhatt, J.S.; Amin, A.F. Getting into the Brain. *CNS Drugs* **2009**, *23*, 35–58. [CrossRef] [PubMed]
12. Touitou, E.; Illum, L. Nasal drug delivery. *Drug. Deliv. Transl. Res.* **2013**, *3*, 1–3. [CrossRef] [PubMed]
13. Duchi, S.; Ovadia, H.; Touitou, E. Nasal administration of drugs as a new non-invasive strategy for efficient treatment of multiple sclerosis. *J. Neuroimmunol.* **2013**, *258*, 32–40. [CrossRef] [PubMed]
14. Touitou, E.; Natsheh, H.; Duchi, S. Buspirone Nanovesicular Nasal System for Non-Hormonal Hot Flushes Treatment. *Pharmaceutics* **2018**, *10*, 82. [CrossRef] [PubMed]
15. Touitou, E.; Duchi, S.; Natsheh, H. A new nanovesicular system for nasal drug administration. *Int. J. Pharm.* **2020**, *580*, 119243. [CrossRef]
16. Natsheh, H.; Touitou, E. Phospholipid Magnesome—a nasal vesicular carrier for delivery of drugs to brain. *Drug Deliv. Transl. Res.* **2018**, *8*, 806–819. [CrossRef]
17. Dhuria, S.V.; Hanson, L.R.; Frey, W.H. Intranasal delivery to the central nervous system: Mechanisms and experimental considerations. *J. Pharm. Sci.* **2010**, *99*, 1654–1673. [CrossRef]
18. Griesman, B.L. Proper and improper administration of oily nasal sprays. *Arch. Otolaryngol. Head Neck Surg.* **1944**, *39*, 124–136. [CrossRef]

19. Touitou, E.; Natsheh, H. Compositions and Methods for Nasal Administration of Drugs to Brain and for Systemic Effect. WO Patent 049145, 14 March 2019.
20. Duchi, S.; Touitou, E.; Pradella, L.; Marchini, F.; Ainbinder, D. Nasal Tramadol delivery system: A new approach for improved pain therapy. *Eur. J. Pain Suppl.* **2011**, *5*, 449–452. [CrossRef]
21. Touitou, E.; Natsheh, H.; Boukeileh, S.; Awad, R. Short Onset and Enhanced Analgesia Following Nasal Administration of Non-Controlled Drugs in Nanovesicular Systems. *Pharmaceutics* **2021**, *13*, 978. [CrossRef]
22. Natsheh, H.; Touitou, E. Phospholipid Vesicles for Dermal/Transdermal and Nasal Administration of Active Molecules: The Effect of Surfactants and Alcohols on the Fluidity of Their Lipid Bilayers and Penetration Enhancement Properties. *Molecules* **2020**, *25*, 2959. [CrossRef] [PubMed]
23. Touitou, E.; Godin, B.; Duchi, S. Compositions for Nasal Delivery. U.S. Patent 8,911,751, 16 December 2014.
24. Sherafudeen, S.P.; Vasantha, P.V. Development and evaluation of in situ nasal gel formulations of loratadine. *Res. Pharm. Sci.* **2016**, *10*, 466–476.
25. Danboyi, T.; Alhassan, A.; Hassan-Danboyi, E.; Jimoh, A. Effect of co-administration of vitamins C and E on reserpine-induced memory impairment in mice. *Niger. J. Sci. Technol.* **2019**, *18*, 261–268.
26. Pereira, A.G.; Poli, A.; Matheus, F.C.; Silva, L.D.B.D.; Fadanni, G.P.; Izídio, G.S.; Latini, A.; Prediger, R. Temporal development of neurochemical and cognitive impairments following reserpine administration in rats. *Behav. Brain Res.* **2020**, *383*, 112517. [CrossRef] [PubMed]
27. De Freitas, C.M.; Busanello, A.; Schaffer, L.F.; Peroza, L.R.; Krum, B.N.; Leal, C.Q.; Ceretta, A.P.C.; Da Rocha, J.B.T.; Fachinetto, R. Behavioral and neurochemical effects induced by reserpine in mice. *Psychopharmacology* **2015**, *233*, 457–467. [CrossRef]
28. Gholizadeh, H.; Messerotti, E.; Pozzoli, M.; Cheng, S.; Traini, D.; Young, P.; Kourmatzis, A.; Caramella, C.; Ong, H.X. Application of a thermosensitive in situ gel of chitosan-based nasal spray loaded with tranexamic acid for localised treatment of nasal wounds. *AAPS Pharm. Sci. Technol.* **2019**, *20*, 299. [CrossRef]
29. Al-Sabahi, B.N.; Fatope, M.O.; Essa, M.M.; Subash, S.; Al-Busafi, S.N.; Al-Kusaibi, F.S.M.; Manivasagam, T. Pomegranate seed oil: Effect on 3-nitropropionic acid-induced neurotoxicity in PC12 cells and elucidation of unsaturated fatty acids composition. *Nutr. Neurosci.* **2016**, *20*, 40–48. [CrossRef]
30. Agnihotri, A.; Aruoma, O.I. Alzheimer's disease and Parkinson's disease: A nutritional toxicology perspective of the impact of oxidative stress, mitochondrial dysfunction, nutrigenomics and environmental chemicals. *J. Am. Coll. Nutr.* **2020**, *39*, 16–27. [CrossRef]
31. Patki, G.; Solanki, N.; Atrooz, F.; Allam, F.; Salim, S. Depression, anxiety-like behavior and memory impairment are associated with increased oxidative stress and inflammation in a rat model of social stress. *Brain Res.* **2013**, *1539*, 73–86. [CrossRef]
32. Fathy, S.M.; El-Dash, H.A.; Said, N.I. Neuroprotective effects of pomegranate (*Punica granatum* L.) juice and seed extract in paraquat-induced mouse model of Parkinson's disease. *BMC Complement. Med. Ther.* **2021**, *21*, 130. [CrossRef]

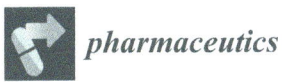

Article

Improving the Efficacy and Accessibility of Intracranial Viral Vector Delivery in Non-Human Primates

Devon J. Griggs [1,2,†], Aaron D. Garcia [2,3,4,5,†], Wing Yun Au [6], William K. S. Ojemann [6], Andrew Graham Johnson [7,8], Jonathan T. Ting [2,4,9], Elizabeth A. Buffalo [2,4] and Azadeh Yazdan-Shahmorad [1,2,6,*]

1. Department of Electrical and Computer Engineering, University of Washington, Seattle, WA 98195, USA; djgriggs@uw.edu
2. Washington National Primate Research Center, Seattle, WA 98195, USA; adg124@uw.edu (A.D.G.); jonathant@alleninstitute.org (J.T.T.); ebuffalo@uw.edu (E.A.B.)
3. Graduate Program in Neuroscience, University of Washington, Seattle, WA 98195, USA
4. Department of Physiology and Biophysics, University of Washington, Seattle, WA 98195, USA
5. Department of Biology, University of Washington, Seattle, WA 98195, USA
6. Department of Bioengineering, University of Washington, Seattle, WA 98195, USA; auwy@uw.edu (W.Y.A.); wojemann@seas.upenn.edu (W.K.S.O.)
7. Department of Earth and Space Sciences, University of Washington, Seattle, WA 98195, USA; grahamgtr@gmail.com
8. Bellevue School District, Bellevue, WA 98005, USA
9. Allen Institute for Brain Science, Seattle, WA 98109, USA
* Correspondence: azadehy@uw.edu
† These authors contributed equally to this work.

Abstract: Non-human primates (NHPs) are precious resources for cutting-edge neuroscientific research, including large-scale viral vector-based experimentation such as optogenetics. We propose to improve surgical outcomes by enhancing the surgical preparation practices of convection-enhanced delivery (CED), which is an efficient viral vector infusion technique for large brains such as NHPs'. Here, we present both real-time and next-day MRI data of CED in the brains of ten NHPs, and we present a quantitative, inexpensive, and practical bench-side model of the in vivo CED data. Our bench-side model is composed of food coloring infused into a transparent agar phantom, and the spread of infusion is optically monitored over time. Our proposed method approximates CED infusions into the cortex, thalamus, medial temporal lobe, and caudate nucleus of NHPs, confirmed by MRI data acquired with either gadolinium-based or manganese-based contrast agents co-infused with optogenetic viral vectors. These methods and data serve to guide researchers and surgical team members in key surgical preparations for intracranial viral delivery using CED in NHPs, and thus improve expression targeting and efficacy and, as a result, reduce surgical risks.

Keywords: non-human primate; convection-enhanced delivery; neurosurgery; optogenetics

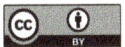

1. Introduction

The development of novel tools to genetically alter the properties of neurons has been instrumental in expanding the scope of neuroscientific questions. Perhaps one of the most popular of these genetic modification methods is optogenetics, through which cells can be made susceptible to rapid, reversible manipulations via light stimulation. This technique was first demonstrated in 2005 [1] and since then has been robustly developed and widely adopted. In particular, optogenetics has become a powerful tool for rodent neuroscience [2,3]. The high-throughput nature of experiments with these models means that researchers can pilot, experiment, and make corrections with new subjects rapidly and with minimal resources. Additionally, the rapid gestational time (~1 month for most research species) and large litter size (4–12 pups/L) of these models extends the genetic modification toolkit of rodent researchers to allow for breeding genetically altered lines and testing transgenic subjects with relative ease. However, transgenic lines are largely unavailable for highly translational non-human primate (NHP) models. In contrast to rodents, the macaque has a gestational period of ~6 months and gives birth to singular offspring, which eliminates the practical viability of transgenic approaches. This leaves viral vector transfection as the primary method of preparing NHPs for experiments requiring genetic modification. However, this experimental approach still proves to be a challenging, and potentially costly, endeavor. Here, we present novel and updated methods that eliminate several of the main dissuading factors of transduction studies in NHPs.

Convection-enhanced delivery (CED) is an infusion technique that has been developed over the past few decades to deliver medicinal agents to the brain [4,5]. Classic neural infusion techniques rely on diffusion, which is based on a concentration gradient and therefore is heavily influenced by molecular weight [6]. Large molecules such as viral vectors are inefficiently spread by diffusion. By contrast, CED capitalizes on a pressure gradient for delivery, which is much less influenced by molecular weight and comes with a number of benefits over diffusion: 1. CED can be performed at higher delivery rates (on the order of 1 µL/min or higher), which speeds up delivery [7–9], 2. CED can distribute agent over greater volumes (hundreds of mm^3) [8,9], 3. CED produces a roughly uniform concentration of agent throughout the distribution volume [6,7,10–14], and 4. as previously alluded, CED is effective at transporting large molecules, such as viral vectors, throughout regions of the brain [7,11–15].

Incentivized by these desirable properties, we have used CED in recent years to deliver optogenetic viral vectors into the brains of non-human primates for neuroscientific experiments [8,9,16,17]. To complement the technique, we utilized a method of real-time infusion validation with magnetic resonance imaging (MRI) technology using a gadolinium-based contrast agent co-infused with the optogenetic viral vector [18]. We previously validated the resulting optogenetic expression with epifluorescence imaging, electrophysiology, and histology [8,9]. However, we recognize that not all institutions have access to an MRI scanner in which live validation of an injection can be visualized. Thus, a separate set of CED experiments without live MRI guidance was performed using novel optogenetic viral vectors co-infused with a manganese-based contrast agent. This allowed us to confirm infusion success the following day with MRI. With these live and next-day in vivo MRI data collected across ten animals and three different brain regions, we were uniquely positioned to develop a model to assist in planning CED procedures in the brains of NHPs. This work is important to the field because not all researchers have access to MRI scanners for next-day imaging, and fewer still are equipped to perform NHP viral infusions in an MRI scanner. We propose a CED modeling method that can assist any researcher in NHP neurosurgical CED planning.

Here, we have developed a quantitative bench-side CED model that provides the users with hands-on CED experience. Our bench-side model builds on our recent qualitative infusion modeling work [19], as well as our in vivo NHP data [8,9]. Bench-side CED models usually comprise dye infused into agar phantom, a clear gel with material properties similar to the brain [20,21]. In this work, we propose a similar model, but to our knowledge, we are the first to base a bench-side model on in vivo MRI data of CED in NHP brains. We provide the MRI data and we present a calibration method for our model using the MRI data to ensure that the reproduction of our quantitative method is practical for the field. Infusions into the primate brain are inherently coupled with surgical and experimental risks; however, the toolkit presented here mitigates the risk factors of these procedures, such as cost, surgical time, and overall subject count, by providing easily accessible ways to plan CED experiments. We also utilize a radiolabel that can be co-infused with viruses that can be imaged in MRI 24 h post-operatively, which empowers researchers without immediate access to an MRI scanner to identify issues and make any necessary surgical corrections in a timely fashion.

2. Materials and Methods

2.1. Subjects

Data from ten macaques were used for this study, as described in Table 1. The cortical and thalamic data (total $n = 5$) come from previously published procedures [8,9,18,22,23], and those data have been used in the present study. In contrast, data from the medial temporal lobe (MTL) group are derived from new injection procedures, which are described in detail below. The ages ranged from 5 to 11 years, and weights ranged from 5.7 to 17.5 kg. Five females and four males were rhesus macaques (*Macaca mulatta*) and one male was a pigtail macaque (*Macaca nemestrina*). MTL subjects were provided by the tissue distribution program available from the Washington National Primate Center (WaNPRC), and no observable differences were seen in our data as a function of age, sex, species, or weight.

Table 1. NHP and surgical data. NHPs are named for their infusion location(s). Medial temporal lobe and caudate nucleus (MTL). Hippocampus (HPC). Entorhinal cortex (EC), Tail of Caudate Nucleus (C).

NHP Name	C1	C2	CT	T1	T2	MTL1	MTL2	MTL3	MTL4	MTL5
Infusion Target	Cortex	Cortex	Cortex, Thalamus	Thalamus	Thalamus	MTL (HPC+C)	MTL (HPC+C)	MTL (EC)	MTL (HPC+C)	MTL (HPC)
NHP Variety	Rhesus Macaque									Pigtail Macaque
Sex	M	M	M	F	F	F	F	F	M	M
Age (y)	7	8	8	9	11	8	9	8	8	5
Weight (kg)	16.5	17.5	8.7	7.5	6.5	8.2	6.4	5.7	8.88	7.2
Cannula Step Tip Length (mm)	1	1	1 (Cortex) and 3 (Thalamus)	3	3	3	3	3	3	3
Left Hemisphere Infusions (µL)	50, 50, 50, 50	50, 50, 50, 50	50 (Cortex)	140, 120	115, 85	15	20	10, 10	15	N/A
Right Hemisphere Infusions (µL)	-	-	246 (Thalamus)	152, 111	-	15	20	10, 10	15	20
Contrast Agent	Gadoteridol					Manganese				
MRI Timing	Live	Live (2 infusions)	Live	Live	Live	Next-day				
Institution	University of California, San Francisco					University of Washington, Seattle				
NHP Alias	Monkey J [8]	Monkey G [8]	NHP-H [9,23]	NHP-A [9]	NHP-B [9]	N/A				

2.2. Animal Procedures and MRI Analysis

Three different neuroanatomical structures were targeted for CED infusions: cortex, thalamus, and the medial temporal lobe together with the caudate nucleus (MTL). Most of the cortical and thalamic infusions were validated with live MRI, while MTL infusions were validated with MRI the day following infusion. Table 1 contains the infusion details for each subject.

Subsequent subsections describe the various methods and MRI analysis related to the cortical, thalamic, and MTL infusions. Because the procedures relating to the cortical and thalamic groups have been previously published, detailed surgical methods are omitted with references to the respective primary studies. However, aspects of the procedures germane to the present study are presented. For the MTL group, details of the surgical methods, euthanasia, and immunohistochemistry are presented in full. For all procedures, vital signs such as heart rate, respiration, and body temperature were monitored throughout.

2.2.1. Cortical Infusion

We have previously described the surgical methods for cortical CED procedures [8,18]. Briefly, the subjects were anesthetized under isoflurane, a craniotomy was made above the sensorimotor cortex in a sterile operating room, and an MR-compatible cannula guide was affixed to the skull with MR-compatible screws and dental acrylic. Afterwards, the subjects were transferred to an MR scanner (Siemens 3T) while remaining under isoflurane anesthesia. We inserted the tip of a stepped-tip cannula about 2 mm below the surface of the brain in the sensorimotor cortex. A syringe pump (WPI UMP3, MICRO2T SMARTouch SGE250TLL, Sarasota, FL, USA) was used to co-infuse a mixture of AAV-CamKIIa-C1V1-EYFP (Table 2; 2.5×10^{12} virus molecules/milliliter (vm UPenn vector core) and a gadolinium-based contrast agent (Table 2; 2 mM Gd-DTPA, ratio of 250:1, Gadoteridol, Prohance, Bracco Diagnostic Inc., Princeton, NJ, USA) into the brain at a starting rate of 1 µL/min, which was increased every few minutes up to 5 µL/min. After the majority of the volume had been delivered, the rate was reduced in the same stair-step method to end with a rate of 1 µL/min. After infusion, we left the cannula in place for 10 min and then removed the cannula. This infusion process was repeated multiple times. During the infusion process, multiple MRI images were taken to track the progress of the infusions. We used fast (2 min) flash T1-weighted images (flip angle = 30°, repetition time/echo time = 3.05, matrix size = 128 × 128, slice thickness = 1 mm, 64 slices, Siemens 3T MR scanner). After recovery and optogenetic expression, Monkeys C1, C2, and CT were euthanized for immunohistochemical analysis of optogenetic expression [8,22,23].

Table 2. Virus information. S1 (primary sensorimotor cortex), M1 (primary motor cortex), AT (anterior thalamus), MT (medial thalamus), PT (posterior thalamus), HPC (hippocampus), C (tail of caudate nucleus), EC (entorhinal cortex). vm/mL (virus molecules per milliliter).

Animal Name	C1	C2	CT	T1	T2	MTL1		MTL2		MTL3	MTL4		MTL5
Hemisphere	Left	Right	Left	Right	Left	Left	Right	Left	Right	Left	Right	Left	Right	Right
Target	S1+M1	S1	MT	AT+PT	HPC		C		HPC	EC	HPC		C	HPC
Vector Serotype	AAV5	AAV2.9	AAV2.2	AAV2.9	AAVRetrograde						PHP.eB	AAV2	PHP.eB
Vector	AAV-CamKIIa-C1V1-EYFP	AAV-CaMKII-ChR2(H134R)-YFP			AAV-CAG-hChR2-H134R-tdTomato	AAV-Syn-Chronos-GFP	AAV-CAG-hChR2-H134R-tdTomato	AAV-CAG-hChR2-H134R-tdTomato	AAV-3xhI56i(core)-minBG-ChR2(CRC)-EYFP-WPRE3-BGHpA	AAV-mDLX5/6-ChrimsonR-tdTomato
Titer (vm/mL)	2.5×10^{12}	5.26×10^{12}	1.02×10^{13}	5.26×10^{12}	7.6×10^{12}	9×10^{12}	7.6×10^{12}	9×10^{12}	3.25×10^{13}	8.7×10^{12}	3.55×10^{12}

2.2.2. Thalamus Infusion

We previously described the surgical details of the thalamic CED infusions [9], which are similar to the cortical infusion procedures described above. Briefly, the subjects were anesthetized with isoflurane and craniotomies were made (15 mm diameter). We implanted cannula guides and secured them with plastic screws and dental acrylic. We allowed the subjects to recover for two weeks before performing CED. After recovery, the subjects were anesthetized, placed in a stereotax and transported to an MR scanner. We used the cannula guides to manually insert a 3 mm stepped-tip cannula (ClearPoint Neuro Inc. (formerly MRI Interventions, Solana Beach, CA, USA) to the targeted regions of the thalamus. We used a syringe pump (WPI UMP3, MICRO2T SMARTouch, SGE250TLL, Sarasota, FL, USA) to co-infuse multiple serotypes of AAV-CamKII-ChR (Table 2; Upenn vector core) with gadolinium-based contrast agent (Table 2; 2 mM Gadoteridol, Prohance, Bracco Diagnostic Inc., Princeton, NJ, USA) at rates between 0.5 µL/min and 3 µL/min while simultaneously performing fast (2 min) flash T1 MR scans (flip angle = 30°, repetition time/echo time = 3.05, matrix size = 128 × 128, slice thickness = 1 mm, 64 slices, Siemens 3T MR scanner). After all infusions were complete, the subjects were transported back to the surgical suite where the cannula guides were explanted and the incision closed. After recovery and optogenetic expression, Monkeys CT, T1, and T2 were euthanized for immunohistochemical analysis of optogenetic expression [9,23].

2.2.3. MTL Infusion

To pilot the efficacy of expression in the medial temporal lobe (MTL), five viral vectors were infused into the brains of five subjects. Subjects MTL1–3 were infused with two retrograde viruses (gifted from Edward Boyden and Karel Svoboda; Addgene viral preps #59170-AAVrg and #29017-AAVrg, respectively) [24,25]. Subjects MTL4 and 5 were infused with three GABA-selective viruses (Allen Institute for Brain Science and University of Washington, Seattle, WA.). See Table 2 for specific information about the vectors and target regions for all animals.

The surgical details of the MTL infusions are described in detail here. The animals were sedated with ketamine. A surgical plane was induced with propofol and maintained with 0.8–1.2% isoflurane, and the subjects were then stereotaxed. Analgesia was administered prior to (meloxicam) and during the procedure (fentanyl CRI transitioned to sustained-release buprenorphine). Sagittal incisions were made to expose the skull, and burr holes were drilled above our intended target. A 3 mm stepped-tip cannula (ClearPoint Neuro Inc. (formerly MRI Interventions, Solana Beach, CA, USA) was stereotactically lowered with a micro-manipulator arm through the burr hole to the targeted region of the MTL (hippocampus or entorhinal cortex), or the tail of the caudate nucleus. We used a syringe pump (WPI UMP3, MICRO2T SMARTouch, SGE250TLL, Sarasota, FL, USA) to co-infuse optogenetic viral vector with manganese-based contrast agent (Mn^{2+}, Millipore Sigma, Burlington, MA) at rates between 1 µL/min and 5 µL/min. The final concentration of Mn^{2+} mixed with virus was 6.5 mM and was specifically chosen as it is well under the limit for neuronal toxicity and interference with viral efficacy, as identified by [26]. After all infusions were complete, the cannula was removed and the incision closed. In one case (MTL5), this procedure was performed using the Brainsight veterinary surgical robot (Rogue Research Inc., Montreal, QC, Canada) instead of micromanipulator arms. A final analgesic was administered in the form of a local anesthetic block (bupivacaine). The day following infusion, the subjects were again anesthetized and placed in an MR-compatible stereotax, and 3D MPRAGE sequences were taken in a 3T MRI scanner to localize the manganese signal (Scanner: Phillips GE, Boston, MA, slice thickness: 0.35 × 0.35 × 0.5 mm anisotropic and 0.5 isotropic voxels, repetition time/echo time = 2, flip angle: 9 degrees). After eight weeks, the animals were euthanized via intraperitoneal pentobarbital injection and transcardially perfused with 4% paraformaldehyde–phosphate buffer solution.

The harvested tissue was stored in sucrose and then sliced into 50 µm sections using a freezing microtome. The resulting slices were treated in a sodium borohydride bath (Millipore Sigma, Burlington, MA, USA) to reduce background fluorescence for 24 h. Afterward, the slices were incubated for 72 h at 4 °C in primary antibodies targeting the respective fluorescent tag of the infused virus (for case MTL4: rabbit-Anti-GFP 1:1000, Abcam #ab290). This was followed by two-hour incubation in fluorescent secondary antibodies (for case MTL4: donkey anti-rabbit 568 1:200, Invitrogen Molecular Probes #A10042) and DAPI stain (1:5000, ThermoFisher Scientific #D21490) before mounting and visualization.

2.2.4. MRI Volume Extraction

The following infusion volume extraction procedure was performed on the MRI scans. For cortical and thalamic trials, the MRIs were taken throughout the infusion period. For MTL infusions, the MRIs were taken the day after infusion. We imported each MRI scan into MRI viewing software (Mango, Research Imaging Institute, UTHSCSA, San Antonio, TX, USA) and identified the location of the infusion—due to the contrast agent, this area had a higher contrast than the surrounding tissue. A spherical region of interest (ROI) was created and adjusted as necessary to encompass the infused volume. We shrink-wrapped the ROI in 3D with a threshold value below the intensity of the infusion location, but above the intensity of the surrounding tissue. The threshold for the ROI was adjusted until it only contained the infusion volume and the final ROI was saved in the NIFTI file format. Next, we reloaded each ROI as its own image and generated an interpolated surface of the infusion volume. Finally, we measured the volume of the bolus using this interpolated surface in the MRI viewing software. In the case of live imaging during infusions, we mapped the infusion trajectories by applying this protocol to successive MRI scans within an infusion trial.

2.3. Bench-Side Modeling

We developed a bench-side CED infusion technique using agar and custom-built cannulas. We also developed an image processing technique and statistical methods to analyze the agar data.

2.3.1. Cannula Production for Agar Infusions

We manufactured 1 mm and 3 mm stepped-tip cannulas (Supplementary Figure S1) with polyimide-coated fused silica capillary tubing (Polymicro Technologies, Phoenix, AZ, USA) for the cortical and deep infusions, respectively. These cannulas were created by sliding the smaller tubing into the larger tubing until the smaller tubing extended out of the larger tubing by 1 mm or 3 mm. This placement was then secured with cyanoacrylate (Super Glue Corporation, liquid super glue, Ontario, CA, USA). For both cannulas, the inner tubing had an inner diameter of 320 µm and an outer diameter of 435 µm (part #1068150204) and the outer tubing had an inner diameter of 450 µm and an outer diameter of 673 µm (part #1068150625). The cannulas were the same as, or similar to, the cannulas used for our NHP CED experiments above.

2.3.2. Agar Phantom Infusion

We prepared a solution of 1× phosphate-buffered saline (PBS) and 0.6% powder mixture, where the powder mixture comprised agar powder (Benchmark Scientific, A1700, Sayreville, NJ, USA) and locust bean gum powder (Modernist Pantry LLC, Eliot, ME, USA) in a 4:1 ratio by mass, respectively. We heated and mixed the solution in a microwave to dissolve the powder and poured it into molds to set. Setting occurred in a refrigerator for at least two hours. The molds were 3D printed with polylactic acid (PLA) filament and were designed to produce agar blocks with a 2 × 2 cm base and either 2 or 4 cm high. The agar phantoms were used shortly after setting or were refrigerated for up to one day for future use.

To prepare for CED infusion, we mounted a pump (WPI UMP3, MICRO2T SMAR-Touch, Sarasota, FL, USA) to a stereotactic arm (KOPF, 1460, Tujunga, CA, USA) attached to a stereotactic frame (KOPF, 1430, Tujunga, CA, USA). We filled the pump's 250 mL syringe (WPI, SGE250TLL, Sarasota, FL, USA) with deionized (DI) water and attached it to the pump. The cannula was attached to the syringe with a catheter connector (B. Braun Medical Inc., part #332283, Bethlehem, PA, USA). All of the DI water was ejected from the syringe to fill the cannula with DI water. Undiluted yellow food coloring (McCormick yellow food coloring, Hunt Valley, MD, USA) was then drawn through the cannula and into the syringe. We positioned the agar phantom under the cannula so that it was centered. The agar phantom was oriented such that the side of the block that was not in contact with the mold during the molding process (i.e., the top side, which was the smoothest side of the phantom) was facing up and would be the side to receive the cannula insertion. The cannula was then lowered until the tip touched the surface of the agar phantom. We lowered the cannula manually with the stereotactic arm to a pre-specified depth, 2 mm deep for cortical infusions and 2 cm deep for thalamic and MTL infusions. We checked that the surface of the agar sealed around the cannula above the stepped-tip before proceeding with the infusion.

To image the infusion process, we positioned a digital single-lens reflex (DSLR) camera (Nikon D5300, Minato City, Tokyo, Japan) with a 35 mm lens (Nikon, AF-S NIKKOR 1:1.8G) and adjusted the camera settings to clearly image the agar phantom edges, needle, and bolus.

The ISO was set at 400, the shutter speed at 1/125, and the aperture at f/6.3. We used interval time shooting. We arranged a white backdrop to help with image processing and placed a ruler near the agar phantom and in-plane with the cannula for scale. We prepared a script in MATLAB (MathWorks Inc., Natick, MA, USA) to run the pump autonomously and in accordance with the infusion rates used in corresponding surgical infusions (Table 3). We started the script and the camera's time interval shooting simultaneously. Representative cortical and thalamic infusion models are compared with MRI data as shown in Figures 1 and 2, respectively. Refinements to infusion techniques during preliminary trials included optimizing lighting conditions, and camera angle and placement with respect to the agar phantom.

Table 3. Gel infusion rates. Medial temporal lobe (MTL).

Cortical Infusion Rates (µL/min)	Duration (min)	Thalamic Infusion Rates (µL/min)	Duration (min)	MTL Infusion Rates (µL/min)	Duration (min)
1	1	1	1	1	1
2	1	2	1	2	1
3	1	3	80	3	3
4	1	2	1	2	1
5	6	1	1	1	1
4	1				
3	1				
2	1				
1	1				
Total infused: 50 µL	Total time: 14 min	Total infused: 246 µL	Total time: 84 min	Total infused: 15 µL	Total time: 7 min

2.3.3. Agar Phantom Image Processing

We estimated volumes of distribution from photographs of the agar phantom infusion. A single-color component was selected from the color images. (Further description of the color component selection process is found below in Section 2.3.4.) Then, we applied a threshold value to the remaining matrix to produce a mask, being a matrix of binary values. (Specific methods for selecting this threshold value are found below in Section 2.3.5.) We manually selected the cluster of binary values representative of the infusion bolus and erased the other clusters from the mask. In some cases, this was enough to isolate the bolus, but in other cases, the mask appeared to depict the cannula together with the bolus. In these cases, the cannula was erased by masking all pixels above a manually selected point in the image such that the mask outlined the bolus alone. Representative images of the agar phantom image processing are shown in Figure 3. Finally, we converted the mask of the bolus to a volume by assuming an ellipsoidal form, where the ellipsoid was radially symmetric about the axis of the cannula. Similar to [27,28], we took the height (h) and width (w) of the bolus and calculated the volume (v) of the associated ellipsoid with the equation

$$v = \left(\frac{\pi}{6}\right) \times h \times w^2 \tag{1}$$

The volume estimation was converted to metric units based on the ruler in the original image.

We performed all agar image processing with MATLAB.

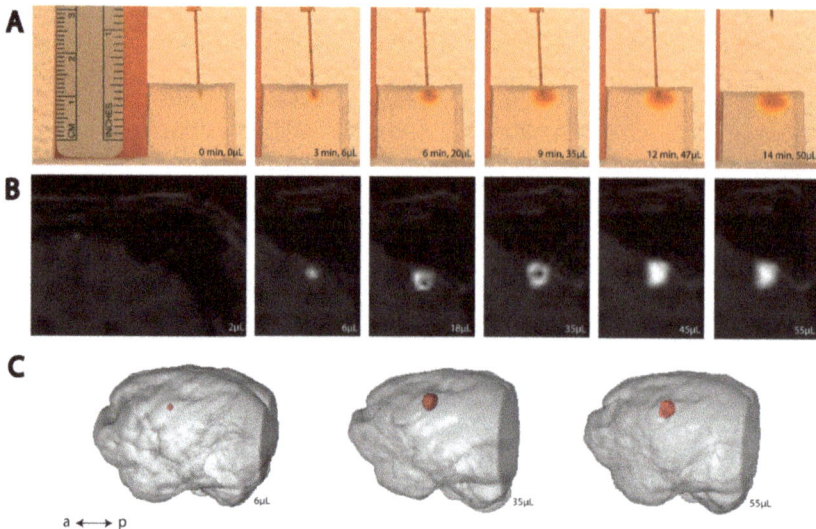

Figure 1. Time-lapse (left to right) of cortical CED. (**A**) Example trial of CED in agar phantom. (**B**) Example MRI visualization of CED in an NHP. (**C**) Post hoc reconstruction of NHP brain (gray) and infusion volume (red).

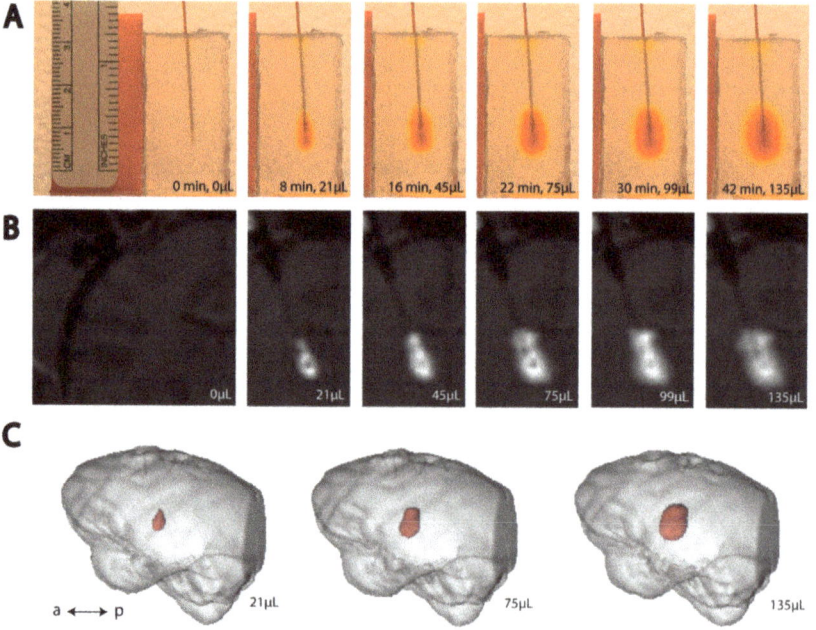

Figure 2. Time-lapse (left to right) of thalamic CED. (**A**) Example trial of CED in agar phantom. (**B**) Example MRI visualization of CED in an NHP. (**C**) Post hoc reconstruction of NHP brain (gray) and infusion volume (red).

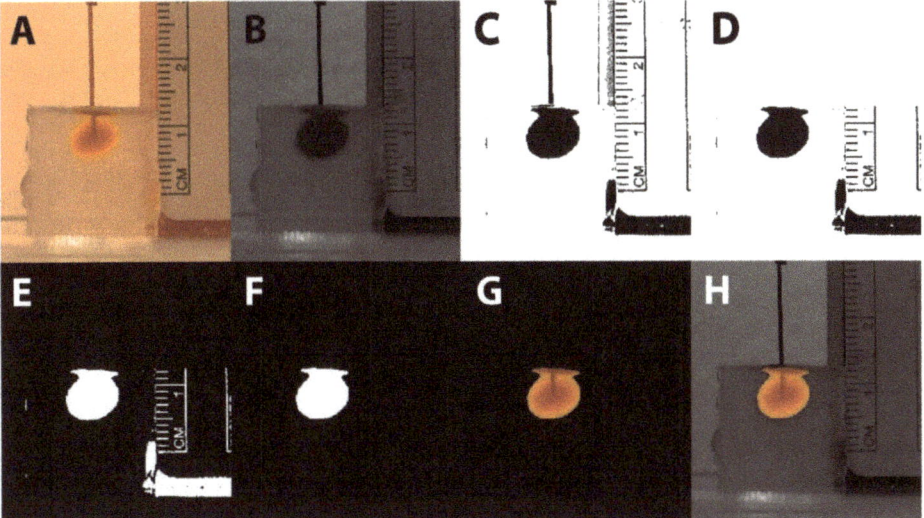

Figure 3. Image processing algorithm. (**A**) Original color image. (**B**) Single-color component image. (**C**) Thresholded image. (**D**) Cannula erasure. (**E**) Binary inversion. (**F**) Deletion of all non-bolus pixels. This is the final image used for volume calculation. (**G**) Color image of bolus overlaid on final image for user reference. (**H**) Color image of bolus overlaid on the single-color component image for user reference.

2.3.4. Color Component Selection

Our color component selection is the process by which a 24-bit RGB color image is converted to an image with one 8-bit value per pixel. We tested the three different color components to determine which aligned the agar data most closely with the MRI data. All data of the same infusion type were processed with one selected color component. While image processing software often have functions built in that will reduce images to a single value per pixel (e.g., the "rgb2gray" function in MATLAB), we found our color component selection process to be more effective.

2.3.5. Threshold Value Selection

After the color component selection, we used a threshold value to distinguish which pixels had strong enough values to be included as part of the bolus. To select the threshold value, we identified a region of the image where heavy coloration faded to no coloration, and then we selected a pixel from this region and used its value as the initial threshold. We performed the entire image processing procedure with this threshold value and plotted the agar data together with the MRI data to observe the quality of alignment. Based on the results, we selected a new threshold and repeated as necessary in an iterative fashion until the MRI data and the agar data were in alignment. Once aligned qualitatively, we compared the NHP volume data quantitatively with the agar volume data by using linear regression to determine the slope of each agar and NHP trial, as described in more detail in Section 2.3.6. All data of the same infusion type were processed with one selected threshold value.

2.3.6. Statistical Methods

To compare the agar and NHP data for the cortical and thalamic trials, we required a quantitative method that would take into account correlations between data points within a given trial, and also compare the different groups of trials. Additionally, we required a method that would not assume a fixed slope between the volume infused by the syringe and the measured bolus volume. To this end, we used a linear mixed-effects model with random slopes to fit each infusion trial, both in agar and in NHP data. All best-fit lines were restricted to passing through the origin (i.e., zero input volume and zero output volume). From this model, we calculated the interaction effect, which is an approximation of the difference in the average slope between the agar and NHP data. All linear mixed-effect model calculations were performed with MATLAB's built-in "fitlme" function.

All other statistical calculations were performed in MATLAB except the average and percent error values of Table 4, which were performed in Excel (Microsoft Corp., Redmond, WA, USA).

Table 4. Cortical and thalamic data.

Cortical Infusion Slopes			
NHP	MRI Slopes (µL/µL)	Trial	Gel Slopes (µL/µL)
C1	2.86	1	3.03
C1	3.90	2	2.69
C1	3.07	3	2.72
C1	4.61	4	4.74
C2	2.67	5	4.11
C2	3.05	6	4.67
CT	3.07	7	4.23
		8	3.10
		9	4.81
		10	3.82
Thalamic Infusion Slopes			
NHP	MRI Slopes (µL/µL)	Trial	Gel Slopes (µL/µL)
T1	3.48	1	2.63
T2	3.59	2	3.71
T2	3.30	3	4.02
CT	6.38	4	2.66
		5	3.17

3. Results

Some agar infusion trials were unsuccessful, and these failed trials were omitted from statistical analyses and reattempted. Failed trials may have been produced by reasons such as dye leaking out through the catheter adapter or damaged agar phantoms.

3.1. Cortical and Thalamic Infusions

We iteratively selected color components and threshold values to align the agar data with our previously published cortical [8] and thalamic [9] NHP data (Figures 4 and 5, respectively). The green component and threshold value of 110 (43% of green component intensity range) were best for the thalamic infusions, and the blue component and threshold value of 67 (26% of blue component intensity range) were best for the cortical infusions.

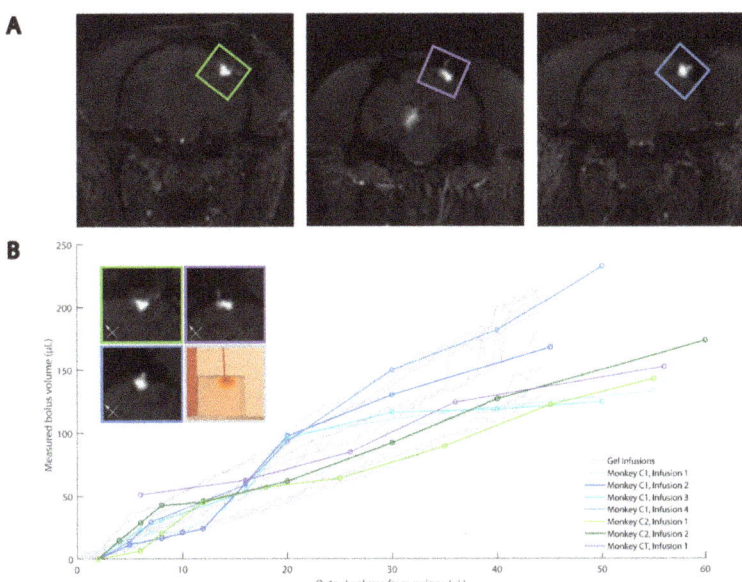

Figure 4. Comparison of agar and MRI cortical CED. (**A**) Example MRIs of cortical infusions. (**B**) Quantitative and example qualitative (inset) comparisons of agar and NHP data. Box colors in inset relate to images in (**A**) and traces in (**B**). Reprinted/adapted with permission from Ref. [8]. Copyright 2016, *Neuron*.

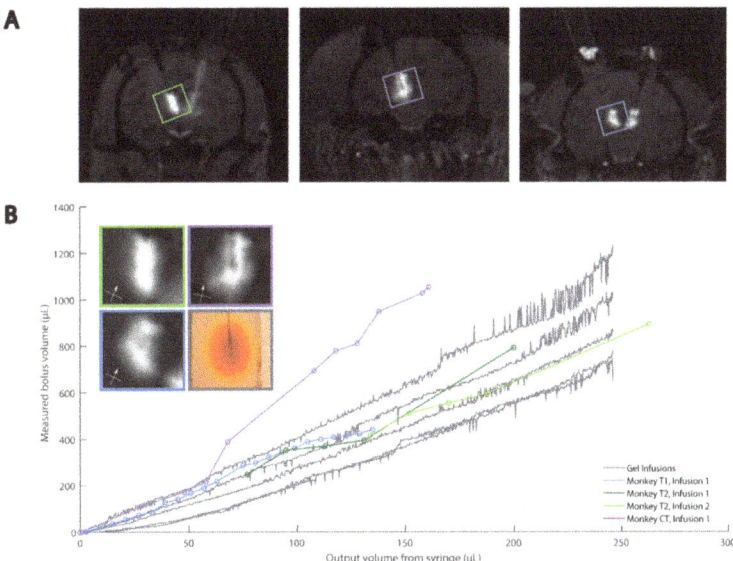

Figure 5. Comparison of agar and MRI thalamic CED. (**A**) Example MRIs of cortical infusions. (**B**) Quantitative and example qualitative (inset) comparisons of agar and NHP data. Box colors in inset relate to images in (**A**) and traces in (**B**). Reprinted/adapted with permission from Ref. [9]. Copyright 2018, *Journal of Neuroscience Methods*.

When comparing the cortical agar data to the thalamic agar data, we observed that the agar and NHP best-fit slopes were similar (Figures 4 and 5). The cortical NHP data had slopes ranging from 2.9–4.6 µL/µL, and the cortical agar data had a range of 2.7–4.8 µL/µL. Meanwhile, the thalamic NHP data had a range of 3.5–6.4 µL/µL and the thalamic agar data had a range of 2.6–4.4 µL/µL (Table 4). There is significant variation in the slopes of the best-fit lines of the agar infusion data; however, this variation reflects the variation in the NHP data (Figures 4B and 5B).

We observed that a reduction of flow rate at the end of the cortical agar trials led to greater increase in bolus volume with respect to infused volume, i.e., the plots steepen near the end of the infusion protocol (Supplementary Figure S2). This is not characteristic of NHP cortical data, so we omitted the agar cortical data from 44 µL to 50 µL from statistical analysis and Figure 4 because it was not characteristic of NHP cortical data. Further descriptions may be found in the discussion (Section 4.4).

For the cortical and thalamic trials, we used a linear mixed-effects model with random slopes to fit each infusion trial, both in agar and in NHPs. This model produces an interaction effect of 1.1 and −0.5 for the cortical and thalamic infusions, respectively. These values are close to zero in comparison with the aforementioned ranges of the slopes, and these values have magnitudes less than the slope ranges, indicating that the agar and NHP data differ only mildly and that our agar phantom is a good representation of the NHP data for cortical and thalamic infusions.

3.2. MTL Infusions

Our MTL NHP data were highly variable, and upon analysis of the MRI scans, we observed that four of the nine infusions displayed a bolus in the MTL as expected (Figure 6A). We only modeled these four successful MTL NHP infusions and omitted the remaining five infusions, which are discussed below (Section 3.2.1).

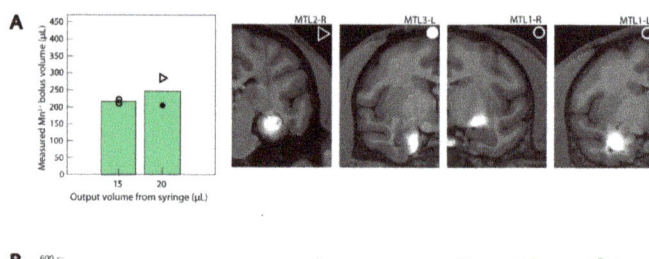

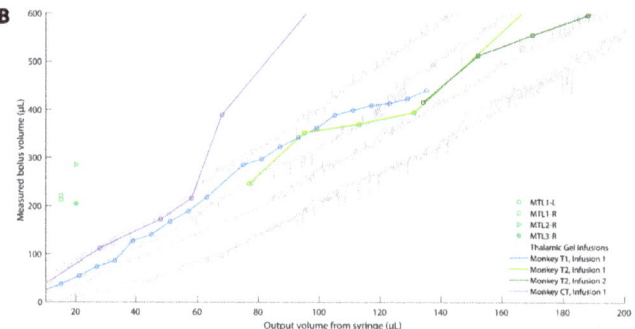

Figure 6. MTL MRI data compared with both agar and MRI thalamic data. (**A**) Deep CED infusions were made into the hippocampus, entorhinal cortex, and the tail of the caudate nucleus. Bar plots show the mean value of measured Mn^{2+} bolus seen in next-day, post-operative MRIs, with individual data points overlaid. Corresponding MRI slices in the coronal plane are shown for infusions into deep brain areas, which are visually similar to cortical and thalamic data. Shape labels correspond to each subject contributing to the data. (**B**) MTL MRI data compared with both agar and MRI thalamic data. Reprinted/adapted with permission from Ref. [9]. Copyright 2018, *Journal of Neuroscience Methods*.

Because the thalamic and MTL NHP infusions used similar cannulas and differed chiefly in the infused volume, we initially compared the thalamic agar bolus volumes with MTL NHP bolus volumes (Figure 6B). Counter to our expectations, the MTL NHP data did not align with either the thalamic NHP or agar data. We recognized that while the cortical and thalamic MRI scans were collected during CED infusion, the MTL MRI scans were collected the next day. Therefore, we reasoned that a CED-generated bolus may diffuse overnight and thus be displayed as a larger bolus in the NHP when MRI is performed the day after infusion. With this in mind, we proposed that the diffusion of food coloring in agar after a standard CED protocol would approximate our MTL data. We collected data following the end of 15 µL infusions into agar and observed that the agar data closely modeled the NHP data after approximately 29 min of diffusion following the completion of the infusion (Figure 7). We calculated the mean of the NHP infusion volumes and the mean of the agar infusion volumes selected approximately 29 min after infusion completion (Table 5), and report a 3.5% percent error between the two datasets. Given the biological context of our model, this error is small enough to safely conclude that 29 min of diffusion in our agar phantom, following CED, approximates the next-day MRI results of NHP MTL infusions.

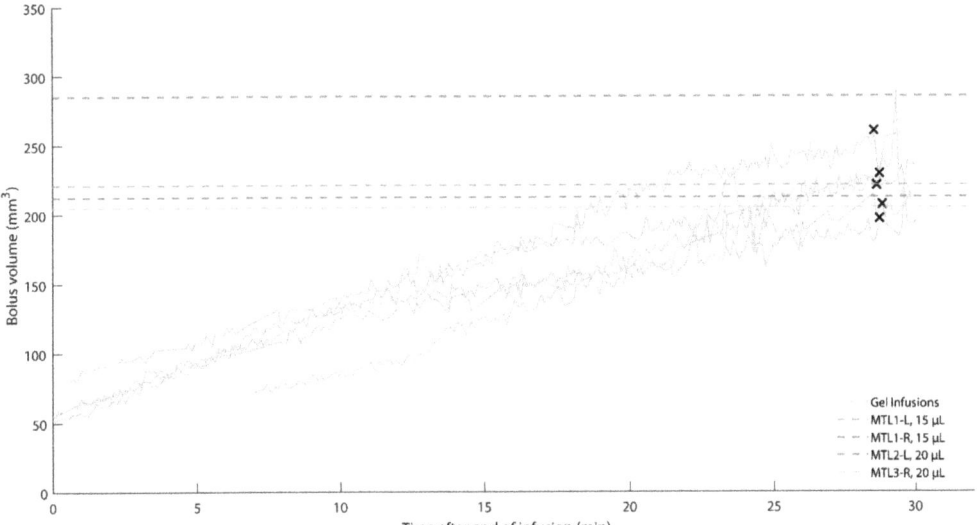

Figure 7. MTL MRI data compared with MTL agar data after CED completion. Some trials lack data early in the diffusion process due to the bolus being difficult to identify. Black Xs indicate the final point used for statistical analysis from each agar trial. The final chosen points may be shifted slightly to avoid noise spikes. All agar infusions were 15 µL.

The green component and threshold value of 100 (39% of green component intensity range) were best to model the MTL infusions. We used a t-test to compare the two NHP data points for the 15 µL infusions and two data points for the 20 µL infusions, and because the two populations were not statistically significant ($p = 0.56$), we pooled the four NHP data points for comparison with the agar data. Significant noise was observed in the MTL agar data, more so than in the cortical and thalamic agar infusions. The additional noise was possibly due to the smaller infusion volumes. We addressed the noise by fitting a line with linear regression to each agar infusion trial and removing data points greater than 1.1 times the corresponding value on the best-fit line.

Table 5. MTL data.

NHP, Hemisphere	Infusion Volume (µL)	Measured Volume (µL)
MTL1, left	15	221.1
MTL1, right	15	212.2
MTL2, left	20	285.3
MTL3, right	20	204.7
Average:		230.8
Gel Trial	Infusion Volume (µL)	Measured Volume (µL)
1	15	196.7
2	15	229.2
3	15	260.2
4	15	220.7
5	15	207.0
Average:		222.8
% Error:		3.5

3.2.1. MTL Data Omitted from Agar Modeling

Five of the nine NHP MTL infusions were excluded from the analysis since the next-day MRI did not confirm infusion into the MTL regions (Figure 6 and Supplementary Figure S3). These failed infusions mostly likely occurred due to the complex shapes of the hippocampus and neighboring structures, which contrast with the structures of the cortex and thalamus. In three of the five unsuccessful MTL cases, the boluses were very small, which suggested either puncturing into the hippocampal fissure, or infusing deep in the dentate gyrus, depending on the injection depth (Supplementary Figure S3). Penetration of the fissure resulted in contrast agent and virus partially escaping our injection target, indicative of unsuccessful CED. By contrast, deep dentate gyrus infusions were limited to a small portion of the hippocampus, limiting the amount of diffusion observed when compared to our gel model. In the remaining unsuccessful case, the bolus was very large and extended well outside of the volume of the hippocampus, indicating that the contrast agent refluxed along the track of the cannula (Supplementary Figure S3). We excluded these five unsuccessful MTL CED data points from our models, but these negative results are presented to highlight the value of in vivo verification of deep injection surgeries.

3.3. Histological Analysis

For cortical and thalamic infusions, the spread of the MR contrast agent modeled the volume of expression of the optogenetic viral vector, as previously analyzed and reported [8,9]. We used different constructs, including retrograde viruses, for our MTL infusions. Because of the variability of the resulting expression, further experiments using a single virus known to express well in these regions is necessary to confirm whether the next-day, Mn^{2+} MRI signal mirrors expression. Nevertheless, the Mn^{2+} MRI confirmed our targeting in vivo. Additionally, preliminary evidence from the successful local infection in case MTL4-L suggests a close match between Mn^{2+} signal and immunofluorescence (Figure 8).

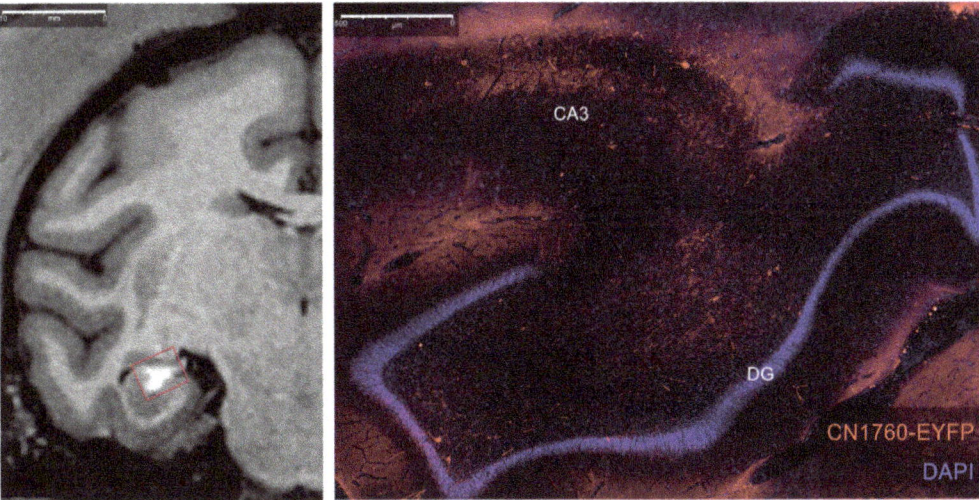

Figure 8. Comparison of Mn^{2+} MRI signal (**left**) and local expression of virus (**right**) after a hippocampal injection in case MTL4-L. Right-imaged region highlighted with red square in MRI (**left**). Our virus used a GABA-specific enhancer to selectively target interneurons, as evidenced by a lack of red pyramidal cell body labeling in CA3 and granule cell body labeling in the dentate gyrus (DG). We tagged infected interneurons and associated fibers with red-shifted fluorophores (anti-EYFP, ThermoFisher, Waltham, MA, USA) and cell bodies were non-selectively labeled using a DAPI stain (ThermoFisher, Waltham, MA, USA). (Viral construct CN1760: trAAV-3xhI56i(core)-minBG-ChR2(CRC)-EYFP-WPRE3-BGHpA (Paul Allen Institute, Seattle, WA., USA)).

4. Discussion

Targeted neural manipulations, such as those achieved via optogenetics, are revolutionary techniques for investigating circuit-level communication in the brain and have the potential to influence novel neurotherapeutic technologies in humans. NHPs are the keystone model for validating these techniques because of their similarity to humans, but they are a scarce resource that does not allow for experiments with many unknowns. As such, the risks associated with the viral infusions necessary for most genetic manipulations have led to a lack of uniformity in experimental design and much trepidation in engaging this type of research [29]. In this work, we developed a simple and efficient pipeline to ameliorate a number of these concerns. Our method improves upon past models [7,20,21] by quantitatively matching agar data with in vivo infusions of viral particles co-infused with MRI contrast agents, which serve as a proxy of the effective infusion volume. Further, we observe that certain contrast agents can signal the location of infusions up to 24 h post-infusion, which is a greater time delay for bolus localization than previously demonstrated [26]. Taken together, the methods presented here serve as an accessible and inexpensive protocol to plan the optimized spread of infusions bench-side and validate the spread and accuracy in vivo, significantly reducing the number of unknowns that hinder confidence during circuit-manipulation experiments. Our presented methods contribute to a body of work supporting large-scale optogenetics in NHPs [8,9,16–19,22,23,30–39].

Agar has been previously established as a model of intraparenchymal neural tissue and is now commonly used as a medium for simulating infusion procedures [7,20,21]. Our work builds on prior studies by presenting a data-driven method developed from in vivo results. To our knowledge, the model proposed here is the first to provide a quantitative method of fitting agar infusion data with NHP CED data collected with live MRI. Because of this, our model serves as a more accurate guide for selecting infusion parameters for future in vivo infusions targeting a wide array of brain areas when compared to other simulations.

Our work lends itself well to case-by-case methodological refinements: for example, researchers may consider alternative cannulas, infusion protocols, etc., to cater to their goals. Additionally, our method is designed to facilitate replication by other labs with its simplicity in both materials and methods. We also recognize that labs replicating our work are unlikely to implement agar infusion imaging setups identical to our own. With this in mind, we designed our image processing technique to be easily adaptable to different imaging setups. We provide NHP MRI bolus volume data (see Supplementary Materials) to which other labs may align their own agar infusion data, using our presented method. We have also made our custom code freely available (see Data Availability Statement), and the code is written in MATLAB, which is widely used by researchers and is straightforward to adapt for applications akin to ours.

4.1. Diversity of Modeled Structures

To maximize the flexibility in accurately predicting spread of CED infusions in a variety of brain areas, we used in vivo data from cortical, thalamic, and MTL infusions of viruses co-infused with MRI contrast agent. Our cortical and thalamic procedures, which represented shallow and deep infusions into large brain structures, utilized live MRI taken during surgery. In addition to the qualitative agreement between these infusion types, the ranges of MRI data best-fit slopes were similar (2.9–4.6 µL/µL for cortical and 3.5–6.4 µL/µL for thalamic), which suggested that the agar models for cortical and thalamic infusions may be similar as well. This proved to be the case. Despite differences in the cannula design, depth of insertion, and infusion protocol, the models for both cortical and thalamic CED were generated with our same presented method and aligned well with the in vivo data (agar model best-fit slopes were 2.7–4.8 µL for cortical and 2.6–4.4 µL/µL for thalamic). The cortical and thalamic models did differ in the parameters used during image processing (cortical: blue component, threshold = 67; thalamic: green component, threshold = 110), but this demonstrates that our method is robust to variations in agar infusion processes. Our successful MTL cases differed from the previous two conditions and represented infusions into more limited and more difficult to access deep structures. Additionally, they differed in their post-operative MRIs in that scans were taken ~20 h after infusion. We found that our initial hypothesis of these data aligning to the thalamic cases was invalidated. However, after accounting for diffusion expected from the delay in imaging, our model successfully aligned to all three conditions.

4.2. Insights from MTL Infusions

Because of its unfurled shape in primates compared to rodents [40], standard injections into the NHP hippocampus are laborious and often require either multiple craniotomies and penetrations [41], or penetrating through the long-axis of the structure and periodically injecting while retracting [42] to try and maximize coverage. To inject into this structure more efficiently, we leveraged the unique ability of CED to deliver a large bolus with a single infusion in our MTL CED group, which, to our knowledge, is the first set of CED infusions delivered to this area in NHPs. Because of the exploratory nature of these experiments, we experienced challenges that made delivery into this structure and subsequent imaging of our contrast agents more difficult. Infusion MTL2-L was a case of mass reflux due to an error made during the infusion delivery. MTL3-R and MTL4-R represent issues in targeting. Because much of the hippocampus is separated from the rest of the brain by ventricular spaces except laterally, targets made too shallow or too deep will leak into those spaces and either dissipate away or reflux upwards. For similar reasons, posterior–medial injections—for example, targeting the intermediate dentate gyrus—produced more isolated boluses (cases MTL4-L, MTL5-R). Our successful cases were qualitatively similar to our cortical and thalamic data because they were delivered to larger, more anterior regions in the genu of the hippocampus, or to large neighboring regions such as the entorhinal cortex or tail of the caudate nucleus. For areas such as MTL, where targeting needs to be very precise, we strongly recommend the use of MRI validation of injection either during infusion or the next day.

4.3. MRI Scan Parameters for Successful Contrast Label Visualization

Our novel MTL infusions were also the first to utilize co-infused manganese to localize viral infusions in MRI scans acquired ~20 h post-operatively. Despite the differences in the employed contrast agent, scan acquisition timing, and even the scanner used between this group and our cortical and thalamic infusions, we observed a few similar parameters for successful contrast imaging in all MRI scans for all groups. Specifically, all scans were T1-weighted scans with a repetition time/echo time ratio around 2 to 3 and flip angles from 9 to 30 degrees. Analysis of other studies employing similar manganese-enhanced MRI protocols either to image viral injections delivered at shorter delays [26] or at much longer delays for in vivo tract tracing [43] also closely mirrored the majority of the parameters used in these experiments, suggesting a range of optimized parameters for imaging T1-weighted MRI contrast agents.

4.4. Diffusion versus Convection Using Agar

It is important to note that while agar is a good model of CED, agar's rate of diffusion differs from the rate of diffusion in the brain. This factor became apparent when we observed that a reduction of flow rate at the end of the cortical agar trials led to a greater increase in the bolus volume with respect to the infused volume, i.e., the plots steepen near the end of the infusion protocol (Supplementary Figure S2). This is consistent with our observation that diffusion will continue to cause the bolus to grow in agar after the end of our infusion trials. With this in mind, we concluded that diffusion and convection both contribute to bolus size in agar to varying degrees during CED. However, we propose the relative contributions of diffusion and convection were skewed when the flow rate was reduced at the end of the protocol, thus allowing diffusion to contribute more heavily to the bolus size in the agar. To prevent the best-fit lines of the cortical agar data from being skewed due to this effect, we omitted the data from 44 µL to 50 µL from the statistical analysis and Figure 4. This effect was not observed in the thalamic agar infusions, likely due to the lower maximum rate of infusion (3 µL for the thalamic agar protocol, as contrasted with 5 µL for the cortical agar protocol) in conjunction with the short duration of infusion at the lower rates and small amount of volume infused during the flow rate reduction at the end of the protocol. This effect was not observed in the in vivo cortical or thalamic injections collected with live MRI. We observed diffusion in our in vivo MTL data, but the data were collected with our next-day imaging technique, thus allowing sufficient time for diffusion. We show that MTL next-day imaging data can be modeled with our agar phantom when we allow 29 min of diffusion following the end of the infusion protocol. This highlights that the speed of diffusion in agar differs from that of the brain. This is also in agreement with our observation that the cortical and thalamic NHP data collected with live MRI did not exhibit high levels of diffusion at the end of the protocols, in contrast to the cortical agar data.

4.5. Technical Considerations

We encountered some issues during the agar infusions. The most common issues faced when refining the infusion techniques were damaging the agar during its extraction from the mold, such that no smooth surface was available for imaging, and reflux of the dye during the infusion. While the agar preparation became more efficient with practice, we suggest that custom, flexible silicone molds be considered in lieu of our 3D-printed molds to more easily produce undamaged agar phantoms. Reflux issues can arise in agar, neural tissue, and other media and are less easily mitigated because the cause of reflux is not always obvious. In some cases, the reflux may be related to the quality of the seal between the media and cannula, which is difficult to assess visually even in transparent media such as agar. Additionally, we hypothesize that, in some cases, the cannula becomes clogged with the media during insertion. To address this potential issue, we suggest a low flow rate during insertion to avoid clogging.

As previously mentioned, the agar data are aligned with the in vivo MRI data with an iterative process of parameter selection. The iterative alignment process allows researchers to fine tune their image processing parameters to overcome potential differences in lighting, camera placement, etc. While our agar image processing techniques are effective, we acknowledge that software refinements may be attained. Our process is currently semi-automated, yet we expect it could be more fully automated in future work. Improvement opportunities may also exist in the refinement of our volume estimation formula, and the characterization of the bolus shape.

4.6. Ethical Considerations

Despite the limitations presented, our methods will allow for the development of more efficient and effective CED procedures. We can inexpensively plan the expected spread of our infusions with our data-driven model and validate our surgical targeting rapidly without the need to perform infusions in an MRI scanner. Critically, our method is not only quantitative and data-based, but also designed to aid surgical planning with its visual, hands-on nature. Our bench-side modeling technique serves to increase the likelihood of success in NHP CED experiments, thus refining animal research processes and reducing the number of animals required for experimentation, both of which are key ethical considerations in animal research and included in the 3Rs [44]. Our model was capable of simulating both cortical and deep infusions (limitations discussed above). Because of this, our method provides a generalized surgical preparation technique to all researchers regardless of region of interest, and particularly to research groups that do not have the facilities or resources required to perform live MRI during CED infusions. Our novel next-day MRI data additionally serve to showcase a post hoc infusion confirmation method that improves upon previous work [26] to highlight the verification of infusion placement ~20 h post-operatively. This method supplements our proposed modeling technique and is a welcome alternative to live MRI, which requires specialized equipment and facilities often unavailable to researchers. In sum, we propose our method as an additional way of applying the principles of replacement, reduction, and refinement (3Rs) to injections in NHPs [44,45]. We recommend NHP CED infusions be modeled in advance of surgery with our proposed method to reduce the number of animals, replace an excess of pilot procedures with artificial simulations, and refine the overall technique to reduce harm. We also suggest the results be confirmed after surgery with MRI if live MRI is not feasible during infusion. Finally, our work is designed to be highly flexible. While our methods are specifically prepared for NHP experiments involving optogenetic actuators, we expect that our method would also be generally effective for modeling the CED of optogenetic sensors, pharmaceutical compounds, and other therapeutic agents in large brains.

Supplementary Materials: The following supporting information can be downloaded at: https://www.mdpi.com/article/10.3390/pharmaceutics14071435/s1. We provide three supplementary figures and a CSV file of the MRI data points.

Author Contributions: Conceptualization, E.A.B. and A.Y.-S.; methodology, D.J.G., A.D.G., W.Y.A., W.K.S.O., A.G.J., E.A.B. and A.Y.-S.; software, D.J.G., A.D.G., W.Y.A. and W.K.S.O.; validation, D.J.G. and A.D.G.; formal analysis, D.J.G., W.Y.A., W.K.S.O. and A.Y.-S.; investigation, D.J.G., A.D.G., W.Y.A., W.K.S.O., A.G.J., E.A.B. and A.Y.-S.; resources, E.A.B., A.Y.-S. and J.T.T.; data curation, D.J.G., A.D.G., W.Y.A., W.K.S.O., A.Y.-S. and A.G.J.; writing—original draft preparation, D.J.G., A.D.G., W.Y.A. and W.K.S.O.; writing—review and editing, D.J.G., A.D.G., W.Y.A., W.K.S.O., A.G.J., E.A.B. and A.Y.-S.; visualization, D.J.G., A.D.G., W.Y.A., E.A.B. and A.Y.-S.; supervision, E.A.B. and A.Y.-S.; project administration, E.A.B. and A.Y.-S.; funding acquisition, E.A.B. and A.Y.-S. All authors have read and agreed to the published version of the manuscript.

Funding: This work was supported by the National Science Foundation Graduate Research Fellowship Program (#1762114, A.D.G.), the National Institutes for Health (NS107609, A.D.G. and E.A.B.; P51 OD010425, all authors; R01 NS119395, D.J.G. and A.Y.; R01 NS116464-01, A.Y.), the University of Washington Mary Gates Research Scholarship (W.Y.A., W.K.S.O.), and the Center for Neurotechnology (CNT, a National Science Foundation Engineering Research Center, EEC-1028725, A.G.J., D.J.G)

Institutional Review Board Statement: All animal care and experiments performed at the University of Washington were approved by the University of Washington's Office of Animal Welfare, the Institutional Animal Care and Use Committee (IACUC protocol information for animals MTL1-5: project identification code: 4316-01, approval date: 1 July 2013), and the Washington National Primate Research Center (WaNPRC). All animal care and experiments performed at the University of California, San Francisco, were performed under the approval of the University of California, San Francisco Institutional Animal Care and Use Committee (IACUC protocol information for animals C1, C2, CT, T1, and T2: approval number: AN080609-03D, approval date: 6 September 2011) and were compliant with the Guide for the Care and Use of Laboratory Animals.

Informed Consent Statement: Not applicable.

Data Availability Statement: MRI files, agar data, and histological data will be made available upon reasonable request. MATLAB code has been made publicly available: https://bitbucket.org/yazdanlab/ced_protocol_and_analysis/src/master/, accessed on 7 July 2022.

Acknowledgments: We would like to thank all of the staff from the University of Washington, Seattle, and University of California, San Francisco, who provided animal care and surgical support. We thank Sabes lab for use of their previously published data. We thank Spencer Hansen, Serge Aleshin-Guendel, and Tianyu Zhang for their help with statistical analyses. We thank the Viral Technology team at the Allen Institute for Brain Science, Ximena Opitz Araya, Shane Gibson, and Greg Horwitz for assistance with virus production. Finally, we thank Toni Haun, Karam Khateeb, and Megan L. Jutras for their technical help.

Conflicts of Interest: The authors declare no conflict of interest.

References

1. Boyden, E.S.; Zhang, F.; Bamberg, E.; Nagel, G.; Deisseroth, K. Millisecond-timescale, genetically targeted optical control of neural activity. *Nat. Neurosci.* **2005**, *8*, 1263–1268. [CrossRef] [PubMed]
2. Yizhar, O.; Fenno, L.E.; Davidson, T.J.; Mogri, M.; Deisseroth, K. Optogenetics in neural systems. *Neuron* **2011**, *71*, 9–34. [CrossRef] [PubMed]
3. Ting, J.T.; Feng, G. Recombineering strategies for developing next generation BAC transgenic tools for optogenetics and beyond. *Front. Behav. Neurosci.* **2014**, *8*, 1–13. [CrossRef] [PubMed]
4. Mehta, A.M.; Sonabend, A.M.; Bruce, J.N. Convection-Enhanced Delivery. *Neurotherapeutics* **2017**, *14*, 358–371. [CrossRef]
5. René, C.A.; Parks, R.J. Delivery of therapeutic agents to the central nervous system and the promise of extracellular vesicles. *Pharmaceutics* **2021**, *13*, 492. [CrossRef]
6. Bobo, R.H.; Laske, D.W.; Akbasak, A.; Morrison, P.F.; Dedrick, R.L.; Oldfield, E.H. Convection-enhanced delivery of macromolecules in the brain. *Proc. Natl. Acad. Sci. USA* **1994**, *91*, 2076–2080. [CrossRef]
7. Krauze, M.T.; Saito, R.; Noble, C.; Tamas, M.; Bringas, J.; Park, J.W.; Berger, M.S.; Bankiewicz, K. Reflux-free cannula for convection-enhanced high-speed delivery of therapeutic agents. *J. Neurosurg.* **2005**, *103*, 923–929. [CrossRef]
8. Yazdan-Shahmorad, A.; Diaz-Botia, C.; Hanson, T.L.; Kharazia, V.; Ledochowitsch, P.; Maharbiz, M.M.; Sabes, P.N. "A Large-Scale Interface for Optogenetic Stimulation and Recording in Nonhuman Primates. *Neuron* **2016**, *89*, 927–939. [CrossRef]
9. Yazdan-Shahmorad, A.; Tian, N.; Kharazia, V.; Samaranch, L.; Kells, A.; Bringas, J.; He, J.; Bankiewicz, K.; Sabes, P.N. Widespread optogenetic expression in macaque cortex obtained with MR-guided, convection enhanced delivery (CED) of AAV vector to the thalamus. *J. Neurosci. Methods* **2018**, *293*, 347–358. [CrossRef]
10. Lieberman, D.M.; Laske, D.W.; Morrison, P.F.; Bankiewicz, K.S.; Oldfield, E.H. Convection-enhanced distribution of large molecules in gray matter during interstitial drug infusion. *J. Neurosurg.* **1995**, *82*, 1021–1029. [CrossRef]
11. Lonser, R.R.; Gogate, N.; Morrison, P.F.; Wood, J.D.; Oldfield, E.H. Direct convective delivery of macromolecules to the spinal cord. *J. Neurosurg.* **1998**, *89*, 616–622. [CrossRef] [PubMed]
12. Lonser, R.R.; Walbridge, S.; Garmestani, K.; Butman, J.A.; Walters, H.A.; Vortmeyer, O.; Morrison, P.F.; Brechbiel, M.W.; Oldfield, E.H. Successful and safe perfusion of the primate brainstem: In vivo magnetic resonance imaging of macromolecular distribution during infusion. *J. Neurosurg.* **2002**, *97*, 905–913. [CrossRef] [PubMed]
13. Sanftner, L.M.; Sommer, J.M.; Suzuki, B.M.; Smith, P.H.; Vijay, S.; Vargas, J.A.; Forsayeth, J.R.; Cunningham, J.; Bankiewicz, K.S.; Kao, H.; et al. AAV2-mediated gene delivery to monkey putamen: Evaluation of an infusion device and delivery parameters. *Exp. Neurol.* **2005**, *194*, 476–483. [CrossRef] [PubMed]

14. Szerlip, N.J.; Walbridge, S.; Yang, L.; Morrison, P.F.; Degen, J.W.; Jarrell, S.T.; Kouri, J.; Kerr, P.B.; Kotin, R.; Oldfield, E.H.; et al. Real-time imaging of convection-enhanced delivery of viruses and virus-sized particles. *J. Neurosurg.* **2007**, *107*, 560–567. [CrossRef]
15. Kells, A.P.; Hadaczek, P.; Yin, D.; Bringas, J.; Varenika, V.; Forsayeth, J.; Bankiewicz, K.S. Efficient gene therapy-based method for the delivery of therapeutics to primate cortex. *Proc. Natl. Acad. Sci. USA* **2009**, *106*, 2407–2411. [CrossRef]
16. Yazdan-Shahmorad, A.; Diaz-Botia, C.; Hanson, T.; Ledochowitsch, P.; Maharabiz, M.M.; Sabes, P.N. Demonstration of a setup for chronic optogenetic stimulation and recording across cortical areas in non-human primates. *SPIE BiOS* **2015**, *9305*, 231–236. [CrossRef]
17. Macknik, S.L.; Alexander, R.G.; Caballero, O.; Chanovas, J.; Nielsen, K.J.; Nishimura, N.; Schaffer, C.B.; Slovin, H.; Babayoff, A.; Barak, R.; et al. Advanced Circuit and Cellular Imaging Methods in Nonhuman Primates. *J. Neurosci.* **2019**, *39*, 8267–8274. [CrossRef]
18. Khateeb, K.; Griggs, D.J.; Sabes, P.N.; Yazdan-Shahmorad, A. Convection Enhanced Delivery of Optogenetic Adeno-associated Viral Vector to the Cortex of Rhesus Macaque Under Guidance of Online MRI Images. *J. Vis. Exp.* **2019**, *147*, e59232. [CrossRef]
19. Ojemann, W.K.; Griggs, D.J.; Ip, Z.; Caballero, O.; Jahanian, H.; Martinez-Conde, S.; Macknik, S.; Yazdan-Shahmorad, A. A mri-based toolbox for neurosurgical planning in nonhuman primates. *J. Vis. Exp.* **2020**, *2020*, e61098. [CrossRef]
20. Chen, Z.J.; Gillies, G.T.; Broaddus, W.C.; Prabhu, S.S.; Fillmore, H.; Mitchell, R.M.; Corwin, F.D.; Fatouros, P.P. A realistic brain tissue phantom for intraparenchymal infusion studies. *J. Neurosurg.* **2004**, *101*, 314–322. [CrossRef]
21. Pomfret, R.; Miranpuri, G.; Sillay, K. The substitute brain and the potential of the gel model. *Ann. Neurosci.* **2013**, *20*, 118–122. [CrossRef] [PubMed]
22. Yazdan-Shahmorad, A.; Silversmith, D.B.; Kharazia, V.; Sabes, P.N. Targeted cortical reorganization using optogenetics in non-human primates. *eLife* **2018**, *7*, e31034. [CrossRef]
23. Yazdan-Shahmorad, A.; Hanson, T.; Tian, N.; He, J.; Sabes, P. A novel technique for infusion of optogenetics viral vectors in nonhuman primates (NHPs) cortex using MR-guided convection enhanced delivery (CED). In Proceedings of the 6th International IEEE/EMBS Conference on Neural Engineering (NER), San Diego, CA, USA, 6–8 November 2013; pp. 5–8.
24. Klapoetke, N.C.; Murata, Y.; Kim, S.S.; Pulver, S.R.; Birdsey-Benson, A.; Cho, Y.K.; Morimoto, T.K.; Chuong, A.S.; Carpenter, E.J.; Tian, Z.; et al. Independent optical excitation of distinct neural populations. *Nat. Methods* **2014**, *11*, 338–346. [CrossRef] [PubMed]
25. Mao, T.; Kusefoglu, D.; Hooks, B.M.; Huber, D.; Petreanu, L.; Svoboda, K. Long-Range Neuronal Circuits Underlying the Interaction between Sensory and Motor Cortex. *Neuron* **2011**, *72*, 111–123. [CrossRef] [PubMed]
26. Fredericks, J.M.; Dash, K.E.; Jaskot, E.M.; Bennett, T.W.; Lerchner, W.; Dold, G.; Ide, D.; Cummins, A.C.; Der Minassian, V.H.; Turchi, J.N.; et al. Methods for mechanical delivery of viral vectors into rhesus monkey brain. *J. Neurosci. Methods* **2020**, *339*, 108730. [CrossRef]
27. Prezelski, K.; Keiser, M.; Stein, J.M.; Lucas, T.H.; Davidson, B.; Gonzalez-Alegre, P.; Vitale, F. Design and Validation of a Multi-Point Injection Technology for MR-Guided Convection Enhanced Delivery in the Brain. *Front. Med. Technol.* **2021**, *3*, 1–12. [CrossRef]
28. Seunguk, O.H.; Odland, R.; Wilson, S.R.; Kroeger, K.M.; Liu, C.; Lowenstein, P.R.; Castro, M.G.; Hall, W.A.; Ohlfest, J.R. "Improved distribution of small molecules and viral vectors in the murine brain using a hollow fiber catheter." *J. Neurosurg.* **2007**, *107*, 568–577. [CrossRef]
29. Tremblay, S.; Acker, L.; Afraz, A.; Albaugh, D.L.; Amita, H.; Andrei, A.R.; Angelucci, A.; Aschner, A.; Balan, P.F.; Basso, M.A.; et al. An Open Resource for Non-human Primate Optogenetics. *Neuron* **2020**, *108*, 1075–1090. [CrossRef]
30. Belloir, T.; Montalgo Vargo, S.; Ahmed, Z.; Griggs, D.; Fisher, S.; Brown, T.; Chamanzar, M.; Yazdan-Shahmorad, A. Large-scale multimodal surface neural interfaces for non-human primates. *iScience. under revision*.
31. Bloch, J.; Shea-brown, E.; Harchaoui, Z.; Shojai, A. E Network structure mediates functional reorganization induced by optogenetic stimulation of non-human primate sensorimotor cortex. *iScience* **2022**, *25*, 104285. [CrossRef]
32. Griggs, D.J.; Belloir, T.; Yazdan-Shahmorad, A. Large-scale neural interfaces for optogenetic actuators and sensors in non-human primates. *SPIE BiOS* **2021**, *1166305*, 17. [CrossRef]
33. Griggs, D.J.; Bloch, J.; Fisher, S.; Ojemann, W.K.S.; Coubrough, K.M.; Khateeb, K.; Chu, M.; Yazdan-Shahmorad, A. Demonstration of an Optimized Large-scale Optogenetic Cortical Interface for Non-human Primates. *IEEE EMBC* **2022**, *119395*, 7–15.
34. Griggs, D.J.; Khateeb, K.; Philips, S.; Chan, J.W.; Ojemann, W.K.S.; Yazdan-Shahmorad, A. Optimized large-scale optogenetic interface for non-human primates. *SPIE BiOS* **2019**, *1086605*, 3. [CrossRef]
35. Griggs, D.J.; Khateeb, K.; Zhou, J.; Liu, T.; Wang, R.; Yazdan-Shahmorad, A. Multi-modal artificial dura for simultaneous large-scale optical access and large-scale electrophysiology in non-human primate cortex. *J. Neural Eng.* **2021**, *18*, 055006. [CrossRef]
36. Komatsu, M.; Sugano, E.; Tomita, H.; Fujii, N. A chronically implantable bidirectional neural interface for non-human primates. *Front. Neurosci.* **2017**, *11*, 514. [CrossRef] [PubMed]
37. Ledochowitsch, P.; Yazdan-Shahmorad, A.; Bouchard, K.E.; Diaz-Botia, C.; Hanson, T.L.; He, J.W.; Seybold, B.A.; Olivero, E.; Phillips, E.A.; Blanche, T.J.; et al. Strategies for optical control and simultaneous electrical readout of extended cortical circuits. *J. Neurosci. Methods* **2015**, *256*, 220–231. [CrossRef] [PubMed]
38. Rajalingham, R.; Sorenson, M.; Azadi, R.; Bohn, S.; DiCarlo, J.J.; Afraz, A. Chronically implantable LED arrays for behavioral optogenetics in primates. *Nat. Methods* **2021**, *18*, 1112–1116. [CrossRef]

39. Yazdan-Shahmorad, A.; Silversmith, D.B.; Sabes, P.N. Novel techniques for large-scale manipulations of cortical networks in non-human primates. In Proceedings of the 40th Annual International Conference of the IEEE Engineering in Medicine and Biology Society (EMBC), Honolulu, HI, USA, 17–21 July 2018; pp. 5479–5482. [CrossRef]
40. Strange, B.A.; Witter, M.P.; Lein, E.S.; Moser, E.I. Functional organization of the hippocampal longitudinal axis. *Nat. Rev. Neurosci.* **2014**, *15*, 655–669. [CrossRef]
41. Zola, S.M.; Squire, L.R.; Teng, E.; Stefanacci, L.; Buffalo, E.A.; Clark, R.E. Impaired recognition memory in monkeys after damage limited to the hippocampal region. *J. Neurosci.* **2000**, *20*, 451–463. [CrossRef]
42. Hampton, R.R.; Buckmaster, C.A.; Anuszkiewicz-Lundgren, D.; Murray, E.A. Method for making selective lesions of the hippocampus in Macaque monkeys using NMDA and a longitudinal surgical approach. *Hippocampus* **2004**, *14*, 9–18. [CrossRef]
43. Simmons, J.M.; Saad, Z.S.; Lizak, M.J.; Ortiz, M.; Koretsky, A.P.; Richmond, B.J. Mapping prefrontal circuits in vivo with manganese-enhanced magnetic resonance imaging in monkeys. *J. Neurosci.* **2008**, *28*, 7637–7647. [CrossRef] [PubMed]
44. Russell, W.; Burch, R. *The Principles of Humane Experimental Technique*; Methuen: London, UK, 1959.
45. Prescott, M.J.; Poirier, C. The role of MRI in applying the 3Rs to non-human primate neuroscience. *Neuroimage* **2021**, *225*, 117521. [CrossRef] [PubMed]

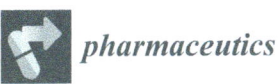

Article

IL-13Rα2 Status Predicts GB-13 (IL13.E13K-PE4E) Efficacy in High-Grade Glioma

Julian S. Rechberger [1,2], Kendra A. Porath [3], Liang Zhang [1], Cody L. Nesvick [1], Randy S. Schrecengost [4], Jann N. Sarkaria [3] and David J. Daniels [1,2,*]

1. Department of Neurologic Surgery, Mayo Clinic, Rochester, MN 55905, USA; rechberger.julian@mayo.edu (J.S.R.); zhang.liang@mayo.edu (L.Z.); nesvick.cody@mayo.edu (C.L.N.)
2. Department of Molecular Pharmacology and Experimental Therapeutics, Mayo Clinic Graduate School of Biomedical Sciences, Rochester, MN 55905, USA
3. Department of Radiation Oncology, Mayo Clinic, Rochester, MN 55905, USA; porath.kendra@mayo.edu (K.A.P.); sarkaria.jann@mayo.edu (J.N.S.)
4. Targepeutics, Inc., Hershey, PA 17033, USA; randys@targepeutics.com
* Correspondence: daniels.david@mayo.edu

Abstract: High-grade gliomas (HGG) are devastating diseases in children and adults. In the pediatric population, diffuse midline gliomas (DMG) harboring H3K27 alterations are the most aggressive primary malignant brain tumors. With no effective therapies available, children typically succumb to disease within one year of diagnosis. In adults, glioblastoma (GBM) remains largely intractable, with a median survival of approximately 14 months despite standard clinical care of radiation and temozolomide. Therefore, effective therapies for these tumors remain one of the most urgent and unmet needs in modern medicine. Interleukin 13 receptor subunit alpha 2 (IL-13Rα2) is a cell-surface transmembrane protein upregulated in many HGGs, including DMG and adult GBM, posing a potentially promising therapeutic target for these tumors. In this study, we investigated the pharmacological effects of GB-13 (also known as IL13.E13K-PE4E), a novel peptide–toxin conjugate that contains a targeting moiety designed to bind IL-13Rα2 with high specificity and a point-mutant cytotoxic domain derived from Pseudomonas exotoxin A. Glioma cell lines demonstrated a spectrum of IL-13Rα2 expression at both the transcript and protein level. Anti-tumor effects of GB-13 strongly correlated with IL-13Rα2 expression and were reflected in apoptosis induction and decreased cell proliferation in vitro. Direct intratumoral administration of GB-13 via convection-enhanced delivery (CED) significantly decreased tumor burden and resulted in prolonged survival in IL-13Rα2-upregulated orthotopic xenograft models of HGG. In summary, administration of GB-13 demonstrated a promising pharmacological response in HGG models both in vitro and in vivo in a manner strongly associated with IL-13Rα2 expression, underscoring the potential of this IL-13Rα2-targeted therapy in a subset of HGG with increased IL-13Rα2 levels.

Keywords: high-grade glioma; diffuse midline glioma; glioblastoma; IL-13Rα2; IL-13; immunotoxin; targeted therapy; GB-13; IL13.E13K-PE4E; receptor expression

1. Introduction

High-grade gliomas (HGG) encompass the majority of malignant tumors within the central nervous system (CNS), and with fewer than 25,000 new cases annually in the US, they are categorized as a rare disease [1]. H3K27-altered diffuse midline glioma (DMG), formerly known as diffuse intrinsic pontine glioma (DIPG), constitute a subset of HGG that predominantly occurs in children and makes up approximately half of the HGGs in this patient population [2,3]. These tumors are localized to the thalamus, brainstem and spinal cord and often lack contrast enhancement on magnetic resonance imaging (MRI), suggesting that they maintain a largely intact blood–brain barrier (BBB), an impediment to systemic drug delivery [4,5]. Despite the recent discovery of key molecular drivers of disease, clinical trials for DMG continue to fail, and palliative external beam radiotherapy remains the mainstay of therapy [6,7]. The prognosis for patients with DMG is dismal, with a median overall survival of 9 months and no long-term survivors [1,8]. In adults, glioblastoma (GBM) is the most prevalent and aggressive HGG subtype. The current standard treatment consists of maximal surgical debulking, radiotherapy, and concomitant and adjuvant temozolomide chemotherapy [9,10]. However, the diffuse, infiltrative nature and proclivity for recurrence render GBM largely intractable [1,2]. While clinical trials are underway utilizing a range of different therapeutic approaches, no treatment has demonstrated a benefit to standard of care by extending survival in this tumor in almost two decades, and the median survival is currently less than two years from diagnosis [11–14]. Consequently, the dire prognosis for patients with HGG and the lack of efficacious, targeted therapies for these tumors demand a novel approach to their treatment.

Interleukin 13 (IL-13) is an immune-regulatory cytokine implicated in both physiologic and tumoral microenvironments through effects on IL-13 receptor alpha 1 (IL-13Rα1) and IL-13 receptor alpha 2 (IL-13Rα2) receptors [15]. Normally, IL-13 binds to IL-13Rα1, with IL-4Rα providing stabilization to this interaction, thereby inducing formation of a receptor dimer [16]. The intracellular signaling axis downstream of IL-13Rα1/IL-4Rα promotes apoptotic signaling cascades via a caspase-dependent mechanism [17]. In contrast, IL-13Rα2 acts as a decoy receptor that directly binds IL-13 as a monomer with greater binding affinity than IL-13Rα1 [18]. When IL-13Rα2 is expressed on the surface of select cell types, IL-13 is sequestered away from IL-13Rα1, thus leading to escape from apoptotic cell death [19,20].

IL-13Rα2 is expressed almost exclusively on cancer cells and is a clinically validated target for biologic therapeutics. Malignant diseases with known IL-13Rα2 upregulation include but are not limited to HGG [16,21–23], malignant peripheral nerve sheath tumors [24], colon cancer [25], pancreatic cancer [26], ovarian cancer [27], and melanoma [28]. Recent studies suggest that overexpression of IL-13Rα2 is detected in up to 83% of malignant pediatric brain tumors, including DMG, and up to 78% of adult GBM [23,29–31]. Furthermore, IL-13Rα2 significantly correlates with poor prognosis in HGG [16]. Given the status of IL-13Rα2 as a promising therapeutic target in HGG, a number of preclinical studies and clinical trials have been conducted, demonstrating the safety and efficacy of chimeric antigen receptor (CAR)-engineered T cell-based therapies and recombinant immunotoxins directed against this target [32,33]. Previously, convection-enhanced delivery (CED) of cintredekin besudotox (IL13-PE38QQR), a wild-type IL-13 pseudomonal exotoxin (PE)-A conjugate that targets both IL-13Rα1 and IL-13Rα2, was evaluated in phase I and phase III clinical trials for DMG and GBM, respectively [33–36]. However, these studies were hampered by ill-defined inclusion criteria and did not consider the IL-13Rα2 expression status in tumors of enrolled subjects, which likely contributed to disappointing survival results [37].

The purpose of this study was to determine the impact of tumor-associated IL-13Rα2 levels on the therapeutic efficacy of IL-13Rα2-targeted therapy in HGG. We screened the novel recombinant chimeric immunotoxin GB-13 (IL13.E13K-PE4E) against a library of select HGG patient-derived cell lines. GB-13 consists of an N-terminal IL-13-targeting moiety with a single engineered point mutation, the C-terminus of which is linked to the N-terminus of a full-length PE molecule containing four point mutations. These modifications greatly enhance the selectivity and affinity for IL-13Ra2 and reduce toxicity to non-malignant cells [24,38,39]. The IL-13 moiety attaches to IL-13Ra2 at the cell surface of malignant target cells and facilitates the internalization of the toxin, which irreversibly disables eukaryotic elongation factor 2 (eEF2) by adenosine diphosphate (ADP)-ribosylation using oxidized nicotinamide adenine dinucleotide (NAD+), causing arrest of protein synthesis and eventual Bak- and caspase-mediated apoptosis [40–42]. Treatment with GB-13 resulted in dose-dependent killing of DMG and adult GBM cells in a manner strongly associated with IL-13Rα2 expression. Moreover, intratumoral administration of GB-13 via CED decreased tumor burden and prolonged survival in both DMG and adult

GBM intracranial murine xenografts with high, but not low levels of IL-13Rα2. Our results illustrate a previously underappreciated role of IL-13Rα2 heterogeneity in HGG and outline the potential of IL-13Rα2-targeted therapies in a subset of these tumors.

2. Materials and Methods

2.1. Materials

The IL-13Rα2-targeted therapy used in this study was GB-13 (IL13.E13K-PE4E), which was a generous gift from Targepeutics Inc. (Hershey, PA, USA). GB-13 was dissolved in PBS and stored as 2.6 mg/mL stock at −80 °C. Human IL-13 recombinant protein (Cat # A42525; Thermo Fisher Scientific, Rockford, IL, USA) was obtained from Invitrogen (Thermo Fisher Scientific). IL-13 was dissolved in ddH$_2$O per the manufacturer's protocol and stored as 5 µg/mL stock at −80 °C.

2.2. Cell Lines and Culture

Informed consent and Institutional Review Board approval were obtained for all patient-derived cell lines. Details regarding cell lines can be found in Table S1. Early-passage HGG lines were used, and all cell lines were validated by short tandem repeat DNA fingerprinting annually and tested for Mycoplasma contamination every 3 months. Cell lines with the H3K27M mutation were validated for K27M-mutant histone expression using Western blot and Sanger sequencing every 3 months. All patient-derived tumor cell lines were maintained in cell-line-appropriate medium, the details of which are provided in Table S2. Cells cultured as neurospheres were passaged every 1–2 weeks. Cells cultured as adherent monolayers were passaged 1–2 times per week.

2.3. RNA Sequencing and Data Analysis

Total RNA was extracted from whole-cell lysates using the RNeasy Plus micro kit (Cat # 74034; QIAGEN, Germantown, MD, USA) according to the manufacturer's instructions. For the purpose of screening a large library of cell lines, RNA-Seq studies were performed as single replicates. RNA library preparation and sequencing were performed by Novogene (Beijing, China). The NEBNext UltraTM RNA Library Prep Kit for Illumina sequencers (New England Biolabs, Ipswich, MA, USA) was used for library preparation, and cDNA libraries were subsequently size selected using AMPure XP magnetic beads (Beckman Coulter, Pasadena, CA, USA). Samples were sequenced on an NovaSeq 6000 sequencer (Illumina, San Diego, CA, USA) using either single- or paired-end sequencing, depending on the timeframe of sample availability and the sequencing technology available. Paired-end sequencing data on adult GBM cell lines were obtained from cBioPortal, a free web-based tool that contains RNA-Seq data on Mayo Clinic's brain tumor patient-derived xenografts [43,44]. Generated FASTQ files underwent quality assessment using FASTQC (https://www.bioinformatics.babraham.ac.uk/projects/fastqc/, accessed on 22 September 2021). Trimmed reads were mapped to hg38 using STARv2.7.3a, and annotated gene counts were obtained using the –quantMode geneCounts function [45]. Transcripts (TPM) or reads per kilo base per million (RPKM) reads values were calculated using RSEM in a manner concordant with the single- or paired-end status of the library [46].

2.4. Immunoblotting

Patient-derived tumor cells for immunoblotting were lysed in Triton X-100 lysis buffer containing protease inhibitors and sonicated. Collected protein lysates were stored at −20 °C. Protein concentrations were determined using the Pierce BCA Protein Assay Kit (Cat #23227; Thermo Fisher Scientific). An amount of 15 µg of total protein was size fractioned by 12.5% SDS-PAGE. Electrophoresis-separated proteins were electrically transferred to a polyvinylidene difluoride (PVDF) membrane, washed in PBST buffer, and blocked in 2% fat-free milk for 1 h at room temperature, then incubated with primary antibodies at 4 °C overnight. Following primary antibody blotting, specific signal was detected with species-appropriate peroxidase-conjugated secondary antibody (Thermo Fisher Scientific) using SuperSignal West Pico PLUS Chemiluminescent Substrate (Cat #34580; Thermo Fisher Scientific) and imaged using an Azure 600 Western blot imaging system (Azure Biosystems, Dublin, CA, USA). Details regarding antibodies used for Western blots can be found in Table S3.

2.5. Cell Proliferation and Viability Assays

Cells in single-cell suspension were plated with culture medium in 96-well clear-bottom black microplates (Cat #3917; Corning Costar, Corning, NY, USA) at a density of 2500 cells per well for adult GBM cell lines (GBM6, GBM 10, GBM14, GBM 39, GBM43, and GBM 108) or 5000 cells per well for DMG cell lines (SU-DIPG XIII-P [47], SU-DIPG XVII [48], SF8628, SF8628-B23 (H3F3A K27M knockout of SF8628), and PED17) and cultured overnight at 37 °C with 5% CO_2. The next day, cells were treated in triplicate with either vehicle (ddH_2O or PBS) or serial dilutions of IL-13 (to final concentrations of 100, 50, 20, 10, 5, 1, and 0.5 ng/mL) or GB-13 (to final concentrations of 320, 100, 32, 10, 3.2, 1, 0.32, 0.1, 0.032, 0.01, 0.0032, and 0.001 ng/mL). Cells were incubated for 72 h and then assayed with CellTiter-Glo Luminescent Cell Viability Assay (Cat #G7570; Promega, Madison, WI, USA) according to the manufacturer's recommendations. Luminescence was measured using an Infinite M200 PRO multimode microplate reader (Tecan Group, Männedorf, Switzerland), normalized to control wells (ddH_2O or PBS only), and relative luminescence treatment was plotted as a function of drug concentration. The potency (50% inhibitory concentration, IC_{50}) of each treatment was calculated by non-linear least-squares curve fitting using Prism 9 (GraphPad, San Diego, CA, USA).

2.6. Immunofluorescence

Cells were plated in single-cell suspensions at a density of 10,000 cells per well on 4 Chamber Cell Culture Slides (Cat # 50-114-9053; CELLTREAT Scientific Products, Pepperell, MA, USA) and cultured overnight at 37 °C with 5% CO_2. After 24 h, cells were treated with either vehicle (PBS) or the IC_{50} concentration of GB-13, as determined by CellTiter-Glo Luminescent Cell Viability Assay (Promega). At specific timepoints (8, 24, 48, and 72 h), cells were then washed in PBS and fixed with 4% paraformaldehyde for 20 min. Cells were washed 3 times for 5 min each in PBS and incubated in 0.5% Triton X-100 in PBS for 5 min. To wash the coverslips of the permeabilization buffer, cells were incubated in PBS 3 times for 5 min each before blocking with 3% BSA in PBS-T (0.1% Tween 20) for 1 h at room temperature. Up to two different primary antibodies were then added in 1% BSA in PBST overnight at 4 °C. Dilution buffer was used in lieu of primary antibody for cell-specific negative controls. The next day, cells were washed 3 times for 5 min each in PBS-T. Cells were then incubated with Alexa Fluor-coupled secondary antibodies (Thermo Fisher Scientific) in 1% BSA in PBS-T for 1 h at room temperature in the dark. To test for cross-reactivity, one control per primary antibody condition was included by applying the other secondary antibody to the primary antibody. After three additional 5 min washes in PBS, chambers were removed and slides were rinsed thrice in ddH_2O. Slides were mounted using ProLong Gold Antifade reagent with DAPI (Cat # P36935; Thermo Fisher Scientific) and stored at 37 °C until microscopy imaging. All slides were examined and images captured using a LSM 780 confocal laser scanning microscope (Carl Zeiss Microscopy, White Plains, NY, USA). Detailed information regarding antibodies used for immunofluorescence can be found in Table S3.

2.7. Patient-Derived Xenografts

All animal experiments were conducted in accordance with the NIH and IACUC guidelines for the use of animals in research and approved by the Mayo Clinic Institutional Committee for Animal Research. HGG cell lines (GBM6, PED17, and SU-DIPG XIII-P [47]) were transduced with a luciferase reporter system (eGFP/fLuc2) that allows bioluminescence readout of tumor volume [49]. Orthotopic tumor inoculation with cultured cells was performed as previously described [49,50]. Briefly, cells were placed in single-cell suspension, and 300,000 cells in 3 μL of sterile PBS were prepared for engraftment into each mouse. A 0.5 mm burr hole was created at the following coordinates: 1 mm posterior and 2 mm to the right of the bregma (GBM6) or 1 mm posterior to the lambdoid suture and 1 mm lateral to the mid-sagittal plane (PED17 and SU-DIPGXIII). Using a 26 gauge (51 mm, point style AS) syringe (Cat. #203185; Hamilton Company, Bonaduz, Switzerland), tumor cells were injected stereotactically at a constant flow rate of 0.5 μL/min into the cerebral hemisphere (GBM6) or pons (PED17 and SU-DIPGXIII) of 6- to 7-week-old female Hsd:Athymic Nude-Foxn1^{nu} mutant mice that were obtained from Charles River Laboratories (Wilmington, MA, USA). The injection depth was 4 mm for all groups. In vivo tumor engraftment and progression were monitored by bioluminescence imaging (BLI). Animals were dosed with an intraperitoneal injection of 10 mg/kg of Cycluc. After 10 min, mice were imaged under isoflurane anesthesia using an IVIS-200 Imaging System (Xenogen Corporation, Berkeley, CA, USA). Image analysis was performed using LivingImage 4.3 (PerkinElmer, Waltham, MA, USA) to quantitate total flux (number of photons per second) within a region of interest.

For brain-targeted drug delivery, animals were randomized to control (PBS) and treatment (GB-13) groups based on BLI signal to ensure equal distribution of tumor sizes at the beginning of the study (when BLI reached approximately 1,000,000 total log flux). Mice were placed under anesthesia with 100 mg/kg of ketamine and 10 mg/kg of xylazine. A 2 cm midline skin incision was made extending from behind the eyes to level of the ears. The previously established burr hole was reopened and mice were secured on a stereotactic stage with automated thermal support using a Rodent Warmer X1 (Cat #53800M; Stoelting, Wood Dale, IL, USA). A 33 gauge internal cannula (Cat #8IC315IS5SPC; P1 Technologies, Roanoke, VA, USA), with a 4 mm projection below the pedestal, was inserted into a 26 gauge guide cannula (Cat #8IC315GS5SPC, P1 Technologies), with a 3.5 mm projection below the pedestal, and both were connected to PE tubing and secured with a single connector assembly (# C313C/SPC; P1 Technologies). The whole unit was secured vertically with a cannula holder (Cat #505254; World Precision Instruments, Sarasota, FL, USA) and connected to a 22 gauge (51 mm, point style AS) syringe (Cat #80400; Hamilton Company) placed in a Legato 130 syringe pump (Cat #788130; KD Scientific, Holliston, MA, USA). Vehicle (PBS) and drug (GB-13 at concentrations of 50 μg/mL (1 μg dose), 15 μg/mL (0.3 μg dose), or 5 μg/mL (0.1 μg dose)) solutions were subsequently primed through the internal cannula and associated tubing. The cannula holder with attached internal cannula was lowered until flush with the mouse skull to reach the desired injection depth of 4 mm (GBM6) or 4.2 mm (PED17 and SU-DIPGXIII). In all study groups, the same ramped CED infusion protocol was performed with a total volume infused of 20 μL and rates of infusion as follows: 3 μL at 0.2 μL/min, 5 μL at 0.5 μL/min, and 12 μL at 0.8 μL/min [51]. To avoid reflux into the injection tract, the cannula was removed 10 min after completion of infusion. Animals were monitored daily and euthanized at indication of progressive neurologic deficit or if found in a moribund condition.

2.8. Immunohistochemistry

Following animal euthanasia by carbon dioxide inhalation, brains were harvested and fixed in 4% paraformaldehyde at room temperature overnight. The brains were then embedded in paraffin and sectioned in the coronal plane (5 μm/section) using a microtome (CM1860 UV; Leica Biosystems, Buffalo Grove, IL, USA). Hematoxylin and eosin (H&E) staining was performed according to standard procedures. For immunohistochemistry (IHC), paraffin-embedded tissue sections were dewaxed in xylene and rehydrated in ethanol. Antigen retrieval was performed by steaming slides in preheated sodium citrate buffer (10 mM tri-sodium citrate, 0.05% Tween 20, pH 6.0) for 30 min. Sections were cooled to room temperature and rinsed with dH20 for 1 min. This was followed by soaking sections in 0.6% hydrogen peroxide in MeOH for 20 min. Sections were then blocked with 10% normal goat serum (NGS) in Tris-buffered saline (TBS) for 30 min at room temperature. Primary antibodies were diluted in TBS with 2% NGS and 0.5%

Triton X-100 and applied to sections overnight at 4 °C. Dilution buffer was used instead of primary antibody for tissue-specific negative controls. The next day, sections were washed 3 times for 5 min in TBS with 2% NGS and 0.5% Triton X-100. The VECTASTAIN Elite ABC kit (Cat # PK-6100; VECTOR Laboratory, Burlingame, CA, USA) containing biotinylated secondary antibody was diluted in TBS with 1.5% NGS and added to the sections according to the manufacturer's recommendations. After 3 additional 5 min washes in TBS, sections were incubated with Avidin/Biotinylated Enzyme Complex (ABC) solution (Cat # PK-6100; VECTOR Laboratory) for 30 min at room temperature. For visualization, the sections were subsequently developed using SignalStain DAB Substrate Kit (Cat # 8059P; Cell Signaling, Danvers, MA, USA) per the manufacturer's protocol, counterstained with hematoxylin, and mounted with Permount^{TM} (Cat # SP15-100, Thermo Fisher Scientific). Images were acquired with a digital slide scanner (Axio Scan.Z1; Carl Zeiss Microscopy) and are presented at a magnification of 40x. Cell quantification was performed using the Cell Counter plugin for ImageJ (NIH). Ten random fields including a total of 300 to 500 cells were captured for each antibody. Results are presented as the percentage of positive cells versus the entire counted cell population. Low-power images are included to demonstrate consistency of staining in tissue sections. Detailed information regarding antibodies used for immunohistochemistry is provided in Table S3.

2.9. Statistical Analysis

The data were collected and presented as the mean ± standard deviation or standard error of the mean when appropriate. Direct statistical comparisons between 2 groups were conducted using two-tailed Student's *t*-tests. Non-linear least-squares curve fitting was used to determine the potency (IC_{50}) of GB-13 treatment in vitro. Survival analysis was performed using the Kaplan–Meier estimate with the Log-Rank test. Statistical tests and analyses were conducted using Prism 9 (GraphPad), with statistical significance set at an α threshold of 0.05, and $p < 0.05$ marked by asterisks in figures.

3. Results

3.1. IL-13Rα2 Is Expressed at Different Levels in HGG Tumor Cell Models

To identify baseline transcript and protein levels of IL-13Rα2 in HGG cells, we performed RNA sequencing and immunoblotting on patient-derived HGG (DMG and adult GBM) cell lines (Figure 1). In accordance with previous investigations [16,52,53], our cohort of sequenced HGG transcriptomes demonstrated highly variable expression of IL-13Rα2 RNA among HGG cell lines (Figure 1A), ranging from low (SU-DIPG XIII-P, GBM39, and GBM108) to intermediate (SU-DIPG XVII, SF8628, GBM43, and GBM6) and high (PED17, GBM10, and GBM14) expression. Next, we evaluated IL-13Rα2 protein levels in available HGG cell lines. IL-13Rα2 protein levels were generally congruent with gene expression in both DMG and adult GBM cell lines (Figure 1B). Several cell models showed high IL-13Rα2 expression, including PED17, GBM10, GBM14, GBM59 and GBM118, while others, such as SU-DIPG XVII, SF8628, SF8628-B23, GBM6, GBM12 and GBM43, showed notably lower (but not absent) IL-13Rα2 levels. IL-13Rα2 expression was not variable between SF8628 and SF8628-B23, indicating expression of this receptor is not impacted by presence of the K27M mutation. A third category of HGG cell lines, including SU-DIPG XIII-P, GBM39, GBM108 and GBM123, demonstrated IL-13Rα2 protein levels that were below the detection threshold of our assay.

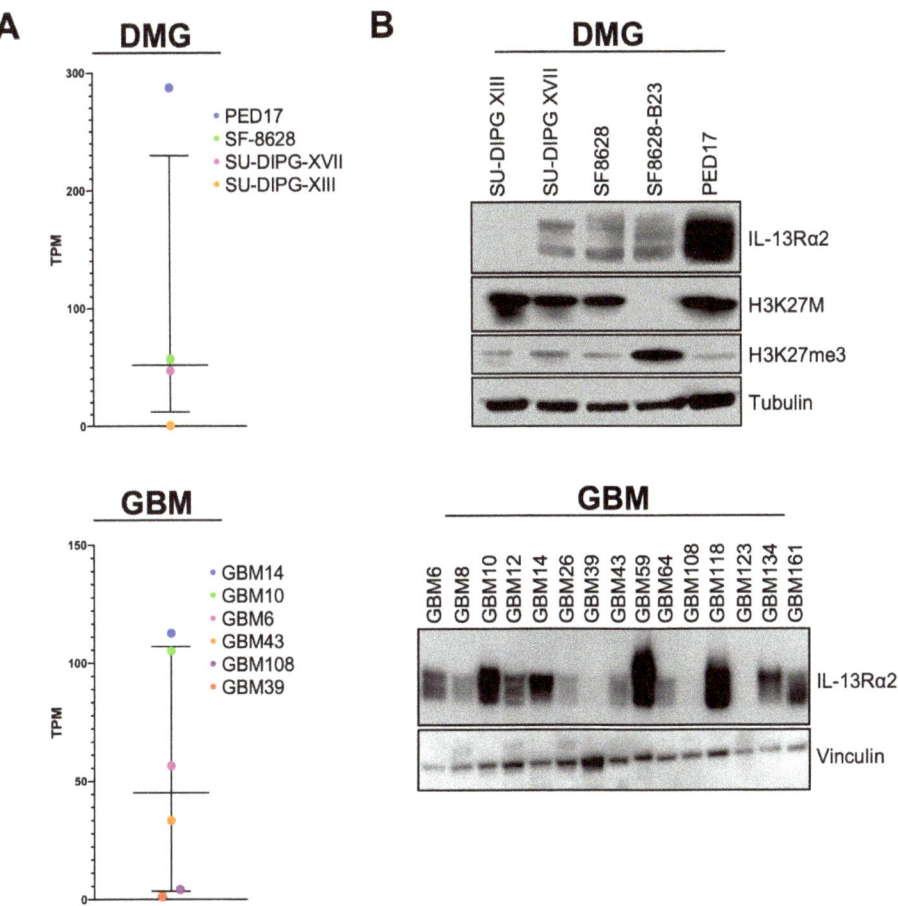

Figure 1. High-grade glioma (HGG) cell lines demonstrate a spectrum of IL-13Rα2 expression on both the mRNA and protein level. (**A**) RNA-Seq and (**B**) immunoblotting of diffuse midline glioma (DMG) and adult glioblastoma (GBM) cell models indicates a correlation between mRNA and protein levels of IL-13Rα2 at baseline. Cell lines differ in terms of IL-13Rα2 expression.

3.2. Functional Impact of IL-13Rα2 on HGG Proliferation and Survival

Given the cell line-dependent overexpression of IL-13Rα2 in our DMG and adult GBM tumor cell models, we investigated the role of IL-13Rα2 signaling in HGG (Figure 2). To determine whether cytokine stimulation by IL-13 impacts cell proliferation in vitro, HGG cells were treated with varying concentrations of the canonical ligand of IL-13Rα2, IL-13. While the lack of SU-DIPG XIII-P response was consistent with the low expression of IL-13Rα2 in the assayed cell models, none of the IL-13Rα2-medium or IL-13Rα2-high cell lines stimulated with IL-13 demonstrated any significant increase in cell proliferation versus media as the control (Figure 2A). Based on previous reports, demonstrating IL-13Rα2 is implicated in cell survival rather than cell growth and invasion [19,52], we hypothesized that cytokine stimulation would be associated with increased IL-13Rα2 expression to enforce this anti-apoptotic effect. To test this, we stimulated HGG cells with IL-13 (10 ng/mL) and investigated protein levels at various time points (Figure 2D). Stimulation with IL-13 resulted in robust upregulation of IL-13Rα2 in IL-13Rα2-medium and IL-13Rα2-high cell lines after 8, 24, 48, and 72 h. Conversely, IL-13Rα1 levels remained unaffected by IL-13 stimulation in all assayed HGG cell models.

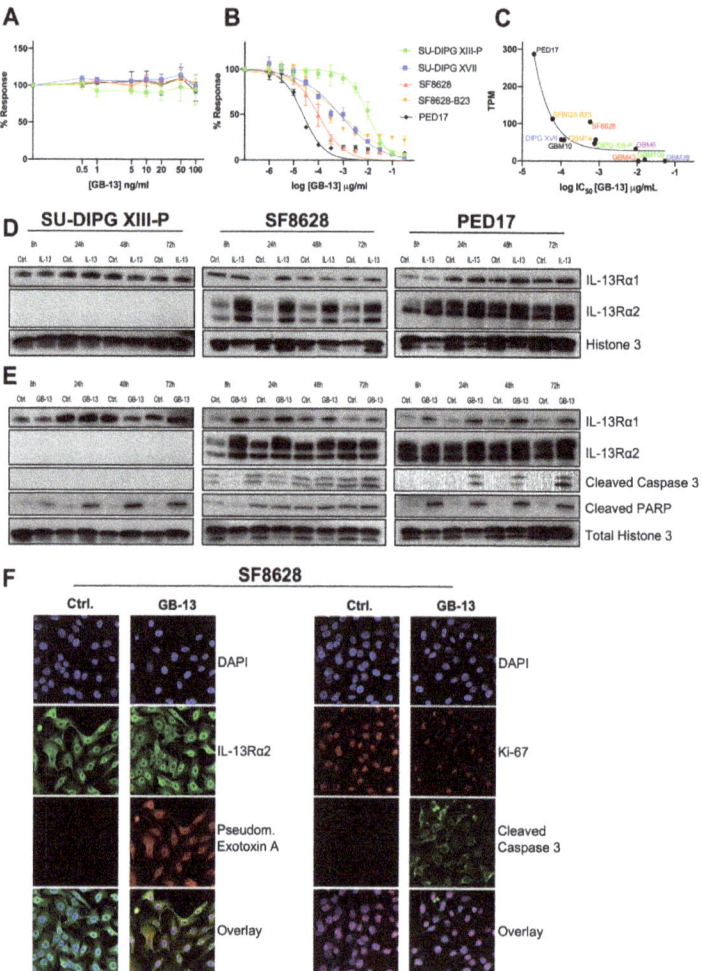

Figure 2. Sensitivity to anti-tumor effects of GB-13 correlates to IL-13Rα2 status and is reflected in apoptosis induction and decreased cell proliferation. (**A,B**) Cell proliferation and viability assay of indicated DMG cell lines at escalating doses of IL-13 and GB-13. IL-13 stimulation does not impact cell proliferation. GB-13 decreases cell viability in a dose and IL-13Rα2 level-dependent manner. IC$_{50}$ values were calculated using non-linear least-squares curve fitting. Each drug was tested in triplicate with three independent experiments (n = 9) in each cell line and assayed at 72 h. (**C**) Inverse relationship between IL-13Rα2 expression and sensitivity towards GB-13 demonstrated by non-linear least-squares curve fitting (r^2 = 0.88). (**D,E**) Immunoblotting of indicated DMG cell lines after 8, 24, 48, and 72 h of IL-13 (10 ng/mL) and GB-13 (cell line-specific IC$_{50}$) exposure. IL-13 can increase IL-13Rα2 expression. Similar to IL-13, GB-13 does not lead to IL-13Rα2 downregulation over time but rather upregulates the receptor in select cell lines. (**F**) Immunofluorescence staining of SF8628 cells following 72 h of treatment with GB-13 at IC$_{50}$. The *Pseudomonas* exotoxin A (PE) moiety of GB-13 colocalizes to IL-13Rα2, while receptor levels are maintained over prolonged durations of treatment (left). Cells demonstrate increased levels of apoptotic cell death (cleaved caspase 3) and decreased cell proliferation (Ki-67) after exposure to GB-13 (right). Images are representative of three independent experiments.

3.3. GB-13 Elicits Potent Anti-Tumor Effects in HGG Cell Models

To assess whether IL-13Rα2 expression confers sensitivity to IL-13Rα2-targeted therapy in vitro, we tested the pharmacological response of HGG cells to GB-13. We selected 11 HGG (5 DMG and 6 adult GBM) cell lines and exposed them to varying concentrations of GB-13, with treatments ranging from 0.001 to 320 ng/mL. The results showed a direct relationship between IL-13Rα2 expression and GB-13 sensitivity (Figures 2B and S1). GB-13 demonstrated strong cytotoxicity in IL-13Rα2-high cell lines versus comparatively insensitive IL-13Rα2-low cell models (Table 1). The IC_{50} values of GB-13 in IL-13Rα2-high cells were: 0.02 ng/mL for PED17 cells, 0.06 ng/mL for GBM14, and 0.58 ng/mL for GBM10. IL-13Rα2-medium cells displayed the following IC_{50} values for GB-13: 0.10 ng/mL for SF8628, 0.75 ng/mL for SU-DIPG XVII, 0.81 ng/mL for SF8628-B23, 0.12 ng/mL for GBM6, 9.08 ng/mL for GBM43. Finally, the IC_{50} values for GB-13 in IL-13Rα2-low cells were: 10.63 ng/mL for SU-DIPG XIII-P, 15.74 ng/mL for GBM108, and 53.82 ng/mL for GBM39. DMG and adult GBM cell models showed similar sensitivity towards GB-13 dependent on IL-13Rα2 status. High and medium expressors were similarly sensitive ($p = 0.43$) and together had significantly different IC_{50} values compared to IL-13Rα2-low cell lines ($p = 0.009$) (Figure S2). Non-linear least-squares curve fitting demonstrated an inverse relationship between IL-13Rα2 expression and GB-13 cytotoxic effect ($r^2 = 0.88$) (Figure 2C).

Table 1. Fifty % inhibitory concentration (IC_{50}) values of GB-13.

Cell Line	IC_{50} Value (ng/mL)
SU-DIPG XIII-P	10.63
SU-DIPG XVII	0.75
SF8628	0.10
SF8628-B23	0.81
PED17	0.02
GBM6	0.12
GBM10	0.58
GBM14	0.06
GBM39	53.82
GBM43	9.08
GBM108	15.74

To gain insight into the effects of GB-13 on IL-13Rα2, we next treated HGG cells with IC_{50} concentrations of the drug and investigated protein levels at 8, 24, 48, and 72 h (Figure 2E). Similar to IL-13 stimulation, GB-13 did not induce IL-13Rα2 downregulation but rather led to stable or increased protein levels over time. Intriguingly, IL-13Rα1 was upregulated in some IL-13Rα2-medium and IL-13Rα2-high cell models exposed to GB-13. Furthermore, while there was some baseline signaling associated with apoptotic cell death in untreated SF8628 cells, apoptosis induction in the GB-13 condition was generally marked by a time-dependent increase in cleaved caspase 3 and/or cleaved PARP levels. These results were confirmed with confocal microscopy (Figures 2F, S3 and S6), where we found prominent IL-13Rα2 levels at baseline, which were retained in cells treated with GB-13 for up to 72 h. By staining for the PE-domain of GB-13, we confirmed colocalization of the drug to the receptor as well as internalization into the cytoplasm and nucleus. In addition to increased levels of apoptosis, cellular proliferation (Ki-67) was decreased in the presence of GB-13.

3.4. Intratumoral Administration of GB-13 Results in Decreased Tumor Burden and Prolonged Survival In Vivo

In order to validate the anti-tumor effects of GB-13 in vivo, we utilized orthotopic patient-derived murine xenograft models of HGG, including IL-13Rα2-low (SU-DIPG XIII-P), IL-13Rα2-medium (GBM6), and IL-13Rα2-high (PED17) models. Tumor-bearing animals were randomized into four cohorts and treated with a single, brain-targeted dose of GB-13 via CED in 4–5 animals per treatment arm (Figure 3A). We initially established our drug delivery system in adult GBM animals by infusing vehicle solution (PBS) or various doses of GB-13 into the hemispheric GBM6 tumor region. All CED systems were placed and tolerated without complications, as previously published [54]. There were no procedure-related deaths, and clinical assessments of animals after completed infusions were all unremarkable with no signs of acute or delayed toxicities or neurological deficits. The tumor volume, measured by BLI, was significantly lower in animals treated with 1 μg of GB-13 ($p = 0.01$) as compared to the 0.3 μg- ($p = 0.14$), 0.1 μg- ($p = 0.08$) and vehicle-treated groups (Figure 3B). A single dose of 1 μg GB-13 significantly prolonged survival, with a median survival of 84 days ($p = 0.01$) in comparison to 64 days in 0.3 μg GB-13 ($p = 0.35$), 68 days in 0.1 μg GB-13 ($p = 0.17$) and 57 days in vehicle groups (Figure 3C).

Histologic evaluation of brains from mice euthanized in a moribund state demonstrated maintained tissue architecture and decreased tumor size after GB-13 treatment (Figure 4A). On-target drug effects were validated in tumors by IHC analysis of IL-13Rα2 levels, apoptosis induction, and cellular proliferation in drug-treated mice compared to control (Figures 4B and S6). In agreement with the in vitro data, high IL-13Rα2 status was retained in GBM6 cells. Cellular proliferation, which was determined by Ki-67 staining, was decreased following exposure to GB-13 ($p = 0.03$). Intriguingly, intense staining for the apoptosis marker cleaved caspase 3 was evidenced throughout the tumor area in all GB-13 groups but largely absent in vehicle-treated animals weeks after GB-13 administration ($p < 0.0001$). To address toxicity considerations that may accompany immunotoxin delivery into the brain, we performed additional IHC analyses for NeuN, a marker of mature neurons, and CD68, which is expressed in high levels by microglia and monocytes. CED of GB-13 did not result in a decrease in NeuN-positive (NeuN+) cells in the infused, ipsilateral hemisphere as compared to vehicle ($p = 0.82$). No CD68+ immune cell infiltration was evidenced in any study group.

We next sought to validate these findings in an IL-13Rα2-upregulated DMG xenograft model. PED17 cells were orthotopically implanted into the pons, and tumor-bearing animals were again treated with vehicle solution, 0.1, 0.3, or 1 μg of GB-13. In line with prior observations, all animals tolerated the CED procedure; however, at the highest dose (a 1 μg CED infusion of GB-13), marked signs of toxicity developed in all five animals within 24 h of infusion (neurological deficits such as hemiparesis or ataxia, hunched body position, dermatitis), and 4 of 5 animals had to be euthanized within 72 h of drug administration. Post-operative clinical assessments were unremarkable for animals treated with 0.1 or 0.3 μg of GB-13. Comparison of BLI signal demonstrated that a single 0.1 or 0.3 μg GB-13 infusion significantly decreased tumor volume ($p = 0.0001$ and 0.0004, respectively; Figure 3D) and significantly extended median survival (147 days for 0.1 μg GB-13 ($p = 0.003$) and 155 days for 0.3 μg GB-13 ($p = 0.003$)) compared to the vehicle group (128 days) (Figure 3E). Similar to the findings in hemispheric GBM6 tumors, none of the 0.1 or 0.3 μg doses had an impact on NeuN+ cell density and CD68+ cell infiltration. Consistent with the observed differential in clinical toxicity, a 1 μg dose of GB-13 resulted in a marked decrease in NeuN-positive cells in the brainstem as compared to lower GB-13 doses or vehicle control ($p = 0.02$). There was no evidence of CD68+ monocyte cell infiltration following exposure to 1 μg GB-13. Detected levels of IL-13Rα2 remained constant among treatment groups. A decrease in DMG-characteristic H3 K27M and increase in H3 K27me3 was evidenced in drug-treated tumors. Additional IHC findings were similar to the results of the first study (Figures S4 and S6).

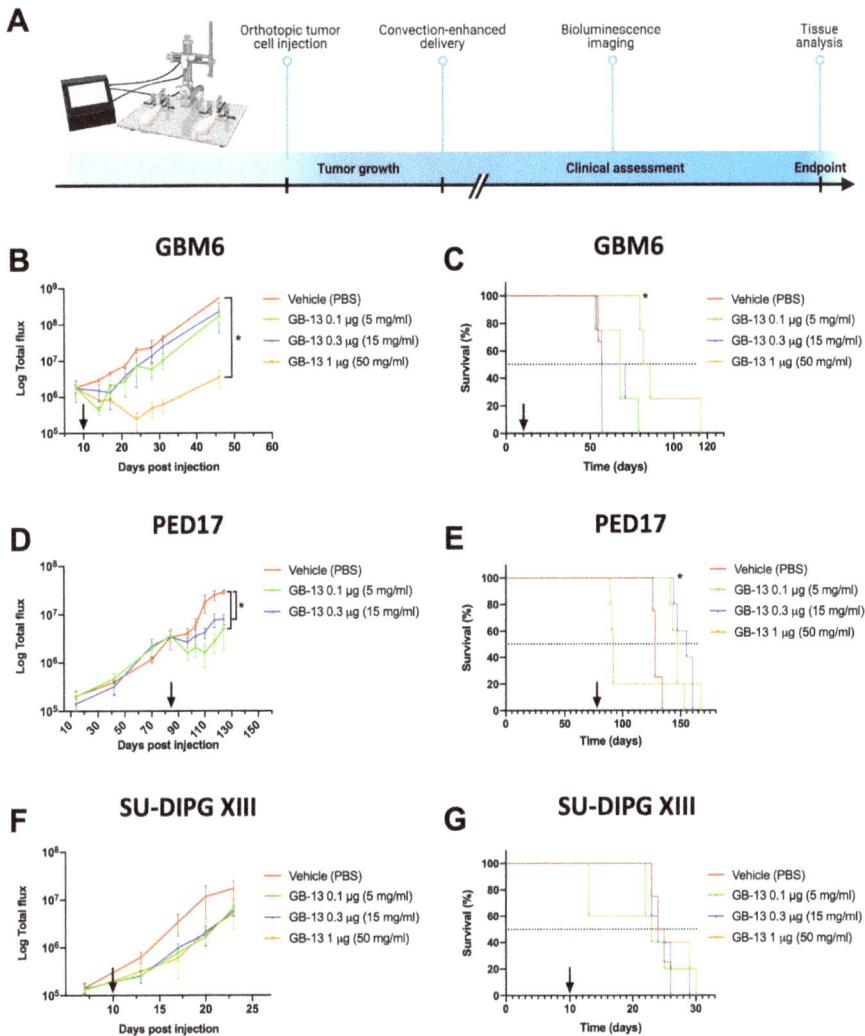

Figure 3. CED infusion of GB-13 results in reduced BLI signals and prolonged survival of IL-13Rα2-upregulated DMG and adult GBM patient-derived xenografts grown as orthotopic tumors. (**A**) Schematic representation of tumor cell injection and CED workflow (created with BioRender.com, accessed on 7 November 2021). Four to five mice were used per treatment group in each cell model (GBM6 is adult GBM with medium IL-13Rα2 levels; PED17 and SU-DIPG XIII-P are DMG with IL-13Rα2-high and IL-13Rα2-low levels, respectively). A single 1 µg dose of GB-13 by CED (arrow) results in decreased (**B**) BLI signals ($p = 0.01$) and (**C**) prolonged survival of GBM6-bearing animals ($p = 0.01$). (**D**) BLI signals in PED17 xenografts are reduced following 0.1 µg ($p = 0.0001$) or 0.3 µg ($p = 0.0004$) of GB-13. (**E**) 0.1 µg ($p = 0.003$) and 0.3 µg ($p = 0.003$) dose levels extend survival without a notable dose–response, but a 1 µg dose of GB-13 is associated with lethal toxicity in 4 out of 5 animals approximately 72 h after the infusion. In SU-DIPG XIII-P animals, CED of GB-13 is not associated with (**F**) reduced BLI signals or (**G**) survival benefit. BLI data are presented as the mean ± standard deviation, and significance between groups was calculated using two-tailed Student's t-tests. Significance of endpoint comparison between treatment groups were calculated using the Log-Rank test.

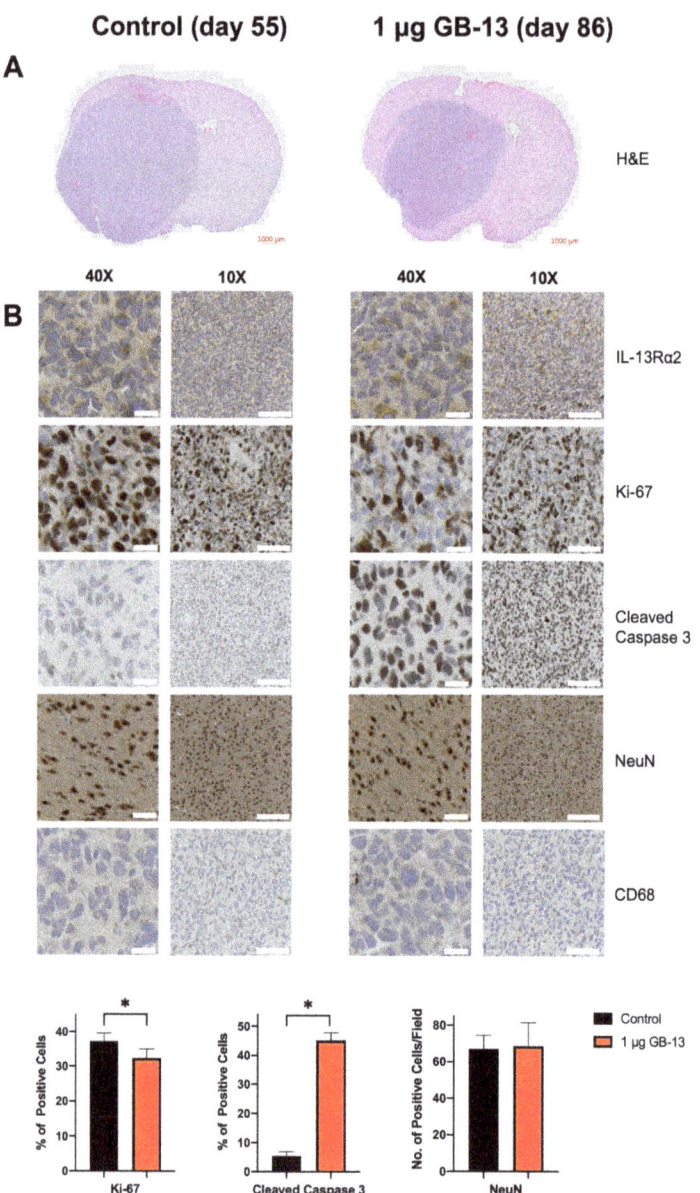

Figure 4. Immunohistochemistry of HGG-bearing mouse brains harvested when moribund. Presented samples were harvested on days 55 and 86 following CED of vehicle solution or GB-13 at a dose of 1 µg, respectively. Images are representative of four mice in each group. (**A**) Corresponding H&E demonstrates maintained tissue architecture and decreased tumor size after GB-13 treatment. (**B**) While IL-13Rα2 status is retained after a single CED infusion of GB-13, treatment leads to decreased cell proliferation ($p = 0.03$) and increases the number of apoptotic cells ($p < 0.0001$). The density of NeuN-positive neuronal (NeuN+) cells is retained in ipsilateral brain regions ($p = 0.82$). CD68+ monocyte infiltrate is not evidenced following GB-13 exposure. Scale bars: 40×: 20 µm, 10×: 100 µm.

Finally, we used the DMG cell line SU-DIPG XIII-P to establish a brainstem HGG xenograft model with low IL-13Rα2 protein levels. Based on the in vitro data, we did not expect GB-13 to impact tumor volume or survival using the previously established dosing regimen. Indeed, CED of 0.1, 0.3, or 1 μg of GB-13 failed to demonstrate significant tumor growth reduction (p = 0.16, 0.18 and 0.27, respectively; Figure 3F) and did not provide profound survival benefit compared to control animals (24.5 days in vehicle, 23 days in 0.1 μg GB-13 (p = 0.92), 24 days in 0.3 μg GB-13 (p = 0.68) and 24 days in 1 μg GB-13 (p = 0.57)) (Figure 3G). While the CED procedure proved to be feasible and safe among all treatment groups, 2 of 5 animals dosed with 1 μg of GB-13 had to be euthanized within 72 h of drug administration. No CD68+ immune cell infiltration or reduction in NeuN-positive cells was observed in mice treated with 0.1 or 0.3 μg of GB-13, there was again evidence of reduced NeuN+ cell density in the brainstem of animals treated with 1 μg of GB-13. IHC did not show increased staining for cleaved caspase 3 in GB-13 drug-treated IL-13Rα2-low xenografts, and a high degree of cellular proliferation was retained in these tumors after GB-13 infusion. In accordance with in vitro protein-level analysis, IHC staining for IL-13Rα2 was absent in SU-DIPG XIII-P xenografts. Furthermore, H3 K27M and H3 K27me3 remained largely unchanged in vehicle versus GB-13-treated tumors (Figures S5 and S6). These results suggest that moderate to high IL-13Rα2 expression is required for targeted therapies such as GB-13 to impart therapeutic effect in HGG orthotopic xenograft models.

4. Discussion

To date, the search for effective treatment against HGGs has not substantially improved outcomes [55–58]. IL-13Rα2 represents a clinically validated target in HGG therapy [33,34,36]. In this study, we identified a favorable correlation between IL-13Rα2 mRNA and protein levels. IL-13Rα2 status predicted the efficacy of a novel IL-13 immunotoxin, GB-13, in cultured HGG cells. Intraparenchymal administration of GB-13 into orthotopically implanted patient-derived xenograft models of HGG was feasible, and a single therapeutic infusion of GB-13 using CED significantly ameliorated tumor burden and resulted in significant prolongation in survival of animals harboring IL-13Rα2-upregulated orthotopic xenografts, underscoring the promise of IL-13Rα2 targeting in the context of HGG with increased IL-13Rα2 expression.

IL-13Rα2 has long been recognized as a prognostic biomarker for poor disease prognosis in brain tumors including HGG [16,32,59]. While the negligible impact of canonical ligand-mediated IL-13Rα2 stimulation on cell proliferation in IL-13Rα2-high versus IL-13Rα2-low cell lines was somewhat surprising, similar results have been previously reported in cell growth and invasion studies [52]. Recent investigations have elucidated the role of IL-13Rα2 as a tumor-associated antigen that mediates aberrant STAT3 signaling, driving increased expression of anti-apoptotic genes and, ultimately, promoting tumor progression by blocking cell death and mediating survival [17,59,60]. These findings mirror those observed in this study, in that IL-13Rα2-upregulated HGG cells selectively increase expression of IL-13Rα2, but not IL-13Rα1, the functional counterpart, when exposed to IL-13, a natural IL-13Rα2-binding partner. We were able to expand these and previous observations by demonstrating that binding of GB-13 equally induces upregulation of IL-13Rα2 in IL-13Rα2-expressing HGG cells [61,62]. Together, this holds promise for IL-13Rα2-targeting agents to achieve repeated and durable response in HGG with increased IL-13Rα2 levels.

Previous efforts to target IL-13Rα2 by various treatment modalities suggest the utility of cellular immunotherapy or immunoconjugates for HGG therapy [32,33,63,64]. The clinical effect of immunotoxins is heavily linked to payload efficacy. Consequently, a pivotal requirement in the design of an immunotoxin is the selection of an exceedingly potent cytotoxic capable of inducing cellular death at low (~10 nM) concentrations [65]. The foundational efforts of Puri and colleagues in developing cintredekin besudotox have demonstrated the feasibility of creating such a molecule for killing of IL-13Rα2-expressing cells by linking a truncated form of PE to human IL-13 [66]. GB-13 is essentially the successor of cintredekin besudotox, featuring refinements to both the targeting moiety and the payload domain [24]. We observed favorable potency with GB-13 compared to previous reports of cintredekin besudotox in IL-13Rα2-upregulated HGG cell lines [42,66–69]. Interestingly, the cytotoxic effect of GB-13 was highly dependent on IL-13Rα2 status, with GB-13 demonstrating dose-depending killing at concentrations more than 100-fold lower in IL-13Rα2-high versus IL-13Rα2-low HGG cells. This observation, whereas potentially underappreciated by previous in vitro investigations of IL-13Rα2-targeting agents, has profound implications for the clinical application of these therapeutics in HGG, where IL-13Rα2 overexpression is detected in a subset of, but not all, tumors [15,23,30,31].

Delivery of immunotoxins via CED is a valuable approach to circumvent the BBB and ensure brain-targeted drug delivery of cytotoxic payloads; however, there is growing evidence that this strategy has unique pitfalls to consider. A phase I study using single-catheter convective infusion of cintredekin besudotox in pediatric patients with DIPG and supratentorial HGG was terminated because the drug did not to reach the predefined distribution volume to cover the entire tumor area on MRI and MR spectroscopy [34]. While several phase I/II studies of CED with cintredekin besudotox for adult patients with HGG showed promise [33,36,64], the only phase III clinical trial, the PRECISE study, failed to demonstrate a 50% improvement in median survival over Gliadel wafers [33]. Extensive post-trial analyses investigated possible explanations for the lack of efficacy observed. While technical issues surrounding catheter placement and drug distribution are surmountable in future studies by optimizing catheter design and positioning of potentially multiple catheters, there was limited consideration of target expression for patient inclusion [37,70]. A large scale analysis of clinical trials utilizing biomarkers found significant improvement in trial success relative to no biomarker inclusion criteria [71]. Consistent with this idea, we compared IL-13Rα2 mRNA and protein levels from homogeneous cell populations, which showed that gene expression correlates with IL-13Rα2 protein status. The herein presented findings in HGG xenograft models with low, medium and high IL-13Rα2 levels demonstrate that GB-13 decreases tumor volume and prolongs survival in a manner strongly associated with IL-13Rα2 status. Although no benefit was observed in animals harboring IL-13Rα2-low HGG, IL-13Rα2-medium and IL-13Rα2-high animals had significantly reduced tumor burden and lived significantly longer than vehicle-treated animals, indicating IL-13Rα2 may not only be a therapeutic target but also a predictive biomarker for future clinical trial patient inclusion.

The moderate anti-tumor efficacy of GB-13 across multiple IL-13Rα2-expressing HGG models provides some support for an early-phase clinical trial in patients with upregulated IL-13Rα2 expressing tumors. However, our study also highlight several limitations. First, high-dose CED infusion into the brainstem of HGG-bearing mice was associated with profound toxicity, which indicates a narrow therapeutic window for this agent when delivered directly into eloquent brain regions. This is especially notable since a previous in vivo study of intra-tumoral GB-13 in a murine model of malignant peripheral nerve sheath tumor did not find dose-limiting toxicities [24]. Furthermore, observed toxicities in a phase I clinical trial of cintredekin besudotox delivered by CED into the brainstem of DIPG patients were limited to transient cranial nerve deficits and lethargy after infusion [72]. While the high local concentrations of infused GB-13 in the comparatively small mouse brainstem likely contributed to the observed peritumoral toxicity in our study, the data presented warrant further investigation before moving into clinical testing. Second, our findings are limited to a single therapeutic infusion of GB-13. Previous studies using CED to deliver small molecules to the brain have shown that these drugs were rapidly cleared from the infusion site [73]. Although large biomolecules such as GB-13 are likely to remain in the brain for longer periods of time, clinical applications may require multiple infusions or longer infusion durations to achieve adequate drug distribution and sustained therapeutic effect. To this extent, a recent clinical trial has demonstrated safety of sequential CED infusions into the pediatric brainstem [74]. Finally, we evaluated GB-13 as a monotherapy, which has obvious limitations considering the long history of negative clinical trials for HGG. The efficacy of IL-13Rα2-targeted therapy has previously been shown to be enhanced by both radiation and cytotoxic chemotherapy [36,75]. Efficacious in HGG with high IL-13Rα2 levels, future studies should investigate GB-13 as part of a comprehensive treatment regimen, including a rational combination of therapeutic strategies that have previously demonstrated to be beneficial in this devastating disease.

5. Conclusions

HGGs encompass a large proportion of malignant tumors within the central nervous system. Up to 80% of HGG overexpress the tumor-associated receptor IL-13Rα2. Despite advances in our understanding of underlying disease mechanisms, the prognosis for HGG remains dismal and efficacious therapies are lacking. As such, there is a dire, unmet, gap in clinical practice for treating this devastating disease. Here, we investigated the pharmacological effects of GB-13, a novel tumor-specific immunotoxin that contains an engineered mutant of human IL-13 fused to a cytotoxic PE molecule. Administration of GB-13 demonstrated a promising pharmacological response in DMG and adult GBM models both in vitro and in vivo in a manner strongly associated with IL-13Rα2 status, underscoring the potential of this IL-13Rα2-targeted therapy in a subset of HGG with increased IL-13Rα2 expression.

Supplementary Materials: The following supporting information can be downloaded at: https://www.mdpi.com/article/10.3390/pharmaceutics14050922/s1, Figure S1: Cell viability and dose–response curve of adult GBM cell models; Figure S2: DMG and adult GBM cell lines demonstrate similar sensitivity towards GB-13 dependent on IL-13Rα2 status; Figure S3: Immunofluorescence of SF8628 cells, a DMG cell line, after 8, 24, 48, and 72 h of GB-13 exposure at IC_{50}; Figure S4: Immunohistochemistry of PED17-bearing mouse brains harvested at endpoint; Figure S5: Immunohistochemistry of SU-DIPG XIII-P-bearing mouse brains harvested at endpoint; Figure S6: Negative staining controls for immunofluorescence and immunohistochemistry experiments; Table S1: Details regarding the cell lines used in this study; Table S2: Media composition for culture of patient-derived cell lines; Table S3: Antibodies used for immunoblotting, immunofluorescence and immunohistochemistry.

Author Contributions: Conceptualization, J.S.R., K.A.P., D.J.D., J.N.S. and R.S.S.; methodology, validation and analysis, J.S.R., K.A.P., L.Z., C.L.N. and R.S.S.; writing—original draft preparation, J.S.R.; writing—review and editing, J.S.R., D.J.D., J.N.S., L.Z., C.L.N. and R.S.S.; visualization, J.S.R., L.Z. and C.L.N.; supervision, D.J.D. and J.N.S. All authors have read and agreed to the published version of the manuscript.

Funding: This research was supported by the foundation Brains Together for a Cure. D.J.D. acknowledges K08 Award Number NS092891 from the National Institute of Neurological Disorders and Stroke (NINDS).

Institutional Review Board Statement: The animal study protocol was approved by the Institutional Committee for Animal Research of Mayo Clinic (protocol code A00004595-19 and A00003911-18-R21).

Informed Consent Statement: Informed consent was obtained for all patient-derived cell lines involved in this study.

Data Availability Statement: All data supporting reported results can be found in the manuscript and Supplementary Materials to the manuscript.

Acknowledgments: The authors gratefully thank Michelle Monje (Stanford University), Edward Hinchcliffe (Hormel Institute) and Charles Day (Hormel Institute) for use of SU-DIPG XIII-P and SF8628-B23 cell lines, respectively. Furthermore, we acknowledge the generous support of Ann Mladek, Shiv Gupta and Jizhi Ge.

Conflicts of Interest: The funders had no role in the design of the study; in the collection, analyses, or interpretation of data; in the writing of the manuscript, or in the decision to publish the results.

References

1. Ostrom, Q.T.; Cioffi, G.; Waite, K.; Kruchko, C.; Barnholtz-Sloan, J.S. CBTRUS Statistical Report: Primary Brain and Other Central Nervous System Tumors Diagnosed in the United States in 2014–2018. *Neuro-Oncol.* **2021**, *23*, iii1–iii105. [CrossRef]
2. Louis, D.N.; Perry, A.; Wesseling, P.; Brat, D.J.; Cree, I.A.; Figarella-Branger, D.; Hawkins, C.; Ng, H.K.; Pfister, S.M.; Reifenberger, G.; et al. The 2021 WHO Classification of Tumors of the Central Nervous System: A summary. *Neuro-Oncol.* **2021**, *23*, 1231–1251. [CrossRef] [PubMed]
3. Hargrave, D.; Bartels, U.; Bouffet, E. Diffuse brainstem glioma in children: Critical review of clinical trials. *Lancet Oncol.* **2006**, *7*, 241–248. [CrossRef]
4. Giagnacovo, M.; Antonelli, M.; Biassoni, V.; Schiavello, E.; Warmuth-Metz, M.; Buttarelli, F.R.; Modena, P.; Massimino, M. Retrospective analysis on the consistency of MRI features with histological and molecular markers in diffuse intrinsic pontine glioma (DIPG). *Childs Nerv. Syst.* **2020**, *36*, 697–704. [CrossRef] [PubMed]
5. Tam, L.T.; Yeom, K.W.; Wright, J.N.; Jaju, A.; Radmanesh, A.; Han, M.; Toescu, S.; Maleki, M.; Chen, E.; Campion, A.; et al. MRI-based radiomics for prognosis of pediatric diffuse intrinsic pontine glioma: An international study. *Neurooncol. Adv.* **2021**, *3*, vdab042. [CrossRef]
6. Wu, G.; Broniscer, A.; McEachron, T.A.; Lu, C.; Paugh, B.S.; Becksfort, J.; Qu, C.; Ding, L.; Huether, R.; Parker, M.; et al. Somatic histone H3 alterations in pediatric diffuse intrinsic pontine gliomas and non-brainstem glioblastomas. *Nat. Genet.* **2012**, *44*, 251–253. [CrossRef] [PubMed]
7. Schwartzentruber, J.; Korshunov, A.; Liu, X.Y.; Jones, D.T.; Pfaff, E.; Jacob, K.; Sturm, D.; Fontebasso, A.M.; Quang, D.A.; Tönjes, M.; et al. Driver mutations in histone H3.3 and chromatin remodelling genes in paediatric glioblastoma. *Nature* **2012**, *482*, 226–231. [CrossRef] [PubMed]
8. Warren, K.E. Diffuse intrinsic pontine glioma: Poised for progress. *Front. Oncol.* **2012**, *2*, 205. [CrossRef] [PubMed]
9. Stupp, R.; Mason, W.P.; van den Bent, M.J.; Weller, M.; Fisher, B.; Taphoorn, M.J.; Belanger, K.; Brandes, A.A.; Marosi, C.; Bogdahn, U.; et al. Radiotherapy plus concomitant and adjuvant temozolomide for glioblastoma. *N. Engl. J. Med.* **2005**, *352*, 987–996. [CrossRef] [PubMed]
10. Wen, P.Y.; Weller, M.; Lee, E.Q.; Alexander, B.M.; Barnholtz-Sloan, J.S.; Barthel, F.P.; Batchelor, T.T.; Bindra, R.S.; Chang, S.M.; Chiocca, E.A.; et al. Glioblastoma in adults: A Society for Neuro-Oncology (SNO) and European Society of Neuro-Oncology (EANO) consensus review on current management and future directions. *Neuro-Oncol.* **2020**, *22*, 1073–1113. [CrossRef]
11. Razavi, S.M.; Lee, K.E.; Jin, B.E.; Aujla, P.S.; Gholamin, S.; Li, G. Immune Evasion Strategies of Glioblastoma. *Front. Surg.* **2016**, *3*, 11. [CrossRef] [PubMed]
12. Fecci, P.E.; Sampson, J.H. The current state of immunotherapy for gliomas: An eye toward the future. *J. Neurosurg.* **2019**, *131*, 657–666. [CrossRef] [PubMed]
13. D'Amico, R.S.; Aghi, M.K.; Vogelbaum, M.A.; Bruce, J.N. Convection-enhanced drug delivery for glioblastoma: A review. *J. Neurooncol.* **2021**, *151*, 415–427. [CrossRef]
14. Faltings, L.; Kulason, K.O.; Patel, N.V.; Wong, T.; Fralin, S.; Li, M.; Schneider, J.R.; Filippi, C.G.; Langer, D.J.; Ortiz, R.; et al. Rechallenging Recurrent Glioblastoma with Intra-Arterial Bevacizumab with Blood Brain-Barrier Disruption Results in Radiographic Response. *World Neurosurg.* **2019**, *131*, 234–241. [CrossRef]
15. Joshi, B.H.; Plautz, G.E.; Puri, R.K. Interleukin-13 receptor alpha chain: A novel tumor-associated transmembrane protein in primary explants of human malignant gliomas. *Cancer Res.* **2000**, *60*, 1168–1172. [PubMed]
16. Zeng, J.; Zhang, J.; Yang, Y.Z.; Wang, F.; Jiang, H.; Chen, H.D.; Wu, H.Y.; Sai, K.; Hu, W.M. IL13RA2 is overexpressed in malignant gliomas and related to clinical outcome of patients. *Am. J. Transl. Res.* **2020**, *12*, 4702–4714. [PubMed]
17. Rahaman, S.O.; Sharma, P.; Harbor, P.C.; Aman, M.J.; Vogelbaum, M.A.; Haque, S.J. IL-13Rα2, a decoy receptor for IL-13 acts as an inhibitor of IL-4-dependent signal transduction in glioblastoma cells. *Cancer Res.* **2002**, *62*, 1103–1109. [PubMed]
18. Lupardus, P.J.; Birnbaum, M.E.; Garcia, K.C. Molecular basis for shared cytokine recognition revealed in the structure of an unusually high affinity complex between IL-13 and IL-13Ralpha2. *Structure* **2010**, *18*, 332–342. [CrossRef]
19. Bhardwaj, R.; Suzuki, A.; Leland, P.; Joshi, B.H.; Puri, R.K. Identification of a novel role of IL-13Rα2 in human Glioblastoma multiforme: Interleukin-13 mediates signal transduction through AP-1 pathway. *J. Transl. Med.* **2018**, *16*, 369. [CrossRef] [PubMed]
20. Cheng, Y.; Dai, Q.; Morshed, R.A.; Fan, X.; Wegscheid, M.L.; Wainwright, D.A.; Han, Y.; Zhang, L.; Auffinger, B.; Tobias, A.L.; et al. Blood-brain barrier permeable gold nanoparticles: An efficient delivery platform for enhanced malignant glioma therapy and imaging. *Small* **2014**, *10*, 5137–5150. [CrossRef] [PubMed]
21. Jarboe, J.S.; Johnson, K.R.; Choi, Y.; Lonser, R.R.; Park, J.K. Expression of interleukin-13 receptor alpha2 in glioblastoma multiforme: Implications for targeted therapies. *Cancer Res.* **2007**, *67*, 7983–7986. [CrossRef]
22. Tu, M.; Wange, W.; Cai, L.; Zhu, P.; Gao, Z.; Zheng, W. IL-13 receptor α2 stimulates human glioma cell growth and metastasis through the Src/PI3K/Akt/mTOR signaling pathway. *Tumour Biol.* **2016**, *37*, 14701–14709. [CrossRef] [PubMed]
23. Berlow, N.E.; Svalina, M.N.; Quist, M.J.; Settelmeyer, T.P.; Zherebitskiy, V.; Kogiso, M.; Qi, L.; Du, Y.; Hawkins, C.E.; Hulleman, E.; et al. IL-13 receptors as possible therapeutic targets in diffuse intrinsic pontine glioma. *PLoS ONE* **2018**, *13*, e0193565. [CrossRef] [PubMed]

24. Mrowczynski, O.D.; Payne, R.A.; Bourcier, A.J.; Mau, C.Y.; Slagle-Webb, B.; Shenoy, G.; Madhankumar, A.B.; Abramson, S.B.; Wolfe, D.; Harbaugh, K.S.; et al. Targeting IL-13Rα2 for effective treatment of malignant peripheral nerve sheath tumors in mouse models. *J. Neurosurg.* **2018**, *131*, 1369–1379. [CrossRef] [PubMed]
25. Bartolomé, R.A.; García-Palmero, I.; Torres, S.; López-Lucendo, M.; Balyasnikova, I.V.; Casal, J.I. IL13 Receptor α2 Signaling Requires a Scaffold Protein, FAM120A, to Activate the FAK and PI3K Pathways in Colon Cancer Metastasis. *Cancer Res.* **2015**, *75*, 2434–2444. [CrossRef]
26. Fujisawa, T.; Joshi, B.; Nakajima, A.; Puri, R.K. A novel role of interleukin-13 receptor alpha2 in pancreatic cancer invasion and metastasis. *Cancer Res.* **2009**, *69*, 8678–8685. [CrossRef] [PubMed]
27. Kioi, M.; Kawakami, M.; Shimamura, T.; Husain, S.R.; Puri, R.K. Interleukin-13 receptor alpha2 chain: A potential biomarker and molecular target for ovarian cancer therapy. *Cancer* **2006**, *107*, 1407–1418. [CrossRef] [PubMed]
28. Okamoto, H.; Yoshimatsu, Y.; Tomizawa, T.; Kunita, A.; Takayama, R.; Morikawa, T.; Komura, D.; Takahashi, K.; Oshima, T.; Sato, M.; et al. Interleukin-13 receptor α2 is a novel marker and potential therapeutic target for human melanoma. *Sci. Rep.* **2019**, *9*, 1281. [CrossRef]
29. Joshi, B.H.; Leland, P.; Puri, R.K. Identification and characterization of interleukin-13 receptor in human medulloblastoma and targeting these receptors with interleukin-13-pseudomonas exotoxin fusion protein. *Croat. Med. J.* **2003**, *44*, 455–462. [PubMed]
30. Kawakami, M.; Kawakami, K.; Takahashi, S.; Abe, M.; Puri, R.K. Analysis of interleukin-13 receptor alpha2 expression in human pediatric brain tumors. *Cancer* **2004**, *101*, 1036–1042. [CrossRef]
31. Debinski, W.; Gibo, D.M.; Hulet, S.W.; Connor, J.R.; Gillespie, G.Y. Receptor for interleukin 13 is a marker and therapeutic target for human high-grade gliomas. *Clin. Cancer Res.* **1999**, *5*, 985–990. [PubMed]
32. Brown, C.E.; Alizadeh, D.; Starr, R.; Weng, L.; Wagner, J.R.; Naranjo, A.; Ostberg, J.R.; Blanchard, M.S.; Kilpatrick, J.; Simpson, J.; et al. Regression of Glioblastoma after Chimeric Antigen Receptor T-Cell Therapy. *N. Engl. J. Med.* **2016**, *375*, 2561–2569. [CrossRef]
33. Kunwar, S.; Chang, S.; Westphal, M.; Vogelbaum, M.; Sampson, J.; Barnett, G.; Shaffrey, M.; Ram, Z.; Piepmeier, J.; Prados, M.; et al. Phase III randomized trial of CED of IL13-PE38QQR vs Gliadel wafers for recurrent glioblastoma. *Neuro-Oncol.* **2010**, *12*, 871–881. [CrossRef] [PubMed]
34. Heiss, J.D.; Jamshidi, A.; Shah, S.; Martin, S.; Wolters, P.L.; Argersinger, D.P.; Warren, K.E.; Lonser, R.R. Phase I trial of convection-enhanced delivery of IL13-Pseudomonas toxin in children with diffuse intrinsic pontine glioma. *J. Neurosurg. Pediatr.* **2018**, *23*, 333–342. [CrossRef]
35. Souweidane, M.M.; Occhiogrosso, G.; Mark, E.B.; Edgar, M.A. Interstitial infusion of IL13-PE38QQR in the rat brain stem. *J. Neurooncol.* **2004**, *67*, 287–293. [CrossRef]
36. Vogelbaum, M.A.; Sampson, J.H.; Kunwar, S.; Chang, S.M.; Shaffrey, M.; Asher, A.L.; Lang, F.F.; Croteau, D.; Parker, K.; Grahn, A.Y.; et al. Convection-enhanced delivery of cintredekin besudotox (interleukin-13-PE38QQR) followed by radiation therapy with and without temozolomide in newly diagnosed malignant gliomas: Phase 1 study of final safety results. *Neurosurgery* **2007**, *61*, 1031–1037; discussion 1037–1038. [CrossRef] [PubMed]
37. Shi, M.; Sanche, L. Convection-Enhanced Delivery in Malignant Gliomas: A Review of Toxicity and Efficacy. *J. Oncol.* **2019**, *2019*, 9342796. [CrossRef] [PubMed]
38. Chaudhary, V.K.; Jinno, Y.; Gallo, M.G.; FitzGerald, D.; Pastan, I. Mutagenesis of Pseudomonas exotoxin in identification of sequences responsible for the animal toxicity. *J. Biol. Chem.* **1990**, *265*, 16306–16310. [CrossRef]
39. Puri, R.K.; Leland, P.; Obiri, N.I.; Husain, S.R.; Kreitman, R.J.; Haas, G.P.; Pastan, I.; Debinski, W. Targeting of interleukin-13 receptor on human renal cell carcinoma cells by a recombinant chimeric protein composed of interleukin-13 and a truncated form of Pseudomonas exotoxin A (PE38QQR). *Blood* **1996**, *87*, 4333–4339. [CrossRef]
40. Jinno, Y.; Ogata, M.; Chaudhary, V.K.; Willingham, M.C.; Adhya, S.; FitzGerald, D.; Pastan, I. Domain II mutants of Pseudomonas exotoxin deficient in translocation. *J. Biol. Chem.* **1989**, *264*, 15953–15959. [CrossRef]
41. Armstrong, S.; Yates, S.P.; Merrill, A.R. Insight into the catalytic mechanism of Pseudomonas aeruginosa exotoxin A. Studies of toxin interaction with eukaryotic elongation factor-2. *J. Biol. Chem.* **2002**, *277*, 46669–46675. [CrossRef]
42. Du, X.; Youle, R.J.; FitzGerald, D.J.; Pastan, I. Pseudomonas exotoxin A-mediated apoptosis is Bak dependent and preceded by the degradation of Mcl-1. *Mol. Cell. Biol.* **2010**, *30*, 3444–3452. [CrossRef] [PubMed]
43. Cerami, E.; Gao, J.; Dogrusoz, U.; Gross, B.E.; Sumer, S.O.; Aksoy, B.A.; Jacobsen, A.; Byrne, C.J.; Heuer, M.L.; Larsson, E.; et al. The cBio cancer genomics portal: An open platform for exploring multidimensional cancer genomics data. *Cancer Discov.* **2012**, *2*, 401–404. [CrossRef]
44. Gao, J.; Aksoy, B.A.; Dogrusoz, U.; Dresdner, G.; Gross, B.; Sumer, S.O.; Sun, Y.; Jacobsen, A.; Sinha, R.; Larsson, E.; et al. Integrative analysis of complex cancer genomics and clinical profiles using the cBioPortal. *Sci. Signal.* **2013**, *6*, pl1. [CrossRef]
45. Dobin, A.; Davis, C.A.; Schlesinger, F.; Drenkow, J.; Zaleski, C.; Jha, S.; Batut, P.; Chaisson, M.; Gingeras, T.R. STAR: Ultrafast universal RNA-seq aligner. *Bioinformatics* **2013**, *29*, 15–21. [CrossRef] [PubMed]
46. Li, B.; Dewey, C.N. RSEM: Accurate transcript quantification from RNA-Seq data with or without a reference genome. *BMC Bioinform.* **2011**, *12*, 323. [CrossRef] [PubMed]
47. Nagaraja, S.; Vitanza, N.A.; Woo, P.J.; Taylor, K.R.; Liu, F.; Zhang, L.; Li, M.; Meng, W.; Ponnuswami, A.; Sun, W.; et al. Transcriptional Dependencies in Diffuse Intrinsic Pontine Glioma. *Cancer Cell* **2017**, *31*, 635–652.e636. [CrossRef]

48. Grasso, C.S.; Tang, Y.; Truffaux, N.; Berlow, N.E.; Liu, L.; Debily, M.A.; Quist, M.J.; Davis, L.E.; Huang, E.C.; Woo, P.J.; et al. Functionally defined therapeutic targets in diffuse intrinsic pontine glioma. *Nat. Med.* **2015**, *21*, 555–559. [CrossRef] [PubMed]
49. Welby, J.P.; Kaptzan, T.; Wohl, A.; Peterson, T.E.; Raghunathan, A.; Brown, D.A.; Gupta, S.K.; Zhang, L.; Daniels, D.J. Current Murine Models and New Developments in H3K27M Diffuse Midline Gliomas. *Front. Oncol.* **2019**, *9*, 92. [CrossRef]
50. Carlson, B.L.; Pokorny, J.L.; Schroeder, M.A.; Sarkaria, J.N. Establishment, maintenance and in vitro and in vivo applications of primary human glioblastoma multiforme (GBM) xenograft models for translational biology studies and drug discovery. *Curr. Protoc. Pharmacol.* **2011**, *52*, 14–23. [CrossRef] [PubMed]
51. Beffinger, M.; Schellhammer, L.; Pantelyushin, S.; Vom Berg, J. Delivery of Antibodies into the Murine Brain via Convection-enhanced Delivery. *J. Vis. Exp.* **2019**, *149*, e59675. [CrossRef]
52. Lian, X.; Kats, D.; Rasmussen, S.; Martin, L.R.; Karki, A.; Keller, C.; Berlow, N.E. Design considerations of an IL13Rα2 antibody-drug conjugate for diffuse intrinsic pontine glioma. *Acta Neuropathol. Commun.* **2021**, *9*, 88. [CrossRef]
53. Nagaraja, S.; Quezada, M.A.; Gillespie, S.M.; Arzt, M.; Lennon, J.J.; Woo, P.J.; Hovestadt, V.; Kambhampati, M.; Filbin, M.G.; Suva, M.L.; et al. Histone Variant and Cell Context Determine H3K27M Reprogramming of the Enhancer Landscape and Oncogenic State. *Mol. Cell* **2019**, *76*, 965–980.e912. [CrossRef]
54. Rechberger, J.S.; Power, E.A.; Lu, V.M.; Zhang, L.; Sarkaria, J.N.; Daniels, D.J. Evaluating infusate parameters for direct drug delivery to the brainstem: A comparative study of convection-enhanced delivery versus osmotic pump delivery. *Neurosurg. Focus* **2020**, *48*, E2. [CrossRef]
55. Rechberger, J.S.; Lu, V.M.; Zhang, L.; Power, E.A.; Daniels, D.J. Clinical trials for diffuse intrinsic pontine glioma: The current state of affairs. *Childs Nerv. Syst.* **2020**, *36*, 39–46. [CrossRef]
56. Vanan, M.I.; Eisenstat, D.D. DIPG in Children—What Can We Learn from the Past? *Front. Oncol.* **2015**, *5*, 237. [CrossRef] [PubMed]
57. Gittleman, H.; Boscia, A.; Ostrom, Q.T.; Truitt, G.; Fritz, Y.; Kruchko, C.; Barnholtz-Sloan, J.S. Survivorship in adults with malignant brain and other central nervous system tumor from 2000–2014. *Neuro-Oncol.* **2018**, *20*, vii6–vii16. [CrossRef] [PubMed]
58. Sarkaria, J.N.; Hu, L.S.; Parney, I.F.; Pafundi, D.H.; Brinkmann, D.H.; Laack, N.N.; Giannini, C.; Burns, T.C.; Kizilbash, S.H.; Laramy, J.K.; et al. Is the blood-brain barrier really disrupted in all glioblastomas? A critical assessment of existing clinical data. *Neuro-Oncol.* **2018**, *20*, 184–191. [CrossRef]
59. Joshi, B.H.; Puri, R.K. IL-13 receptor-alpha2: A novel target for cancer therapy. *Immunotherapy* **2009**, *1*, 321–327. [CrossRef]
60. Rahaman, S.O.; Vogelbaum, M.A.; Haque, S.J. Aberrant Stat3 signaling by interleukin-4 in malignant glioma cells: Involvement of IL-13Ralpha1. *Cancer Res.* **2005**, *65*, 2956–2963. [CrossRef]
61. Utsuyama, M.; Hirokawa, K. Differential expression of various cytokine receptors in the brain after stimulation with LPS in young and old mice. *Exp. Gerontol.* **2002**, *37*, 411–420. [CrossRef]
62. Xiao, L.; Li, T.; Ding, M.; Yang, J.; Rodríguez-Corrales, J.; LaConte, S.M.; Nacey, N.; Weiss, D.B.; Jin, L.; Dorn, H.C.; et al. Detecting Chronic Post-Traumatic Osteomyelitis of Mouse Tibia via an IL-13Rα2 Targeted Metallofullerene Magnetic Resonance Imaging Probe. *Bioconjug. Chem.* **2017**, *28*, 649–658. [CrossRef]
63. Candolfi, M.; Xiong, W.; Yagiz, K.; Liu, C.; Muhammad, A.K.; Puntel, M.; Foulad, D.; Zadmehr, A.; Ahlzadeh, G.E.; Kroeger, K.M.; et al. Gene therapy-mediated delivery of targeted cytotoxins for glioma therapeutics. *Proc. Natl. Acad. Sci. USA* **2010**, *107*, 20021–20026. [CrossRef] [PubMed]
64. Kunwar, S.; Prados, M.D.; Chang, S.M.; Berger, M.S.; Lang, F.F.; Piepmeier, J.M.; Sampson, J.H.; Ram, Z.; Gutin, P.H.; Gibbons, R.D.; et al. Direct intracerebral delivery of cintredekin besudotox (IL13-PE38QQR) in recurrent malignant glioma: A report by the Cintredekin Besudotox Intraparenchymal Study Group. *J. Clin. Oncol.* **2007**, *25*, 837–844. [CrossRef] [PubMed]
65. Nejadmoghaddam, M.R.; Minai-Tehrani, A.; Ghahremanzadeh, R.; Mahmoudi, M.; Dinarvand, R.; Zarnani, A.H. Antibody-Drug Conjugates: Possibilities and Challenges. *Avicenna J. Med. Biotechnol.* **2019**, *11*, 3–23.
66. Debinski, W.; Obiri, N.I.; Pastan, I.; Puri, R.K. A novel chimeric protein composed of interleukin 13 and Pseudomonas exotoxin is highly cytotoxic to human carcinoma cells expressing receptors for interleukin 13 and interleukin 4. *J. Biol. Chem.* **1995**, *270*, 16775–16780. [CrossRef] [PubMed]
67. Kawakami, M.; Kawakami, K.; Puri, R.K. Intratumor administration of interleukin 13 receptor-targeted cytotoxin induces apoptotic cell death in human malignant glioma tumor xenografts. *Mol. Cancer Ther.* **2002**, *1*, 999–1007.
68. Husain, S.R.; Puri, R.K. Interleukin-13 receptor-directed cytotoxin for malignant glioma therapy: From bench to bedside. *J. Neurooncol.* **2003**, *65*, 37–48. [CrossRef]
69. Husain, S.R.; Joshi, B.H.; Puri, R.K. Interleukin-13 receptor as a unique target for anti-glioblastoma therapy. *Int. J. Cancer* **2001**, *92*, 168–175. [CrossRef]
70. Mueller, S.; Polley, M.Y.; Lee, B.; Kunwar, S.; Pedain, C.; Wembacher-Schröder, E.; Mittermeyer, S.; Westphal, M.; Sampson, J.H.; Vogelbaum, M.A.; et al. Effect of imaging and catheter characteristics on clinical outcome for patients in the PRECISE study. *J. Neurooncol.* **2011**, *101*, 267–277. [CrossRef] [PubMed]
71. Parker, J.L.; Kuzulugil, S.S.; Pereverzev, K.; Mac, S.; Lopes, G.; Shah, Z.; Weerasinghe, A.; Rubinger, D.; Falconi, A.; Bener, A.; et al. Does biomarker use in oncology improve clinical trial failure risk? A large-scale analysis. *Cancer Med.* **2021**, *10*, 1955–1963. [CrossRef]

72. Lieb, S.; Blaha-Ostermann, S.; Kamper, E.; Rippka, J.; Schwarz, C.; Ehrenhöfer-Wölfer, K.; Schlattl, A.; Wernitznig, A.; Lipp, J.J.; Nagasaka, K.; et al. Werner syndrome helicase is a selective vulnerability of microsatellite instability-high tumor cells. *eLife* **2019**, *8*, e43333. [CrossRef] [PubMed]
73. Singleton, W.G.B.; Bienemann, A.S.; Woolley, M.; Johnson, D.; Lewis, O.; Wyatt, M.J.; Damment, S.J.P.; Boulter, L.J.; Killick-Cole, C.L.; Asby, D.J.; et al. The distribution, clearance, and brainstem toxicity of panobinostat administered by convection-enhanced delivery. *J. Neurosurg. Pediatr.* **2018**, *22*, 288–296. [CrossRef] [PubMed]
74. Bander, E.D.; Ramos, A.D.; Wembacher-Schroeder, E.; Ivasyk, I.; Thomson, R.; Morgenstern, P.F.; Souweidane, M.M. Repeat convection-enhanced delivery for diffuse intrinsic pontine glioma. *J. Neurosurg. Pediatr.* **2020**, *26*, 661–666. [CrossRef]
75. Kawakami, K.; Kawakami, M.; Liu, Q.; Puri, R.K. Combined effects of radiation and interleukin-13 receptor-targeted cytotoxin on glioblastoma cell lines. *Int. J. Radiat. Oncol. Biol. Phys.* **2005**, *63*, 230–237. [CrossRef] [PubMed]

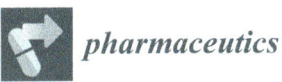

Article

An On-Demand Drug Delivery System for Control of Epileptiform Seizures

Takashi Nakano [1,†], Shakila B. Rizwan [2,†], David M. A. Myint [3], Jason Gray [4], Sean M. Mackay [3], Paul Harris [5], Christopher G. Perk [4], Brian I. Hyland [6], Ruth Empson [6], Eng Wui Tan [3], Keshav M. Dani [7], John NJ Reynolds [4] and Jeffery R. Wickens [1,*]

1. Neurobiology Research Unit, Okinawa Institute of Science and Technology Graduate University, Okinawa 904-0495, Japan; nakano.takashi@gmail.com
2. School of Pharmacy, University of Otago, Dunedin 9016, New Zealand; shakila.rizwan@otago.ac.nz
3. Department of Chemistry, University of Otago, Dunedin 9016, New Zealand; dmyint@atascientific.com.au (D.M.A.M.); sean.mackay@otago.ac.nz (S.M.M.); ewtan@chemistry.otago.ac.nz (E.W.T.)
4. Department of Anatomy, University of Otago, Dunedin 9016, New Zealand; jason.gray@otago.ac.nz (J.G.); cperk@umass.edu (C.G.P.); john.reynolds@otago.ac.nz (J.N.R.)
5. Callaghan Innovation, Wellington 5010, New Zealand; paul.harris@callaghaninnovation.govt.nz
6. Department of Physiology, University of Otago, Dunedin 9016, New Zealand; brian.hyland@otago.ac.nz (B.I.H.); ruth.empson@otago.ac.nz (R.E.)
7. Femtosecond Spectroscopy Unit, Okinawa Institute of Science and Technology Graduate University, Okinawa 904-0495, Japan; kmdani@oist.jp
* Correspondence: wickens@oist.jp; Tel.: +81-98-966-8875
† These authors contributed equally to this work.

Abstract: Drug delivery systems have the potential to deliver high concentrations of drug to target areas on demand, while elsewhere and at other times encapsulating the drug, to limit unwanted actions. Here we show proof of concept *in vivo* and *ex vivo* tests of a novel drug delivery system based on hollow-gold nanoparticles tethered to liposomes (HGN-liposomes), which become transiently permeable when activated by optical or acoustic stimulation. We show that laser or ultrasound simulation of HGN-liposomes loaded with the $GABA_A$ receptor agonist, muscimol, triggers rapid and repeatable release in a sufficient concentration to inhibit neurons and suppress seizure activity. In particular, laser-stimulated release of muscimol from previously injected HGN-liposomes caused subsecond hyperpolarizations of the membrane potential of hippocampal pyramidal neurons, measured by whole cell intracellular recordings with patch electrodes. In hippocampal slices and hippocampal–entorhinal cortical wedges, seizure activity was immediately suppressed by muscimol release from HGN-liposomes triggered by laser or ultrasound pulses. After intravenous injection of HGN-liposomes in whole anesthetized rats, ultrasound stimulation applied to the brain through the dura attenuated the seizure activity induced by pentylenetetrazol. Ultrasound alone, or HGN-liposomes without ultrasound stimulation, had no effect. Intracerebrally-injected HGN-liposomes containing kainic acid retained their contents for at least one week, without damage to surrounding tissue. Thus, we demonstrate the feasibility of precise temporal control over exposure of neurons to the drug, potentially enabling therapeutic effects without continuous exposure. For future application, studies on the pharmacokinetics, pharmacodynamics, and toxicity of HGN-liposomes and their constituents, together with improved methods of targeting, are needed, to determine the utility and safety of the technology in humans.

Keywords: liposome; nanoparticle; seizure; laser; ultrasound

Citation: Nakano, T.; Rizwan, S.B.; Myint, D.M.A.; Gray, J.; Mackay, S.M.; Harris, P.; Perk, C.G.; Hyland, B.I.; Empson, R.; Tan, E.W.; et al. An On-Demand Drug Delivery System for Control of Epileptiform Seizures. *Pharmaceutics* 2022, 14, 468. https://doi.org/10.3390/pharmaceutics14020468

Academic Editor: Flávia Sousa

Received: 20 December 2021
Accepted: 17 February 2022
Published: 21 February 2022

Publisher's Note: MDPI stays neutral with regard to jurisdictional claims in published maps and institutional affiliations.

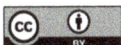

Copyright: © 2022 by the authors. Licensee MDPI, Basel, Switzerland. This article is an open access article distributed under the terms and conditions of the Creative Commons Attribution (CC BY) license (https://creativecommons.org/licenses/by/4.0/).

1. Introduction

Conventional drug treatments aim to minimize the side-effects of drugs by targeting specific receptors or bodily compartments. For diseases with episodic, paroxysmal expression, another way to limit side-effects is to reduce exposure to active drugs inside the body by delivering the drug only when and where it is needed [1]. Time-selective focal triggering of drug release has the potential to reduce side-effects by limiting drug exposure to the specific time period and location at which therapeutic effects occur [2]. Such a possibility requires the development of on-demand drug delivery devices that sequester drugs so that they remain inert until required, and trigger release when necessary. We here report the electrophysiological effects of on-demand release of the gama aminobuturic acid (GABA) agonist, muscimol, from hollow gold nanoparticle-tethered liposomes (HGN-liposomes) and its effectiveness in attenuating seizures in experimental animal models.

Liposomes are phospholipid-based vesicles composed of a lipid bilayer, in which a wide range of drugs can be encapsulated [3]. Drug release from liposomes can be triggered by external stimulation, such as hyperthermia [4]. Earlier studies aimed at discharging the entire contents of the liposomes in a single release event [5]. Later studies investigated the possibility of repeated release from liposomes over an extended life-time in the body. Our recently developed HGN-liposome system provides repetitive, on-demand release *ex vivo*, with the temporal profile and quantity of release controlled by varying laser power and exposure duration or pulses of low-intensity, therapeutic ultrasound (US) [6]. Here, we apply these technologies to release muscimol from liposomes within the extracellular matrix of the mammalian brain.

We used muscimol (3-hydroxy-5-aminomethylisoxazole) in the present study because it is a potent and selective $GABA_A$ receptor agonist, used extensively in electrophysiological studies of GABAergic inhibitory neurotransmission. Muscimol potently and reversibly inhibits neuronal activity, and thus has been considered to have the potential to suppress an epileptic seizure [7]. The metabolism of muscimol in both the brain and periphery is largely through the removal of an amino group by transamination [8]. In the mouse, about 1/3 is excreted as muscimol, 1/3 as a cationic conjugate, and 1/3 as an oxidation product [9]. The rapid clearance of muscimol in the periphery, and its slow passage across the blood–brain barrier (BBB), mean that high doses are needed when given intravenously, causing adverse effects, and making it unsuitable for systemic use in the treatment of epilepsy [10,11].

In contrast to systemic administration, when delivered transmeningeally in experimental animals, muscimol has antiepileptic effects, without the adverse effects associated with systemic delivery [12–15]. Direct injection of muscimol into the brain is orders-of-magnitude more effective than intravenous injection. For example, nanomomolar concentrations injected into brain produce similar effects to micromolar concentrations injected intravenously [16,17]. When injected locally into the brain in low μg quantities, muscimol produced no sedation or other central side-effects [18,19]. Similarly, studies of convection enhanced delivery of muscimol into the brain of non-human primates and patients with drug-resistant epilepsy, as well as other disorders, have shown that it is safe, with no adverse effects [20–22]. Thus, muscimol is a potential anti-epileptic treatment with few side-effects, provided it can be delivered directly to the brain. Muscimol is, therefore, a suitable candidate for proof of concept of the HGN-liposome delivery system.

Here, we used muscimol-loaded HGN-liposomes to produce repetitive on-demand release of muscimol within the extracellular matrix of the brain. We aimed to determine whether release of muscimol from HGN-liposomes by laser or ultrasound stimulation in live brain tissue was effective in attenuating seizure activity. We used three well-known models of seizure activity: two *ex vivo* models that rely on removal of Mg^{2+} ions and repetitive stimulation [23–25]; and *in vivo* pentylenetetrazol (PTZ), to cause seizures that propagate to status epilepticus [26]. We found that when muscimol-containing HGN-liposomes were present in brain slices, laser or US stimulation released muscimol on-demand and caused neural inhibition and arrest of seizure activity. Similarly, in whole animals, we found that US stimulation of the brain after intravenous injection of muscimol loaded HGN-liposomes was effective in reducing seizure activity.

2. Methods

2.1. Animals

A total of 11 mice and 58 rats were used in the research. Animals were handled in accordance with protocols approved by the Okinawa Institute of Science and Technology Animal Care and Use Committee (*ex vivo* hippocampal seizure model) and the University of Otago Animal Ethics Committee (*ex vivo* entorhinal cortex seizure model, and *in vivo* seizure model). In the *ex vivo* hippocampal experiments, brain slices were obtained from $n = 6$ male, 3 to 8-week-old Swiss Webster mice. Mice were group housed with littermates on reversed light cycle, with free access to standard chow and water. An additional $n = 5$ male 3 to 5-week-old Swiss Webster mice were used to test liposome ability to sequester contents in absence of stimulation. After injection, these mice were individually housed until perfused for histology. In the *ex vivo* entorhinal cortex experiments, brain slices were obtained from 40 male and female 4 to 8-week-old Wistar rats. In the *in vivo* experiments a total of $n = 18$ male Wistar rats were used, group housed in standard open top cages under reverse light cycle, and fed standard rat chow and water *ad libitum*. The targeted weight range was 250 to 300 g. These were allocated to four groups, unbiased by any animal-related factors (PTZ-only, $n = 3$; PTZ plus HGN-liposome, $n = 3$; US without liposomes, $n = 4$; and PTZ plus HGN-liposome plus US, $n = 8$).

2.2. HGN-Liposome Preparation

Liposomes and hollow gold nanoshells were prepared and assembled, as previously described [6,27,28], by conjugation using a terminal thiol-derived phospholipid (DSPE-PEG2000-SH) to produce a biocompatible drug delivery system that could encapsulate muscimol, a GABA agonist. DSPE-PEG2000-SH was synthesized by combining 1,2-distearoyl-sn-glycero-3-phosphoethanolamine-N-[amino(polyethylene glycol)-2000] (ammonium salt) (DSPE-PEG2000-NH$_2$) (100 mg; 35.8 µmol with 2-iminothiolane (10 mg, 73 µmol) in phosphate buffer (3 mmol L^{-1}; pH 9.5; 15 mL) for 30 min at room temperature. Sodium chloride (approx. 1 g) was dissolved in the reaction mixture, and the product was subsequently extracted into chloroform and dried over magnesium sulfate. The solvent was then removed by rotary evaporation, and the product was further dried under vacuum for 5 h.

Hollow gold nanoparticles were synthesized by the galvanic replacement of a silver nanoparticle template, as previously reported, resulting in a hydrodynamic diameter of approximately 30 nm and strong absorption in the visible to near-infrared region [29]. HGN-liposomes were prepared using a phospholipid composition previously described by our group [6,27,28]. Chloroform solutions of 1.2-distearoyl-sn-glycero-3-phosphcholine (DSPC), cholesterol, sphingomyelin, 1,2-distearoyl-sn-glycero-3-phosphoethanolamine-N-[methoxy(polyethylene glycol)-2000] (DSPE-PEG2000), DSPE-PEG2000-SH were combined in a molar ratio of 100:5:5:4:3.5. The solvent was removed under vacuum to form a thin lipid film, which was rehydrated using a phosphate-buffered solution (20 mmol L^{-1} Na$_2$HPO$_4$; pH 5.5) containing either 100 mmol L^{-1} muscimol or 25 mM kainic acid. The lipid suspension was then extruded through 400-nm polycarbonate membranes, to maximize the passive encapsulation of muscimol, producing uniformly sized liposomes for laser studies. However, as liposomes of smaller sizes are generally regarded as more suitable for intravenous administration, liposomes of 200 nm were prepared for ultrasound studies. The suspension of concentrated HGNs (Au concentration 6–10 mg mL^{-1} by inductively coupled plasma mass spectrometry) was added incrementally to the liposome suspension, until a final HGN:liposome ratio of approximately 1:1 was reached (as determined by transmission electron microscopy (Figure 1A). Approximately 200 µL of HGNs with an Au concentration of 7 mg mL^{-1} to 1 mL of 200 nm liposomes, with a total lipid concentration of 10 mmol L^{-1}, or approximately $\frac{1}{4}$ the amount of gold was added to 400 nm liposomes, with an equivalent 10 mmol L^{-1} phospholipid concentration. The HGN-liposome suspension was subsequently dialyzed against phosphate buffered saline (100 mmol L^{-1} NaCl; 20 mmol L^{-1} Na$_2$HPO$_4$; pH 7.4; 2 L) for 24 h to remove the unencapsulated muscimol.

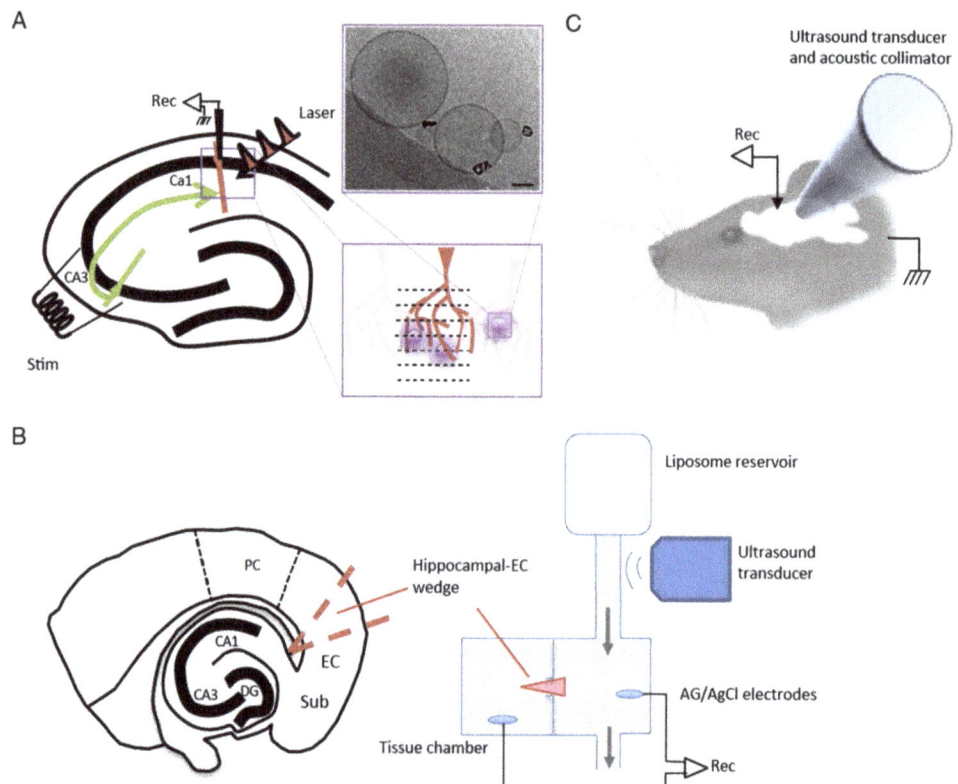

Figure 1. Experimental setups for three different models. (**A**) Hippocampal slice experiments. Schematic of hippocampal slice shows location of electrical field stimulating electrode (Stim) in area CA3, and whole cell intracellular recording electrode (Rec) in area CA1. Femtosecond pulses (Laser) were applied via the use of a 2-Photon microscope. Expanded schematic of CA1 shows location of dendrites (red) and liposomes (purple) in relation to sequential laser scan lines (dashes), forming a grid pattern in the dendritic zone. Example cryo-transmission electron microscope image shows liposomes tethered to hollow gold nanoshells (black; scale bar = 50 nm). (**B**) Entorhinal cortex wedge experiments. Schematic shows position of entorhinal cortex wedge, and wedge positioned in two-compartment grease gap chamber. Liposomes were stimulated with ultrasound as they passed into the tissue chamber. Grey arrows indicate flow of ACSF. (**C**). *In vivo* preparation. Field potential signals were obtained via an extracellular recording electrode (Rec) in the left frontal cortex. Liposomes were stimulated using an ultrasound transducer coupled to an acoustic collimator and positioned on the dura above the cortex.

We have previously reported on release measurements of dopamine, as well as carboxyfluorescein, from ultrasound and laser activated HGN liposomes [6,27]. In the present study, we were unable to do in vitro release studies for muscimol, because we were unable to identify a chemical, electrochemical, or spectroscopic assay that could distinguish between encapsulated and non-encapsulated muscimol and that was sensitive enough to measure its release in real time. Hence, we used the biological assays described below. Further details of the preparation and analysis of liposomal nanostructures and hollow gold nanoshells are given in Supplementary Materials Figures S1–S5.

2.3. Ex Vivo Hippocampal Seizure Model

Mice were deeply anesthetized with isoflurane and decapitated, and the brain was rapidly removed. Horizontal slices, 300 mm thick, containing the hippocampus were cut on a vibratome (VT1200S, Leica Microsystems, Wetzlar, Germany) in cold cutting solution containing the following (in mM): 92.0 N-methyl-D-glucamine (NMDG), 2.5 KCl, 10.0 $MgCl_2$, 0.5 $CaCl_2$, 1.25 NaH_2PO_4, 30.0 $NaHCO_3$, 20.0 HEPES, 2.0 thiourea, 5.0 sodium ascorbate, 3.0 sodium pyruvate, and 25.0 glucose, and saturated with 95% O_2—5% CO_2, Slices were then incubated in oxygenated artificial cerebrospinal fluid (ACSF) maintained at a temperature of 36 °C for 1 h. The standard ACSF had the following composition (mM): 118.0 NaCl, 2.5 KCl, 2.0 $CaCl_2$, 1.0 $MgCl_2$, 26.0 $NaHCO_3$, 1.25 NaH_2PO_4, 1.5 myo-inositol, 0.5 sodium ascorbate, 2.0 sodium pyruvate, and 10.0 Glucose. The composition of low Mg^{2+}/high K^+ ACSF was the same, except for (mM) 5.0 K^+ and 0.5 Mg^{2+}.

After incubation, a single slice was transferred to a recording chamber placed on the stage of an upright microscope, and perfused (3–4 mL/min) with oxygenated ACSF at 32 °C. HGN-liposomes were injected directly into the slice in the region of interest. The remaining slices were kept in a holding chamber containing oxygenated ACSF at room temperature until required.

The experimental setup for the hippocampal slice experiments is shown in Figure 1A. Whole-cell recordings were made from CA1 pyramidal neurons using patch pipettes (4–6 MΩ) filled with internal solution containing the following (mM): 132.0 K gluconate, 6.0 KCL, 6 $NaCl_2$, 10.0 HEPES, 2 $MgCL_2$, 2.0 NaATP, 0.4 NaGTP, 0.5 EGTA; pH 7.2–7.4. Local field potentials (LFPs) were recorded in the same location using extracellular electrodes positioned in the CA1 stratum pyramidal layer of the subiculum. LFPs were measured using borosilicate glass pipettes (1–2 MΩ) filled with ACSF. Signals were amplified by MultiClamp 700B (Molecular Devices, Union City, CA, USA), digitized at 10,000 Hz, and band-pass filtered over 1–2000 Hz by pCLAMP 10 (Molecular Devices, Silicon Valley, CA, USA). Offline analysis was conducted using MATLAB (MathWorks, Natick, MA, USA).

Optical stimulation of liposomes was delivered using infrared (890 nm) femtosecond (fs) pulsed laser of a 2-photon microscope. Pulse duration was 100 fs, and repetition rate was 80 MHz. Laser pulses were transmitted through a 60× objective lens and made a 430-nm diameter spot in the brain slice. The light source (MaiTai, Coherent, Santa Clara, CA, USA) provided continuous laser power at the source of approximately 2 W, which was attenuated by an acousto-optic modulator. The laser stimulation was set using software (FluoView, Olympus, Tokyo, Japan) to a scan area of 211.14 μm × 211.14 μm and a sampling speed of 10 μs/pixel.

In the hippocampal slice model system, seizures were induced by perfusion with low Mg^{2+}/high K^+ ACSF. Spontaneous seizure-like events (SLEs) seldom occurred in response to this treatment alone. When SLEs did not occur spontaneously they were induced by repetitive electrical stimulation. Electrical stimulation (600–1200 μA, 100 μs, monophasic) was applied through a bipolar stimulating electrode placed in CA3, in order to stimulate Schaffer collaterals. The intensity of the stimulation for each slice was adjusted to a value that evoked SLEs in the CA1 area. After initial adjustment, the stimulation intensity remained fixed. To test the effect of muscimol release from liposomes, HGN-liposomes containing muscimol (100 mM, Tocris Bioscience, Tokyo, Japan), were pressure-injected directly into slices via a glass micropipette (tip diameter 50–100 μm) over a period of 1 s.

2.4. Ex Vivo Entorhinal Cortex Seizure Model

Experiments using an entorhinal cortex (EC) seizure model were performed on brain slice wedges obtained from 40 male and female 1–2 month-old Wistar rats. Electrophysiological recordings in the EC were made using methods described previously [23]. Briefly, horizontal combined hippocampal EC slices (500 μm thick) were cut using a Vibroslice (Campden Instruments, Leicester, UK). From these slices, a wedge-shaped segment of the EC tissue, 2–3 mm wide, was dissected and transferred to a custom designed two-compartment grease gap chamber (see experimental setup in Figure 1B) continuously perfused with ACSF at room temperature (~1.5 mL/min). The ACSF contained (in mM): NaCl 135, KCl 3, NaH$_2$PO$_4$ 1.25, MgCl$_2$ 2, CaCl$_2$ 2, glucose 10, and NaHCO$_3$ 26 (all from Sigma, NZ), saturated with 95% O$_2$/5% CO$_2$. For Mg^{2+}-free ACSF, the MgCl$_2$ was omitted. An HGN-liposome reservoir was plumbed in and out of the perfusion flow and an ultrasound probe was positioned at the base of the HGN-liposome reservoir to trigger release of muscimol.

Differential recordings were made across the grease gap using Ag/AgCl pellet electrodes (Harvard Apparatus, Waterbeach, UK) located in both chambers (Figure 1B) with an NL102 amplifier (Neurolog, Welwyn Garden City, UK) (×100 gain, high-pass filter with 8.9 Hz cut-off) and a chart recorder (Semat, London, UK). After placing the slice on the grease gap, the slice was perfused with ACSF for 30 min, and thereafter with ACSF lacking Mg^{2+}. Removal of Mg^{2+} from the ACSF led to the appearance of repetitive SLEs 40 to 120 min after the switch. A solution of muscimol-containing HGN-liposomes was applied for 15 min, after which the ultrasound (US) trigger was applied to the liposome reservoir (Figure 1B). Slices were perfused with this ultrasonicated liposomal formulation for 30 min before being washed-out with Mg^{2+}-free ACSF and the frequency of seizure-like events (SLEs) and late recurrent discharges (LRDs) was measured before and during drug application.

2.5. In Vivo Seizure Model

Rats were anesthetized (urethane, 1500 to 1800 mg/kg) and mounted in a stereotaxic frame (Figure 1C). Craniotomies were made on the superior surface of frontal bone (2.7 mm in diameter) and on the lateral side caudal to the left orbit (4.0 mm in diameter). A 4-mm collimator was inserted through the lateral craniotomy and pressed gently against the dura over the lateral aspect of the left frontal lobe, with a layer of acoustic coupling gel between. A silver wire epidural electroencephalogram (EEG) recording electrode was secured using dental cement in the uppermost craniotomy. Epileptiform EEG was induced using 60 mg/kg PTZ administered intravenously via a cannula in the left jugular vein. Animals were divided into four groups (PTZ-only, $n = 3$; PTZ plus HGN-liposome, $n = 3$; US without liposomes, $n = 4$; and PTZ plus HGN-liposome plus US, $n = 8$). In groups exposed to muscimol-loaded HGN-liposomes (90 mM), the formulation was administered intravenously via the jugular cannula and allowed to circulate for 5 min, after which ultrasound was delivered in bursts of 30 sec at 30% duty cycle at 1 MHz. No more than three applications of ultrasound occurred in any given 5 min recording interval.

For analysis, individual power spectra were constructed and normalized, such that the total area under the curve of each plot was 1. The fraction of total area in the EEG frequency bands 0–1 Hz, 1–3 Hz, and 3–5 Hz was calculated. For each rat mean post-PTZ values for the intervals 10–19, 20–29, 30–39, and 40–49 min were derived by averaging the values for the 1st and 2nd 5-min period in each interval. These averaged time epoch data for each rat were then normalized to the values for the 5-min period following PTZ application.

2.6. Test of Liposome Ability to Sequester Contents in Absence of Stimulation

For this control experiment, designed to test whether a drug will remain in HGN-liposomes until released by an external trigger, HGN-liposomes containing kainic acid (KA) were injected into the primary somatosensory cortex of mice at stereotaxic coordinates (AP: −1.0 mm, ML: +/−1.5 mm, DV: 1.5 mm) in a volume of 1.0 µL. Positive control injections of KA directly into brain tissue were made in other mice, using a volume of 1 µL in a concentration of 10 nM. One week after the injection of HGN-liposomes, animals were perfused with 4% paraformaldehyde and were brains extracted and post-fixed in the same fixative. Coronal sections (80 µm) using a vibratome (VT1000S; Leica, Wetzlar, Germany) were prepared and sections divided into four vials. NeuN staining for neuronal nuclei was performed by Neu-N primary antibody (AB104224; Abcam, Tokyo, Japan) and a secondary antimouse IgG-conjugated biotin (Invitrogen, Tokyo, Japan). NeuN signals were enhanced by an avidin–biotin complex method (ABC Elite; Vector Laboratories,

Tokyo, Japan) and visualized using a metal-enhanced DAB Substrate Kit (#34065; Thermo Scientific, Tokyo, Japan). Images of sections were obtained using a digital microscope (BZ-9000; Keyence, Osaka, Japan) and inspected for obvious qualitative signs of neuronal loss.

2.7. Statistical Analysis

For statistical analysis of group differences in the *ex vivo* wedge experiments, we used one-way analysis of variance (ANOVA) to test for overall group differences and Tukey's multiple comparisons post hoc test for contrasts. For statistical analysis of group differences in the *in vivo* experiments, we used general linear model mixed model (GLMM) [30,31] analysis of data, further dissected by Fisher's least significant difference post hoc analyses. In the *in vivo* experiments GLMM analysis was used, due to the use of multiple control groups of smaller size.

3. Results

3.1. Induction of Seizure Activity in Three Different Models

Seizure-like activity was reliably induced in all three preparations, as illustrated in Figure 2. In hippocampal brain slices, repetitive electrical stimulation of Schaffer collaterals in area CA1 in the presence of high K^+, Mg^{2+}-free conditions produced SLEs reliably in six slices from six animals. An example trace from these slices showing induction of SLEs by electrical stimulation in hippocampal area CA is shown in Figure 2A.

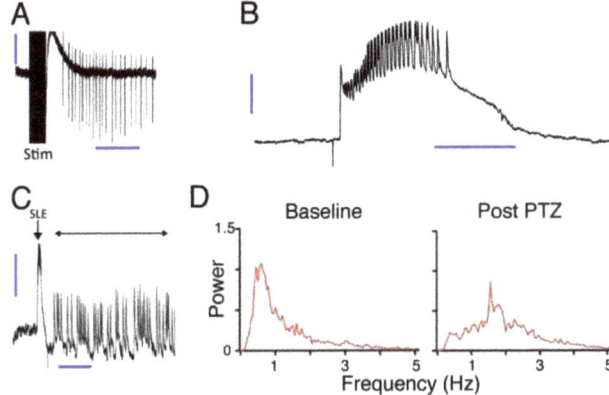

Figure 2. Example data from experiments showing induction of SLEs in three different models. (**A**) *Ex vivo* hippocampal slice preparation. Trace shows field potentials recorded from area CA1. Repetitive electrical stimulation (Stim) induced clonic afterdischarges. Vertical and horizontal scale bars (thick blue lines) show 0.2 mV and 5 s. (**B,C**) *Ex vivo* entorhinal cortex grease gap recordings. (**B**) Trace shows spontaneous SLE after removal of extracellular Mg^{2+} from the perfusing ACSF. Vertical and horizontal scale bars (thick blue lines) show 0.5 mV and 20 s. (**C**) Longer timescale trace shows transition of SLE (arrow) to late recurrent discharges (double headed arrow). Vertical and horizontal scale bars (thick blue lines) show 0.2 mV and 5 min. (**D**) *In vivo* anaesthetized animal preparation. Traces show EEG power spectrum before (Baseline) and after (Post PTZ) application of PTZ. Frequency (Hz) in D refers to EEG frequency.

In wedges of entorhinal cortex, K^+, Mg^{2+}-free solution induced spontaneous SLEs. These began 40 to 120 min after switching to high K^+, Mg^{2+}-free solution. An example trace of a spontaneous SLE from this set of wedges is shown in Figure 2B. In 20 cases out of 43 wedges from 32 animals (i.e., in 47% of wedges) the SLEs spontaneously transitioned to faster, shorter, and more continuous LRDs. An example of this transition is shown in Figure 2C.

In the whole animal (Figure 2C,D), PTZ application induced seizure activity, indicated by a shift in the EEG power spectrum to higher frequencies. In particular, the power in the 0–1 Hz EEG frequency band, which is normally high under control conditions due to urethane anesthesia (Figure 2D, Baseline), decreased markedly 5 min after PTZ injection (Figure 2D, After PTZ). Conversely, the power in the 1–3 Hz EEG frequency band, which is usually very low at baseline, markedly increased after PTZ, with a prominent peak in the group average across all 18 animals.

To confirm that the muscimol release from muscimol-containing HGN-liposomes in normal brain tissue is sufficient to evoke a physiological effect, we used laser stimulation during whole-cell recording from CA1 pyramidal cells in the presence muscimol-containing HGN-liposomes in brain slices. Laser exposure caused transient hyperpolarizations of the membrane potential that were similar to GABAegic inhibitory postsynaptic potentials (Figure 3A,B). The repeatability and accuracy of the laser-induced release is shown in the repeated hyperpolarizations induced over multiple stimuli, which showed a distinct time-course with repeated stimuli (Figure 3C). The membrane potential time course indicates that the half-life of the electrophysiological effects of muscimol after release from HGN-liposomes is extremely short, on the order of seconds. Thus, our intracellular recordings of the timecourse of the response to release of muscimol from HGN-liposomes reveal a rapid, reversible, and repeatable action, on a timescale of seconds. The effects that we observed of applying small amounts locally were very fast.

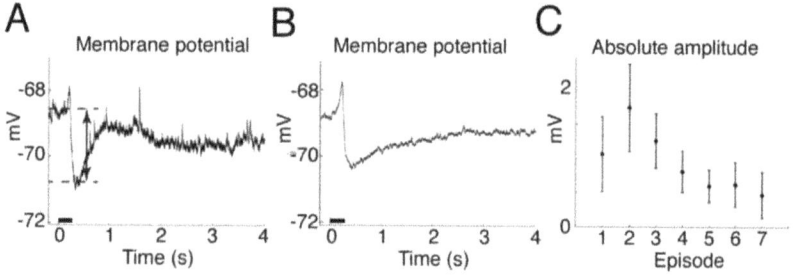

Figure 3. Effects of laser-induced muscimol release on hippocampal CA1 pyramidal neuron membrane potential measured in whole-cell recording, current-clamp mode. (**A**) Trace shows single trial example. Laser stimulation (horizontal black bar) induces transient hyperpolarization. Double-headed arrow indicates amplitude of hyperpolarization measured between baseline and peak average values. (**B**) Average of first 10 episodes from same neuron, as in (**A**). (**C**) Graph shows absolute value of group average hyperpolarization responses to first seven laser stimulation episodes (n = 3 animals, mean ± SEM).

3.2. Amelioration of Seizure Activity by Muscimol Release from Liposomes Ex Vivo

We found that muscimol release from HGN-liposome reduced seizure activity in the three seizure models. In the hippocampal brain slice, laser stimulation of HGN-liposomes that did not contain muscimol had no effect on evoked SLEs (Figure 4A). In contrast, in the presence of muscimol-containing HGN-liposomes, laser stimulation applied at the onset of the electrical stimulus train blocked the SLEs (Figure 4B). As illustrated in the example in Figure 4B, this effect was consistently evoked with repeated laser stimulation in the same slice. Analysis of pooled data across all experiments confirmed that, on average, the number of epileptiform events per minute was reduced on each occasion that laser stimulation was applied in the presence of muscimol-containing HGN-liposomes, but not with control HGN-liposome containing no muscimol (Figure 4C). Laser stimulated release of muscimol also reduced spontaneous SLE frequency (Figure 4D).

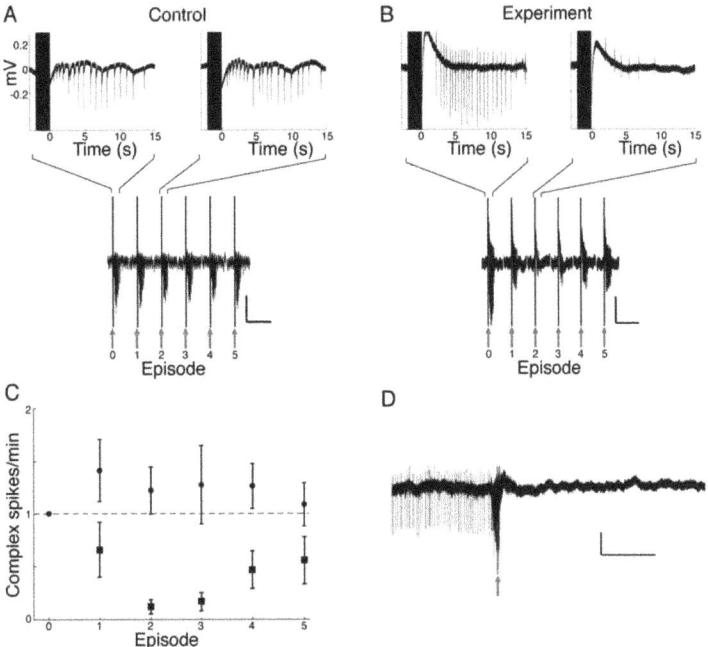

Figure 4. Effect of laser-stimulated release of muscimol on SLEs recorded in hippocampal area CA1. (**A**) No muscimol control. Top traces, two typical responses to electrical stimulation. Lower trace shows the series of six successive SLE-inducing electrical stimuli on a compressed time scale, from which the top traces are taken (Scale bars show 0.2 mV and 1 min). Blue arrows show episodes where only electrical stimulation was applied. Red arrows show episodes where electrical and laser stimulation was combined. In the presence of liposomes containing no muscimol, repeated laser stimulation had no effect on electrical stimulation-evoked SLE. (**B**) Effect of laser-stimulated muscimol release on SLE. Conventions, as for A, in the presence of muscimol-containing HGN-liposomes. Note the reduction in electrically-evoked complex spikes after muscimol release. (Scale bars show 0.2 mV and 1 min). (**C**) Group average baseline normalized complex spike activity in control (circles, $n = 3$ animals) and experimental (squares, $n = 3$ animals) conditions. (**D**). Effect of laser-induced muscimol release (red arrow) on spontaneous SLE. Trace shows example in which spontaneously occurring complex spikes (thin lines) were eliminated by laser release of muscimol (red arrow). Scale bars in (**A**,**B**,**D**) show 0.1 mV and 10 s.

Having established the efficacy of laser induced muscimol release from HGN-liposome for reducing electrical-stimulation induced seizure activity, we then measured the effect of ultrasound release of muscimol on the frequency of spontaneous SLEs. Figure 5A shows a representative recording from an entorhinal-wedge expressing spontaneous epileptiform activity under Mg^{2+}-free conditions. Exposure of the preparation to ultrasound-stimulated HGN-liposome was associated with a dramatic reduction in SLE frequency. In contrast, wash-in of unstimulated muscimol-containing HGN-liposomes caused little change. Group analysis (Figure 5B) revealed an overall effect of treatment (one-way ANOVA, $p < 0.0001$, $F_{(2,25)} = 21.0$). Post hoc tests confirmed a significant reduction in the frequency of epileptiform activity after the application of ultrasound to the formulation, compared to both the pre-ultrasound wash in period ($p < 0.0001$; Tukey's multiple comparisons post hoc test) and to the equivalent post-wash in period with no US applied ($p = 0.0035$). There was no significant difference between the wash-in and post-wash-in, no US periods.

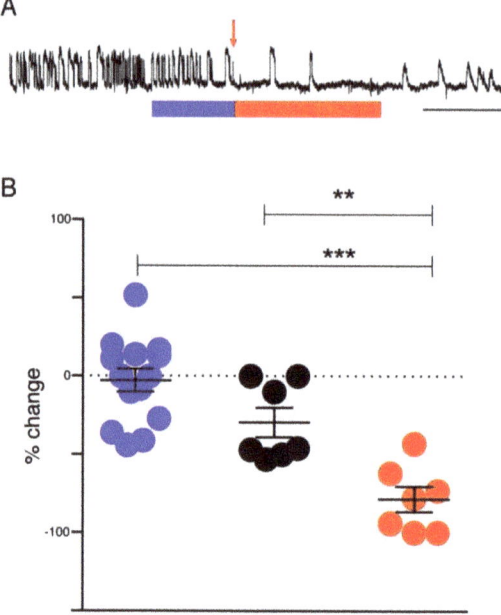

Figure 5. Effect of ultrasound-stimulated release of muscimol on SLEs in hippocampal–entorhinal wedge preparation. (**A**) Example recording shows typical reduction of seizure activity following ultrasound stimulation. Blue bar, wash-in period of unstimulated muscimol-containing liposomes. Red arrow, time of ultrasound stimulation of liposomes in the reservoir supplying ACSF to the tissue chamber. Red bar, duration of subsequent exposure to solution containing ultrasound stimulated liposomes. Scale bar, 15 min. (**B**) Graph shows group mean ± standard error for percent change of seizure activity (SLE + LRD). Filled circles show individual animal data. Blue circles, wash-in period data; black circles, post wash-in data from no-ultrasound stimulation controls; red circles, post wash-in data from ultrasound stimulated slices (US). ** $p < 0.01$ and *** $p < 0.0001$, Tukey's post hoc comparisons.

3.3. Amelioration of Seizure Activity by Muscimol Release from Liposomes In Vivo

The foregoing experiments indicated that seizure activity could be arrested by release of muscimol from HGN-liposomes *ex vivo*. In order to determine whether the treatment would be effective *in vivo*, experiments were conducted in anesthetized whole animals expressing seizure activity induced by PTZ applications. HGN-liposomes were intravenously injected and ultrasound stimulation was applied via an extradural collimator (Figure 1C). Four groups were compared (PTZ, PTZ plus HGN-liposome, US, and PTZ plus HGN-liposome plus US). The key finding of these experiments concerned the effect of US-activated release of muscimol on the PTZ-induced seizure signatures in the EEG.

As shown in Figure 6, before any treatment, all groups showed changes in the power of the EEG post-PTZ (5–9 min period) relative to the pre-PTZ baseline (0 min) in all EEG frequency bands. In the 0 to 1 Hz EEG band (Figure 6A) there was a decrease, with increases in the 1 to 3 Hz and 3–5 Hz EEG bands (Figure 6B,C). These effects of PTZ treatment, reflecting successful generation of the model, were confirmed by statistical analyses using GLMM procedures, which revealed significant main effects of time in all bands (0 to 1 Hz, $F(1,31) = 63.49$, $p < 0.001$; 1 to 3 Hz, $F(1,31) = 177.24$, $p < 0.001$; 3–5 Hz, $F(1,31) = 29.07$, $p < 0.001$, respectively).

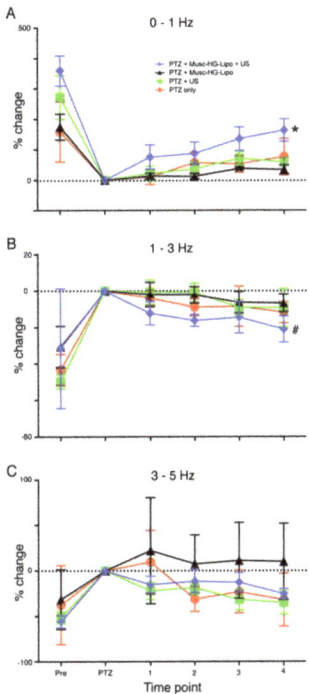

Figure 6. Ultrasound stimulation of liposomes reduces seizure activity *in vivo*. Line plots show effect of experimental and control treatments on EEG power measured in different EEG frequency bands. In all groups PTZ treatment causes a significant difference from pre-treatment measures. (**A**) * indicates significant main effect of treatment ($p = 0.004$) on power measured in the 0–1 Hz EEG band. Post hoc contrasts showed that the group that received US application to muscimol-containing HGN-liposomes (PTZ + Musc-HG-Lipo + US, blue line and symbols, $n = 8$) was significantly different from all control groups ($p < 0.022$ in all cases), while there were no differences between the control groups that received either, application of muscimol-containing HGN-liposome without US application (PTZ + Musc-HG-Lipo, black line and symbols; $n = 3$); ultrasound application only with no liposomes present (PTZ + US, green lines and symbols; $n = 4$); or PTZ-only with no subsequent manipulation (PTZ only, red lines and symbols; $n = 3$). (**B**) # indicates significant main effect of treatment in 1–3 Hz EEG band ($p = 0.043$). In this band the group that received US application to muscimol-containing HGN-liposomes was significantly different from the group that received US only ($p = 0.02$) and the group treated with muscimol-containing HGN-liposomes only ($p = 0.026$), but the contrast with the group receiving no treatment did not reach significance ($p = 0.126$). (**C**) There was no significant effect of treatment on power measured in the 3–5 Hz band ($p = 0.079$). Data are normalized to power measured over 5 min, following PTZ administration and expressed as percentage change. See text for details of statistical analysis.

As expected, before treatment there was no significant difference in the effect of PTZ between rats allocated to receive either US application to muscimol-containing HGN-liposomes (blue lines and symbols in Figure 6A,B; $n = 8$); muscimol-containing HGN-liposome without US application, (black lines and symbols; $n = 3$); ultrasound application only, with no liposomes present (green lines and symbols; $n = 4$); or PTZ-only, with no subsequent manipulation (red lines and symbols; $n = 3$); overall ANOVA by EEG frequency bands (0–1Hz, $F(3,31) = 1.97$, $p = 0.39$, 1–3 Hz $F(3,31) = 1.94$, $p = 0.144$, 3–5 Hz $F(3,31) = 0.401$, $p = 0.753$), GLMM. This shows that the experimental and control groups were not significantly different in the way they responded to PTX prior to treatment.

After treatment, effects differed by group and EEG bands. For the 0–1 Hz EEG band, in the group that received US application to muscimol-containing HGN-liposomes (blue lines and symbols in Figure 6A,B; $n = 8$), the EEG power reverted towards pre-PTZ levels. In contrast, there was little change over the same time period in the control groups. These control groups received either, application of muscimol-containing HGN-liposome without US application, (black lines and symbols; $n = 3$); ultrasound application only, with no liposomes present (green lines and symbols; $n = 4$); or PTZ-only, with no subsequent manipulation (red lines and symbols; $n = 3$). Similar effects were seen in the 1–3 Hz band (Figure 6B). These differential effects led to a visible separation of the traces for the test group versus the controls. There was no visible effect in the 3–5 Hz band (Figure 6C). These effects were confirmed by the GLMM analyses of post-PTZ data, which for both 0–1 and 1–3 Hz EEG bands revealed a significant main effect of group (0–1 Hz, F (3) = 5.007, $p = 0.004$; 1–3 Hz, F (3) = 2.907, $p = 0.043$), but not for the 3–5 Hz band (F (3) = 2.387, $p = 0.079$). There were no main effects of time, and no significant group x time interactions. The significant effects were further dissected using Fisher's least significant difference post hoc analyses. For the 0–1 Hz band, Group 4 (treatment with muscimol-containing HGN-liposomes + ultrasound) was significantly different from all other groups ($p < 0.022$ in all cases), while there were no differences between the other groups. For the 1–3 Hz band, Group 4 was significantly different from group 2 (US only; $p = 0.02$) and group 3 (muscimol-containing HGN-liposomes only; $p = 0.026$), but the contrast with group 1 (no treatment) did not reach significance ($p = 0.126$).

3.4. Unstimulated HGN-Liposome Effectively Sequester Bioactive Compounds In Vivo

One of the potential advantages of HGN-liposome drug delivery is that drugs can be sequestered in the body without activity, until released on demand. That this occurs is suggested by the lack of effect of infusion of muscimol-containing HGN-liposome in the absence of ultrasound stimulation (Figures 5 and 6). To further test the ability of the HGN-liposome used here to sequester bioactive compounds, we loaded HGN-liposome with a neurotoxin, kainic acid (KA), which causes widespread cell death when injected into brain, and injected it into the cerebral cortex. Following one week of survival we examined the effects of the injection on neural tissue. As shown in Figure 7, injection of HGN-liposome containing KA had no effect (Figure 7B), whereas injection of unencapsulated KA solution caused damage to neural tissue, indicated by the pale areas in Figure 7C. Together, these results indicate that the HGN-liposome used here are able to sequester drugs until release is triggered.

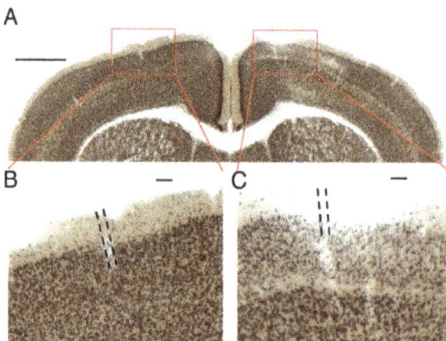

Figure 7. Liposomes effectively sequester drugs *in vivo*. (**A**) Transverse section of brain stained for cell bodies (NeuN), showing injection sites of KA-containing liposomes (**left**) and unencapsulated KA solution (**right**). Red rectangles show location of enlarged images in (**B,C**). Scale bar, 1 mm. (**B,C**) Enlargements of sites shown in (**A**). Dashed lines indicate injection tracks. Scale bar 100 μm.

4. Discussion

The main finding of this study was that on-demand release of muscimol using a HGN-liposome drug delivery system effectively reduced seizure activity in *ex vivo* and *in vivo* experimental models. In brain slices, patch-clamp recordings from hippocampal pyramidal cells showed that laser-triggered release of the GABA agonist muscimol from HGN-liposome caused hyperpolarization of the membrane potential and blockade of action potentials. This remotely-controlled release of muscimol also arrested seizure activity (SLEs, LRDs) in the hippocampus and entorhinal cortex wedges. In anaesthetized animals, *in vivo* US stimulation of previously intravenously injected HGN-liposomes caused attenuation of PTZ-induced SLEs, observed as increased power in the high frequency spectrum of the EEG. Finally, HGN-liposomes protected brain tissue from damage by intra-liposome neurotoxin for at least one week, demonstrating effective containment. Together, these findings demonstrate the potential for effective reduction of seizure activity *in vivo*, with reduced toxicity, by remotely controlled release of drugs sequestered in HGN-liposome.

We used muscimol in these proof-of-concept experiments, rather than approved medications, for several reasons. First, we were aiming for immediate seizure suppression, on demand, and focally at the site of seizure generation. Muscimol is both potent and rapidly-acting, thus is suitable for this approach. As shown in the present paper, and earlier studies [12–15], muscimol is immediately effective in attenuating seizures when applied locally at the site of the seizures. In contrast, the approved drugs are optimized for systemic treatment with minimal side effects, require several dosing cycles to make them effective at stopping seizures, and do not act as quickly when locally applied. Thus, because they are not optimal for local application and generally effective given systemically, there is less value in using them in HGN-liposome delivery. Second, about one-third of people with epilepsy have seizures refractory to systemic pharmacotherapy with approved medications [32]. For these people in particular, new approaches are needed. Third, as noted by Gernert [32], targeted intracranial delivery, by providing higher drug concentrations in localized target regions, and lower concentrations in other brain or peripheral areas, allows the use of drugs that are otherwise unsuitable for systemic administration because of their toxicity or poor uptake into the brain. Since intracranial delivery of muscimol, in small quantities, has been shown to be safe in previous studies [11–15,18–20], we used it as a test of the delivery system.

In the present study, we used laser stimulation to cause release of muscimol from HGN-liposomes in brain slices. Several previous studies have established that substances can be released from HGN-liposome nanostructures on a rapid timescale by laser stimulation in non-biological assays [27,33–35]. These studies demonstrated the feasibility of drug delivery on a rapid timescale using laser stimulation. We have also previously shown that release and dosage can be controlled by varying the number and intensity of femtosecond pulses of light [27]; and, furthermore, that on-demand release of different neurochemicals and drugs from HGN-liposome in live brain tissue has rapid, repeatable, and reliable physiological effects [28]. However, at present, laser-stimulated release from HGN-liposomes is not suitable for *in vivo* use, because light does not penetrate far through the skull or brain parenchyma, and miniature femtosecond pulsed lasers are not available for chronic implantation. On the other hand, focused US can be transmitted through the skull and brain tissue. Recent work has demonstrated the feasibility of US-stimulated release of drugs from liposomes *in vivo* [2]. We have also shown that in vitro, US can evoke multiple release events of a constant amount over 25 individual applications [6]. The present study extends this work, by showing that transcranial US-stimulation, both *ex vivo* and *in vivo*, can cause sufficient release of muscimol from HGN-liposomes, to arrest ongoing seizure activity.

Our intracellular recordings of the timecourse of the membrane potential hyperpolarization show that the timecourse of the inhibitory effect of muscimol after release from HGN-liposomes is extremely short, on the order of seconds. This finding is consistent with previous reports of rapid, subsecond to second clearance of other neurotransmitters such as dopamine [27] and glutamate [28], measured after release from laser-stimulated HGN-liposomes. The amount of release and, hence, peak concentration of the drug obtained with each stimulation is linearly related to duration and intensity for both laser [27] and US [6] stimulation. Since only a small percentage of content is released with each stimulus, dose can be titrated against clinical effect by increasing intensity or duration of stimulation, and terminated immediately by turning off stimulation. These properties of the drug delivery system provide a means for precise control over drug actions.

The very small quantities of muscimol contained in, and released from, HGN-liposomes are unlikely to cause adverse effects. The amount of muscimol needed to produce therapeutic effects by local application in the brain is small compared to the amount that would cause side effects after diffusion into the cerebrospinal fluid and distribution throughout the bloodstream. Studies in non-human primates showed that administration of muscimol into the subarachnoid space suppressed seizures locally, but otherwise led to no detectable levels of muscimol in blood or cisternal CSF [15]. Delivery of 1.0–2.5 mM muscimol into the neocortex of rodent and nonhuman primate models has been shown to have powerful antiepileptic effects, without adverse effects on the animal's behavior [13,36]. Muscimol is metabolized in the brain and periphery and excreted in the urine in roughly equal proportions as unchanged muscimol, a cationic conjugate, or an oxidation product [9,37]. Experiments with [3H] muscimol showed that it rapidly disappears from the blood [8].

The biocompatibility, distribution and eventual fate of the liposome constituents and HGNs is less clear and possibly more of a concern than the distribution of muscimol. After intravenous injection liposomes in circulation might be sequestered in liver or spleen. They might also cause immune reactions peripherally or cellular changes after crossing the BBB. Some of the pitfalls have been reviewed recently [38]. Gold, the constituent of the HGN component, has been used medically in ionic form in the treatment of human rheumatoid arthritis, and the literature concerning adverse reactions to ionic gold has been reviewed recently [39]. In rats, gold nanoparticles were found to be biocompatible and relatively innocuous after intravenous injection, but the highest accumulation was in spleen and lowest in brain [40]. Laser-synthesized gold nanoparticles are considered to be purer and safe for biomedical applications [41], without causing liver damage. However, studies of gold nanoparticle effects in mice have revealed an increased rate of abortion and fetal abnormalities if given in the early pregnancy [42]. Reviews of this topic highlight the limited available evidence and need for more knowledge concerning the toxicity of HGN after injection [43]. Excretion of accumulated particles from the liver and spleen can take up to 3 to 4 months, indicating that further studies of the toxicity of HGNs are needed.

Even if biocompatibility issues can be overcome, clinical application of muscimol-containing HGN-liposomes will not be feasible until future technological developments provide a practical means to infiltrate them into the brain parenchyma. In the present study, HGN-liposomes may have gained access to the brain as a result of the seizure activity itself [44], or by momentary disruption of the BBB by the US stimulation, allowing liposome penetration [45]. The combination of systemic injection of HGN-liposomes with focal US stimulation might, thus, achieve a high local concentration of muscimol in the brain or brain vasculature, with relatively low concentration in the periphery, due to encapsulation within liposomes and dilution of the cerebrally released muscimol. However, procedures such as carotid or intracerebral injections, as used in the present study, are invasive neurosurgical procedures that might only be considered in intractable drug resistant epilepsy [32]. For routine use, less invasive methods will be required to move HGN-liposomes across the BBB and into the brain. Trojan horse liposomes (THLs) may be a future possibility. THLs are pegylated liposomes with a receptor-specific monoclonal antibody targeted to receptors that can transport liposomes across the blood–brain barrier, such as the transferrin receptor [46,47]. The antibody is conjugated to the surface of the THL and the transferrin receptor ferries the liposome across the BBB. Further work is needed to determine if HGN-liposomes can be transported intact from the blood into the brain by hijacking existing transport mechanisms.

To be considered as a possible treatment, liposomes injected *in vivo* must also retain the ability to release their contents over a useful time period following administration. Previous work measuring release in brain slices from previously injected animals has shown that liposomes retain their ability to repeatedly release drug after one week *in vivo* [28]. Further work is needed to determine the time course over which liposomal nanostructures remain intact and responsive to ultrasound stimulation after injection *in vivo*. Another challenge is to minimize leakage from liposomes, while preserving the ability to trigger release. In the current work, we show that the HGN-liposomes successfully encapsulated KA and could be injected into the brain and remain there for one week, without causing damage to surrounding tissue. Leakage can be minimized by increasing the stability of the liposome formulation. However, there is a trade-off between the stability of liposomes and sensitivity to stimulation, which requires systematic study to arrive at optimal formulations.

Ideally, treatment for epilepsy should prevent seizures before they occur. However, in one third of patients existing treatments are not effective in preventing seizures, and treatment-resistant epilepsy is associated with significant morbidity and mortality [48,49]. Existing technology is not yet capable of predicting seizures with clinically useful reliability. However, the technology for seizure detection already exists. For example, Kim et al. [50] concluded from a review of the literature that '... the state-of-the-art seizure detection system performance is sufficient to build a robust and reliable wearable device that could be used for daily seizure monitoring and classification.' What is needed, therefore, is a means to deliver the drug immediately on the first sign of a seizure. Here we aimed to demonstrate proof of principle that seizures can be arrested almost instantaneously provided HGN-liposomes are preloaded in the brain. However, the practical use of this approach will require the future development of tools for applying US or laser stimulation in an ambulatory patient setting, as well as new technology for infiltrating the HGN-liposomes into the brain. Extensive studies of pharmacokinetics, pharmacodynamics, and toxicity will also be needed to determine the utility and safety of the technology in humans.

5. Conclusions

The present experiments demonstrated that the HGN-liposome formulation we have developed is able to encapsulate and contain muscimol, and release it in the brain in response to femtosecond laser or US stimulation. Release is rapid and immediate, causing fast and repeatable hyperpolarizations of neurons, similar to physiological inhibitory postsynaptic potentials. In *ex vivo* seizure models, stimulation of muscimol loaded HGN-liposomes caused immediate suppression of spontaneous and electrically-evoked seizure activity. Experiments also showed that ultrasound stimulation applied to the brain through the dura attenuated seizure activity induced by PTZ in rats given intravenous injection of muscimol-loaded HGN-liposomes. We also showed that intracerebrally injected HGN-liposomes loaded with toxic concentrations of KA did not cause damage to surrounding tissue. Thus, we demonstrated the feasibility of precise temporal control over exposure of neurons to the drug, potentially enabling therapeutic effects without continuous exposure. Overall, these findings suggest that HGN-liposomes combined with ultrasound triggering have potential for the development of innovative treatment strategies for neurological disorders, using on-demand release of pharmaceuticals.

The present study focused on epileptic seizures in particular, because of the challenges of long-term treatment with systemic antiepileptic drugs, and the large number of patients with drug-resistant epilepsy. The ability to deliver high concentrations of drug to target areas on demand, while keeping drug concentrations low at other sites and times may enable the use of drugs that are effective when applied locally, but unsuitable for systemic use, because of their effects on other systems. Muscimol is one example of such a drug, which has been found unsuitable for systemic application, but potentially effective when applied locally. For such applications, the development of technology to move HGN-liposomes across the BBB and anchor them with the brain parenchyma would be necessary. Further work is needed to determine the utility and safety of the technology in humans, particularly concerning the pharmacokinetics, pharmacodynamics, and toxicity of HGN-liposomes and their constituents. Technology for detection of seizures and application of US stimulation in ambulatory patients will also be needed. If these problems can be solved, HGN-liposomes have the potential to be developed into a new treatment for responsive forms of epilepsy.

Supplementary Materials: The following supporting information can be downloaded at: https://www.mdpi.com/article/10.3390/pharmaceutics14020468/s1, Figure S1: DLS of typical HGN suspensions indicating the hydrodynamic diameter of HGNs, Figure S2: Typical UV-vis spectrum of a HGN suspension showing maximum absorbance around 750–800 nm, Figure S3: DLS of typical liposome suspensions indicating their size distributions, Figure S4: DLS indicating the hydrodynamic diameter of HGNs, liposomes, and HGN-liposome conjugate suspensions, and Figure S5: Cryo-TEM of HGN-liposome conjugates at different tilt angles.

Author Contributions: Conceptualization, T.N., S.B.R., P.H., R.E., E.W.T., K.M.D. and J.N.R.; Data curation, C.G.P.; Formal analysis, T.N., S.B.R., D.M.A.M., J.G., S.M.M., P.H., C.G.P., B.I.H., R.E., E.W.T., K.M.D. and J.N.R.; Investigation, T.N., S.B.R., D.M.A.M., J.G., S.M.M., P.H. and C.G.P.; Methodology, D.M.A.M., S.M.M., P.H. and K.M.D.; Project administration, J.N.R.; Resources, R.E., E.W.T., K.M.D., J.N.R. and J.R.W.; Supervision, J.R.W.; Writing—original draft, T.N., S.B.R., B.I.H., E.W.T. and J.R.W.; Writing—review & editing, S.B.R., D.M.A.M., J.G., S.M.M., P.H., C.G.P., B.I.H., R.E., J.N.R. and J.R.W. All authors have read and agreed to the published version of the manuscript.

Funding: This work was supported by a University of Otago Doctoral Scholarship to SMM, a Royal Society of New Zealand Rutherford Discovery Fellowship to JNJR, and grants from the Okinawa Institute of Science and Technology, Japan; the Ministry of Science and Innovation (NERF Grant No. UOOX0807) (NZ); the Ministry of Business, Innovation and Employment (Smart Ideas Phase 1; No. UOOX1403) (NZ), the Otago Medical Research Foundation (NZ), and Otago Innovation Ltd. (NZ).

Institutional Review Board Statement: Animals were handled in accordance with protocols approved by the Okinawa Institute of Science and Technology Animal Care and Use Committee Approval Code: 2014-102; Approval Date: 14 November 2014 and the University of Otago Animal Ethics Committee University of Otago Animal Ethics Committee AEC 85/11 (approved 11 November 2011), and University of Otago Animal Ethics Committee approval code: 60/08 (approved 15 September 2008).

Informed Consent Statement: Not applicable.

Data Availability Statement: Data is contained within the article and Supplementary Materials.

Acknowledgments: We thank Richard Easingwood at the Otago Centre for Electron Microscopy for TEM assistance, and David Barr at the Trace Elements Centre, University of Otago, for assistance with ICP-MS.

Conflicts of Interest: Aspects of technology presented in this article are described in patent applications WO2015088042, methods for controlled release with femtosecond laser pulses, for which T.N., K.M.D. and J.R.W. are co-inventors, and WO2017034418, acoustic driven drug delivery systems, for which S.M.M., E.W.T., J.N.J.R. and J.R.W. are co-inventors. The authors declare no conflict of interest.

References

1. Bennewitz, M.F.; Saltzman, W.M. Nanotechnology for delivery of drugs to the brain for epilepsy. *Neurotherapeutics* **2009**, *6*, 323–336. [CrossRef]
2. Ozdas, M.S.; Shah, A.S.; Johnson, P.M.; Patel, N.; Marks, M.; Yasar, T.B.; Stalder, U.; Bigler, L.; von der Behrens, W.; Sirsi, S.R.; et al. Non-invasive molecularly-specific millimeter-resolution manipulation of brain circuits by ultrasound-mediated aggregation and uncaging of drug carriers. *Nat. Commun.* **2020**, *11*, 4929. [CrossRef]
3. Torchilin, V.P. Recent advances with liposomes as pharmaceutical carriers. *Nat. Rev. Drug Discov.* **2005**, *4*, 145–160. [CrossRef]
4. Ponce, A.M.; Vujaskovic, Z.; Yuan, F.; Needham, D.; Dewhirst, M.W. Hyperthermia mediated liposomal drug delivery. *Int. J. Hyperth.* **2006**, *22*, 205–213. [CrossRef] [PubMed]
5. Salkho, N.M.; Turki, R.Z.; Guessoum, O.; Martins, A.M.; Vitor, R.F.; Husseini, G.A. Liposomes as a promising ultrasound-triggered drug delivery system in cancer treatment. *Curr. Mol. Med.* **2018**, *17*, 668–688. [CrossRef] [PubMed]
6. Mackay, S.; Mo Aung Myint, D.; Easingwood, R.; Hegh, D.; Wickens, J.R.; Hyland, B.; Jameson, G.; Reynolds, J.; Tan, E. Dynamic control of neurochemical release with ultrasonically-sensitive nanoshell-tethered liposomes. *Commun. Chem.* **2019**, *2*, 122. [CrossRef]

7. Enna, S.J.; Maggi, A.; Worms, P.; Lloyd, K.G. Muscimol—Brain penetration and anticonvulsant potency following gaba-t inhibition. *Brain Res. Bull.* **1980**, *5*, 461–464. [CrossRef]
8. Baraldi, M.; Grandison, L.; Guidotti, A. Distribution and metabolism of muscimol in the brain and other tissues of the rat. *Neuropharmacology* **1979**, *18*, 57–62. [CrossRef]
9. Ott, J.; Wheaton, P.S.; Chilton, W.S. Fate of muscimol in the mouse. *Physiol. Chem. Phys.* **1975**, *7*, 381–384. [PubMed]
10. Mares, P.; Ticha, K.; Mikulecka, A. Anticonvulsant and behavioral effects of muscimol in immature rats. *Brain Res.* **2014**, *1582*, 227–236. [CrossRef]
11. Shoulson, I.; Goldblatt, D.; Charlton, M.; Joynt, R.J. Huntington's disease: Treatment with muscimol, a gaba-mimetic drug. *Ann. Neurol.* **1978**, *4*, 279–284. [CrossRef] [PubMed]
12. Collins, R.C. Anticonvulsant effects of muscimol. *Neurology* **1980**, *30*, 575–581. [CrossRef] [PubMed]
13. Baptiste, S.L.; Tang, H.M.; Kuzniecky, R.I.; Devinsky, O.; French, J.A.; Ludvig, N. Comparison of the antiepileptic properties of transmeningeally delivered muscimol, lidocaine, midazolam, pentobarbital and gaba, in rats. *Neurosci. Lett.* **2010**, *469*, 421–424. [CrossRef] [PubMed]
14. Ludvig, N.; Tang, H.M.; Artan, N.S.; Mirowski, P.; Medveczky, G.; Baptiste, S.L.; Darisi, S.; Kuzniecky, R.I.; Devinsky, O.; French, J.A. Transmeningeal muscimol can prevent focal eeg seizures in the rat neocortex without stopping multineuronal activity in the treated area. *Brain Res.* **2011**, *1385*, 182–191. [CrossRef]
15. Ludvig, N.; Tang, H.M.; Baptiste, S.L.; Medveczky, G.; Vaynberg, J.K.; Vazquez-DeRose, J.; Stefanov, D.G.; Devinsky, O.; French, J.A.; Carlson, C.; et al. Long-term behavioral, electrophysiological, and neurochemical monitoring of the safety of an experimental antiepileptic implant, the muscimol-delivering subdural pharmacotherapy device in monkeys. *J. Neurosurg.* **2012**, *117*, 162–175. [CrossRef]
16. Biggio, G.; Brodie, B.B.; Costa, E.; Guidotti, A. Mechanisms by which diazepam, muscimol, and other drugs change the content of cgmp in cerebellar cortex. *Proc. Natl. Acad. Sci. USA* **1977**, *74*, 3592–3596. [CrossRef]
17. Naik, S.R.; Guidotti, A.; Costa, E. Central gaba receptor agonists: Comparison of muscimol and baclofen. *Neuropharmacology* **1976**, *15*, 479–484. [CrossRef]
18. Penn, R.D.; Kroin, J.S.; Reinkensmeyer, A.; Corcos, D.M. Injection of gaba-agonist into globus pallidus in patient with parkinson's disease. *Lancet* **1998**, *351*, 340–341. [CrossRef]
19. Pahapill, P.A.; Levy, R.; Dostrovsky, J.O.; Davis, K.D.; Rezai, A.R.; Tasker, R.R.; Lozano, A.M. Tremor arrest with thalamic microinjections of muscimol in patients with essential tremor. *Ann. Neurol.* **1999**, *46*, 249–252. [CrossRef]
20. Heiss, J.D.; Argersinger, D.P.; Theodore, W.H.; Butman, J.A.; Sato, S.; Khan, O.I. Convection-enhanced delivery of muscimol in patients with drug-resistant epilepsy. *Neurosurgery* **2019**, *85*, E4–E15. [CrossRef]
21. Heiss, J.D.; Walbridge, S.; Argersinger, D.P.; Hong, C.S.; Ray-Chaudhury, A.; Lonser, R.R.; Elias, W.J.; Zaghloul, K.A. Convection-enhanced delivery of muscimol into the bilateral subthalamic nuclei of nonhuman primates. *Neurosurgery* **2019**, *84*, E420–E429. [CrossRef] [PubMed]
22. Heiss, J.D.; Walbridge, S.; Asthagiri, A.R.; Lonser, R.R. Image-guided convection-enhanced delivery of muscimol to the primate brain. *J. Neurosurg.* **2010**, *112*, 790–795. [CrossRef] [PubMed]
23. Avsar, E.; Empson, R.M. Adenosine acting via a1 receptors, controls the transition to status epilepticus-like behaviour in an in vitro model of epilepsy. *Neuropharmacology* **2004**, *47*, 427–437. [CrossRef] [PubMed]
24. Dreier, J.P.; Heinemann, U. Late low magnesium-induced epileptiform activity in rat entorhinal cortex slices becomes insensitive to the anticonvulsant valproic acid. *Neurosci. Lett.* **1990**, *119*, 68–70. [CrossRef]
25. Rafiq, A.; Zhang, Y.F.; DeLorenzo, R.J.; Coulter, D.A. Long-duration self-sustained epileptiform activity in the hippocampal-parahippocampal slice: A model of status epilepticus. *J. Neurophysiol.* **1995**, *74*, 2028–2042. [CrossRef]
26. Bialer, M.; White, H.S. Key factors in the discovery and development of new antiepileptic drugs. *Nat. Rev. Drug Discov.* **2010**, *9*, 68–82. [CrossRef]
27. Nakano, T.; Chin, C.; Myint, D.M.; Tan, E.W.; Hale, P.J.; Krishna, M.B.; Reynolds, J.N.; Wickens, J.; Dani, K.M. Mimicking subsecond neurotransmitter dynamics with femtosecond laser stimulated nanosystems. *Sci. Rep.* **2014**, *4*, 5398. [CrossRef]
28. Nakano, T.; Mackay, S.M.; Wui Tan, E.; Dani, K.M.; Wickens, J. Interfacing with neural activity via femtosecond laser stimulation of drug-encapsulating liposomal nanostructures. *eNeuro* **2016**, *3*, ENEURO.0107-16.2016. [CrossRef]
29. Prevo, B.G.; Esakoff, S.A.; Mikhailovsky, A.; Zasadzinski, J.A. Scalable routes to gold nanoshells with tunable sizes and response to near-infrared pulsed-laser irradiation. *Small* **2008**, *4*, 1183–1195. [CrossRef]
30. Dean, C.B.; Nielsen, J.D. Generalized linear mixed models: A review and some extensions. *Lifetime Data Anal.* **2007**, *13*, 497–512. [CrossRef]
31. Tuerlinckx, F.; Rijmen, F.; Verbeke, G.; de Boeck, P. Statistical inference in generalized linear mixed models: A review. *Br. J. Math. Stat. Psychol.* **2006**, *59 Pt 2*, 225–255. [CrossRef]
32. Gernert, M.; Feja, M. Bypassing the blood-brain barrier: Direct intracranial drug delivery in epilepsies. *Pharmaceutics* **2020**, *12*, 1134. [CrossRef] [PubMed]
33. Wu, G.; Mikhailovsky, A.; Khant, H.A.; Fu, C.; Chiu, W.; Zasadzinski, J.A. Remotely triggered liposome release by near-infrared light absorption via hollow gold nanoshells. *J. Am. Chem. Soc.* **2008**, *130*, 8175–8177. [CrossRef] [PubMed]
34. Leung, S.J.; Romanowski, M. Light-activated content release from liposomes. *Theranostics* **2012**, *2*, 1020–1036. [CrossRef]

35. Huang, H.L.; Lu, P.H.; Yang, H.C.; Lee, G.D.; Li, H.R.; Liao, K.C. Fiber-optic triggered release of liposome in vivo: Implication of personalized chemotherapy. *Int. J. Nanomed.* **2015**, *10*, 5171–5184.
36. Ludvig, N.; Baptiste, S.L.; Tang, H.M.; Medveczky, G.; von Gizycki, H.; Charchaflieh, J.; Devinsky, O.; Kuzniecky, R.I. Localized transmeningeal muscimol prevents neocortical seizures in rats and nonhuman primates: Therapeutic implications. *Epilepsia* **2009**, *50*, 678–693. [CrossRef] [PubMed]
37. Maggi, A.; Enna, S.J. Characteristics of muscimol accumulation in mouse brain after systemic administration. *Neuropharmacology* **1979**, *18*, 361–366. [CrossRef]
38. Inglut, C.T.; Sorrin, A.J.; Kuruppu, T.; Vig, S.; Cicalo, J.; Ahmad, H.; Huang, H.C. Immunological and toxicological considerations for the design of liposomes. *Nanomaterials* **2020**, *10*, 190. [CrossRef]
39. Balfourier, A.; Kolosnjaj-Tabi, J.; Luciani, N.; Carn, F.; Gazeau, F. Gold-based therapy: From past to present. *Proc. Natl. Acad. Sci. USA* **2020**, *117*, 22639–22648. [CrossRef]
40. Pannerselvam, B.; Devanathadesikan, V.; Alagumuthu, T.S.; Kanth, S.V.; Pudupalayam Thangavelu, K. Assessment of in-vivo biocompatibility evaluation of phytogenic gold nanoparticles on wistar albino male rats. *IET Nanobiotechnol.* **2020**, *14*, 314–324. [CrossRef]
41. Bailly, A.L.; Correard, F.; Popov, A.; Tselikov, G.; Chaspoul, F.; Appay, R.; Al-Kattan, A.; Kabashin, A.V.; Braguer, D.; Esteve, M.A. In vivo evaluation of safety, biodistribution and pharmacokinetics of laser-synthesized gold nanoparticles. *Sci. Rep.* **2019**, *9*, 12890. [CrossRef] [PubMed]
42. Yang, H.; Du, L.; Wu, G.; Wu, Z.; Keelan, J.A. Murine exposure to gold nanoparticles during early pregnancy promotes abortion by inhibiting ectodermal differentiation. *Mol. Med.* **2018**, *24*, 62. [CrossRef] [PubMed]
43. Khlebtsov, N.; Dykman, L. Biodistribution and toxicity of engineered gold nanoparticles: A review of in vitro and in vivo studies. *Chem. Soc. Rev.* **2011**, *40*, 1647–1671. [CrossRef]
44. Friedman, A. Blood-brain barrier dysfunction, status epilepticus, seizures, and epilepsy: A puzzle of a chicken and egg? *Epilepsia* **2011**, *52* (Suppl. S8), 19–20. [CrossRef] [PubMed]
45. Mesiwala, A.H.; Farrell, L.; Wenzel, H.J.; Silbergeld, D.L.; Crum, L.A.; Winn, H.R.; Mourad, P.D. High-intensity focused ultrasound selectively disrupts the blood-brain barrier in vivo. *Ultrasound Med. Biol.* **2002**, *28*, 389–400. [CrossRef]
46. Pardridge, W.M. Drug and gene targeting to the brain with molecular trojan horses. *Nat. Rev. Drug Discov.* **2002**, *1*, 131–139. [CrossRef] [PubMed]
47. Pardridge, W.M. Brain delivery of nanomedicines: Trojan horse liposomes for plasmid DNA gene therapy of the brain. *Front. Med. Technol.* **2020**, *2*, 602236. [CrossRef]
48. DeGiorgio, C.M.; Curtis, A.; Hertling, D.; Moseley, B.D. Sudden unexpected death in epilepsy: Risk factors, biomarkers, and prevention. *Acta Neurol. Scand.* **2019**, *139*, 220–230. [CrossRef] [PubMed]
49. Laxer, K.D.; Trinka, E.; Hirsch, L.J.; Cendes, F.; Langfitt, J.; Delanty, N.; Resnick, T.; Benbadis, S.R. The consequences of refractory epilepsy and its treatment. *Epilepsy Behav.* **2014**, *37*, 59–70. [CrossRef]
50. Kim, T.; Nguyen, P.; Pham, N.; Bui, N.; Truong, H.; Ha, S.; Vu, T. Epileptic seizure detection and experimental treatment: A review. *Front. Neurol.* **2020**, *11*, 701. [CrossRef]

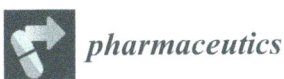

Article

Micro- and Nano-Systems Developed for Tolcapone in Parkinson's Disease

Yaquelyn Casanova [1], Sofía Negro [1,2], Karla Slowing [3], Luis García-García [4], Ana Fernández-Carballido [1,2], Mahdieh Rahmani [1] and Emilia Barcia [1,2,*]

[1] Department of Pharmaceutics and Food Technology, School of Pharmacy, Universidad Complutense de Madrid, Ciudad Universitaria s/n, 28040 Madrid, Spain; ycasanov@ucm.es (Y.C.); soneal@ucm.es (S.N.); afernand@ucm.es (A.F.-C.); mahdiera@ucm.es (M.R.)

[2] Institute of Industrial Pharmacy, Universidad Complutense de Madrid, Ciudad Universitaria s/n, 28040 Madrid, Spain

[3] Department of Pharmacology, Pharmacognosy and Botany, School of Pharmacy, Universidad Complutense de Madrid, Ciudad Universitaria s/n, 28040 Madrid, Spain; karlas@ucm.es

[4] Brain Mapping Lab, Pluridisciplinary Research Institute, Universidad Complutense de Madrid, Ciudad Universitaria s/n, 28040 Madrid, Spain; lgarciag@ucm.es

* Correspondence: ebarcia@ucm.es; Tel.: +34-913941741

Abstract: To date there is no cure for Parkinson's disease (PD), a devastating neurodegenerative disorder with levodopa being the cornerstone of its treatment. In early PD, levodopa provides a smooth clinical response, but after long-term therapy many patients develop motor complications. Tolcapone (TC) is an effective adjunct in the treatment of PD but has a short elimination half-life. In our work, two new controlled delivery systems of TC consisting of biodegradable PLGA 502 (poly (D,L-lactide-co-glycolide acid) microparticles (MPs) and nanoparticles (NPs) were developed and characterized. Formulations MP-TC4 and NP-TC3 were selected for animal testing. Formulation MP-TC4, prepared with 120 mg TC and 400 mg PLGA 502, exhibited a mean encapsulation efficiency (EE) of 85.13%, and zero-order in vitro release of TC for 30 days, with around 95% of the drug released at this time. Formulation NP-TC3, prepared with 10 mg of TC and 50 mg of PLGA 502, exhibited mean EE of 56.69%, particle size of 182 nm, and controlled the release of TC for 8 days. Daily i.p. (intraperitoneal) doses of rotenone (RT, 2 mg/kg) were given to Wistar rats to induce neurodegeneration. Once established, animals received TC in saline (3 mg/kg/day) or encapsulated within formulations MP-TC4 (amount of MPs equivalent to 3 mg/kg/day TC every 14 days) and NP-TC3 (amount of NPs equivalent to 3 mg/kg/day TC every 3 days). Brain analyses of Nissl-staining, GFAP (glial fibrillary acidic protein), and TH (tyrosine hydroxylase) immunohistochemistry as well as behavioral testing (catalepsy, akinesia, swim test) showed that the best formulation was NP-TC3, which was able to revert PD-like symptoms of neurodegeneration in the animal model assayed.

Keywords: tolcapone; microparticles; nanoparticles; PLGA; Parkinson's disease

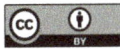

1. Introduction

Parkinson's disease (PD) represents the second most prevalent neurodegenerative disorder in the elderly population after Alzheimer's disease. PD is a disabling progressive disorder presenting tremors, slow movements, stiffness, and postural instability as neurodegeneration progresses [1]. The incidence of PD is rapidly increasing, it being estimated that it is the fastest growing neurodegenerative disease worldwide [2].

Over the last decades, the main treatment for PD in monotherapy is based on the administration of levodopa, which in the early stages of the disease provides a smooth clinical response. However, after a few years of treatment many PD patients develop motor complications. Regarding complex PD in which patients suffer from moderate to severe disability and cognitive impairment, it can be treated with combination therapy including catechol-O-methyltransferase inhibitors (ICOMTs), along with dopamine (DA) precursors [3].

COMT is a selective and widely distributed enzyme involved in the catabolism of levodopa, with tolcapone (TC) being a selective and potent COMT inhibitor able to slow down levodopa metabolism thereby leading to a prolongation of its effect [4]. TC inhibits COMT activity, in both the brain and the peripheral tissues [5], and has been approved as an adjunctive therapy for PD patients who are treated with levodopa/carbidopa.

Although several years ago rare reports of severe hepatotoxicity limited its use, a reappraisal of the data for TC in PD has determined that this risk is very small if proper hepatic monitoring is conducted [4]. Moreover, various studies on TC have indicated that the drug may have a wider safety window than previously believed [6,7]. Current recommendations indicate the need to perform tests on liver function before starting the patient on TC and avoiding its use in patients with impaired liver functionality. According to the European Medicines Agency (EMA), EMEA/H/C/000132 [8], in any case, once patients begin treatment with TC, their liver function should be monitored.

TC has a short elimination half-life of around 1.6 to 3.4 h [9,10], with the area under the plasma concentration vs. time curve being dose-dependent [11]. After oral administration, the overall bioavailability of TC is around 65%, the usual dosage schedule being t.i.d. (three times a day). These frequent dosing intervals have an important impact on adherence thereby, resulting in less effective treatments for the disease. It should also be noted that poor treatment adherence/compliance can be a very important problem when managing chronic diseases such as PD.

For this, the development of controlled release systems can significantly minimize poor patient compliance as dosage intervals can be extended. In this regard, polymeric micro- and nano-systems prepared with biocompatible and biodegradable polymers such as PLGA may enable achieving sustained drug release at the targeted site over long periods of time.

The potential applications of MPs and NPs for PD therapy have been explored in the last few years for different drugs, such as levodopa [12,13], rasagiline [14,15], puerarin [16], schisantherin A [17], glial cell line-derived neurotrophic factor (GDNF) [18], ropinirole [19], and apomorphine [20].

Due to their sizes ranging from 1 to 1000 μm microparticles (MPs), they are unlikely to cross most biological barriers; however, they present the possibility to accurately control the release rate of the encapsulated drugs over long periods of time (hours to months), thereby facilitating less frequent dosing intervals.

The blood brain barrier (BBB), due to the tight junctions between the endothelial membranes, represents the main obstacle for drugs to enter the CNS. To overcome this fact, polymeric nanoparticles (NPs) are being extensively investigated for their potential use in neurodegenerative diseases as they can facilitate the passage of drugs across the BBB. NPs are sub-micrometer-sized carrier materials designed to improve the biodistribution of encapsulated agents by delivering them more selectively and effectively to the target site [21–23].

In our study, two new drug delivery systems are developed for TC, consisting of PLGA microparticles and nanoparticles. After characterization, the best formulations are evaluated in a rotenone-induced animal model of PD.

2. Materials and Methods

2.1. Materials

Tolcapone (TC) was obtained from Jinan Haohua Industry Co., Ltd., (Jinan Haohua Industry Co., Ltd., Jinan, China); the neurotoxin rotenone (RT) was obtained from Sigma-Aldrich (Madrid, Spain); PVA (polyvinyl alcohol) of Mw = 72 kDa was purchased from Merck (Madrid, Spain); and the polymer PLGA (poly (D,L-lactide-co-glycolide acid) Resomer® RG 502 (ratio 50:50 with inherent viscosity of 0.2 dL/g) was obtained from Evonik Industries (Darmstadt, Germany). The other reagents/solvents used were of analytical grade and obtained from Panreac (Madrid, Spain). Purified water from a Milli-Q filtration system (Merck Millipore, Burlington, MA, USA) was employed in the preparation of solutions/buffers.

2.2. Preparation of TC-Loaded Microparticles

The method used for the preparation of TC microparticles was that of solvent extraction–evaporation from an O/W emulsion. For this, 400 mg of polymer PLGA 502 were weighed and dissolved in 1.5 mL of dichloromethane (DCM) with vortex stirring for 2 min. A fixed amount of TC (70–120 mg) (Table 1) was added to this solution and stirred for 2 min until a homogeneous mixture of the active ingredient was obtained. The dispersion formed was added to 10 mL of 1% PVA and homogenized with a polytron at 5000 rpm for 3 min until the emulsion was formed. Then, the emulsion was transferred to a beaker containing 50 mL of 0.1% PVA solution and kept with gentle agitation for 3 h at room temperature until complete evaporation of the organic solvent. The microspheres were then filtered through 0.45 μm filters and washed with Milli-Q water. Finally, the microparticles were freeze-dried to remove the remaining moisture. All batches of microparticles were prepared in triplicate (Table 1).

Table 1. Formulations prepared. MP (microparticles). NP (nanoparticles). TC (tolcapone). EE (encapsulation efficiency).

Formulation	Amount of TC (mg)	Process Yield (%) ± SEM	EE (%) ± SEM	Mean Particle Size ± SEM
MP-TC1	70	62.33 ± 15.10	73.92 ± 10.17	27.73 ± 2.59 μm
MP-TC2	80	78.30 ± 11.96	79.63 ± 3.55	23.05 ± 3.53 μm
MP-TC3	100	84.58 ± 5.75	83.17 ± 4.82	16.35 ± 0.10 μm
MP-TC4	120	87.69 ± 7.04	85.13 ± 2.08	17.00 ± 0.04 μm
NP-TC1	6	55.78 ± 16.87	56.16 ± 4.65	197.39 ± 43.19 nm
NP-TC2	8	75.28 ± 5.73	55.99 ± 21.41	202.08 ± 48.70 nm
NP-TC3	10	70.35 ± 14.19	53.69 ± 9.09	182.59 ± 23.94 nm
NP-TC4	12	73.29 ± 4.50	46.16 ± 5.99	210.20 ± 7.92 nm

2.3. Preparation of TC-Loaded PLGA Nanoparticles

Tolcapone nanoparticles were prepared by the nanoprecipitation technique [24], which requires low energy, allowing for the use of an organic solvent such as acetone with better toxicity profile than others [25]. The amount of PLGA 502 used in the preparation of all NPs formulations was 50 mg, and that of TC ranged from 6 mg to 12 mg (Table 1). For this procedure, both the drug (TC) and the polymer (PLGA 502) were dissolved in acetone (4 mL) under agitation (2 min). Then, the solution obtained was added to 0.5% PVA (12 mL) under constant agitation (15 min) to form the NPs. To completely remove the organic solvent, the suspension was evaporated for 2 h at 25 °C and 70 mBar in a Büchi rotavapor-R (BÜCHI Labortechnik AG, Flawil, Switzerland). The resulting suspension was washed with Milli-Q water and centrifuged (Avanti J-301, Beckman Coulter Inc., Brea, CA, USA) at 15,000× g rpm to eliminate all PVA. Liophillization of the dispersed solution obtained was performed for 24 h, employing 3% sucrose as a cryoprotectant agent (Lyo Quest®, Telsta Technologies S.L, Barcelona, Spain).

2.4. Characterization of Microparticles and Nanoparticles

2.4.1. Morphological Characterization and Size Distribution

SEM (scanning electron microscopy) was used to analyze the morphology of the microparticles (MPs) and nanoparticles (NPs) in a JEOL JEM 6335F system (Jeol Ltd., Tokyo, Japan). For this procedure, samples were coated with colloidal gold applied in a cathodic vacuum evaporator. SEM analysis was carried out at 20 KV. Moreover, laser diffraction measurements were carried out in a Microtrac-S3500 analyzer (Micro-trak Inc., Largo, FL, USA) to estimate mean diameters and size distributions of MPs and NPs. Before each measurement, the lyophilized samples were suspended in Milli-Q water and sonicated for 30 s to avoid clumping. Data were expressed as mean diameter and standard deviation (SD).

2.4.2. Calculation of Process Yield and Encapsulation Efficiency

Estimation of encapsulation efficiency (EE%) was performed according to the ratio between the amount of TC encapsulated within the MPs/NPs and the amount of TC used in their preparation according to the following equation:

$$EE\% = \text{amount of TC encapsulated within MPs/NPs(mg)} \times 100/\text{initial amount of TC used in the preparation of MPs/NPs (mg)}$$

The ratio between the weight of MPs/NPs obtained after preparation and the weight of drug/polymer used was employed for estimating process yield (%).

To determine the amount of TC incorporated within the MPs/NPs, the following procedure was used: 10 mg of MPs/NPs were weighed, to which 1 mL of DCM and 16 mL of ethanol were added to precipitate the polymer. Then, samples were centrifuged at $3000 \times g$ rpm for 5 min. The supernatant obtained after centrifugation at $5000 \times g$ for 5 min was then filtered through 0.45 mm filters and analyzed by an HPLC method previously validated by the authors.

2.4.3. Quantification of Tolcapone by HPLC

Quantification of TC was performed by high-performance liquid chromatography (HPLC). The apparatus consisted of an HPLC Waters chromatograph with a model 510 pump, a model 1490 E UV detector, a 717 auto sampler, and an Empower Login HPLC System Manager Software (Waters Corporation, Milford, MA, USA). A Mediterranean C18 column (5 µm, 250 mm × 4 mm) (Teknokroma S. Coop., Barcelona, Spain) was used. The mobile phase was composed of phosphate buffer:acetonitrile (30:70, v/v). The 0.05 M phosphate buffer was prepared from monobasic potassium phosphate (KH_2PO_4) and adjusted to pH 2 with phosphoric acid. Before use, the mobile phase was filtered through 0.45 µm filters and degassed. The flow rate was 1 mL/min and the injection volume was 20 µL. For analysis, a wavelength of 268 nm was used with the sensitivity adjusted to 0.250 aufs. All analyses were performed at $25.0 \pm 0.5\ °C$. The method was linear within the concentration range of 0.5–20 µg/mL, with a limit of detection (LOD) of 0.12 µg/mL and limit of quantification (LOQ) of 0.36 µg/mL.

PLGA did not interfere with the chromatographic method.

2.4.4. Zeta Potential

A Laser-Doppler anemometry with a Malvern Zetasizer (Malvern Panalytical, Malvern, UK) was employed for measuring the zeta potential of the NPs. Analyses were carried out at 25 °C in aqueous medium with the effective voltage set at 150 V. Briefly, an exact amount (5 mg) of each formulation was placed in a flask, diluted with distilled water (50 mL), and sonicated for a period of 5 min. For zeta potential estimations, each sample was placed in a capillary cell (Cell Enhances Capillary®, Malvern Panalytical, Malvern, UK). All formulations were analyzed in triplicate.

2.4.5. In Vitro Release Study

In vitro release of the drug (TC) from all the formulations developed (MPs and NPs) was performed by suspending 20 mg of each formulation in PBS (3 mL). The tests were carried out in a water bath (Memmert, Schwabach, Germany) kept at $37 \pm 0.2\ °C$ and constant agitation (100 rpm). At pre-fixed times, all sample volume was withdrawn and the supernatant was removed and filtered through 0.45 µm filters for MPs. For NPs, samples were ultracentrifuged at 15,000 rpm for 20 min and filtered through 0.05 µm filters. The volumes withdrawn were then replaced with fresh medium. Tests lasted 42 days for MPs and 27 days for NPs. Quantification of TC was performed by direct spectrophotometry at 266 nm. In vitro release tests were carried out in triplicate.

2.5. Animal Testing

Animal experiments were carried out in male Wistar rats weighing 180–220 g and obtained from Harlan (Harlan France SARL, Gannat, France). Animal experiments complied with the 3R principles (reduction, replacement, and refinement). Animals were housed at 22 ± 2 °C under normal laboratory conditions on a standard light–dark cycle. Food and water were supplied ad libitum. To minimize pain and discomfort, all adequate measures were taken with efforts made to minimize the number of animals used. All experimental procedures were approved by the Ethics Committee for animal testing of the Universidad Complutense de Madrid (permit number PROEX: 14/18) and carried out according to the Spanish RD 1201/2005 regarding the care and use of experimental animals.

2.5.1. Treatments and Animal Groups

The neurotoxin rotenone (RT) was given intraperitoneally (i.p.) to the animals dissolved in sunflower oil [26]. The following animal groups were included in the study:

- Group 1 (G1): Control group. Animals (n = 8) receiving the vehicles; sunflower oil (subgroup G1A, n = 4) or saline (subgroup G1B, n = 4).
- Group 2 (G2): Animals (n = 8) receiving only the neurotoxin RT (2 mg/kg/day) for 43 days.
- Group 3 (G3): Animals (n = 8) receiving RT (2 mg/kg/day) for 43 days and the amount of MPs equivalent to 3 mg/kg/day of TC every 14 days from day 15.
- Group 4 (G4): Animals (n = 8) receiving RT (2 mg/kg/day) for 43 days and the amount of NPs equivalent to 3 mg/kg/day of TC every 3 days from day 15.
- Group 5 (G5): Animals (n = 8) receiving RT (2 mg/kg/day) for 43 days and TC in saline (3 mg/kg/day) from day 15.

Doses assayed were chosen based upon previous experiments carried out in our laboratory. For this, appropriate amounts of MPs/NPS adapted to animal weight and encapsulation efficiency were injected i.p. MPs/NPs were dispersed in saline for administration. After 44 days, animals were sacrificed by decapitation with a guillotine.

2.5.2. Body Weight Evaluation

On pre-established times (1, 5, 10, 14, 20, 26, 30, 35, 40, and 44 days) animals were weighed to determine changes occurring throughout the study.

2.5.3. Behavioral Testing

Catalepsy test. This test consists of placing the animal in an unusual posture and then recording the time taken for the animal to correct this posture. In our study, both the "grid test" and the "bar test" were performed to measure catalepsy. Catalepsy tests were performed on days 16, 25, 35, and 44 of the study. After a period of adaptation to the test, animals were placed either on a bar (bar test) situated 10 cm above and parallel from a horizontal base or hung by all four paws (grid test) on a vertical grid (25.5 cm × 44 cm). For the bar test, latency with removal of the paw was recorded. For the grid test, the time (latency) needed for the animal to make the first move was recorded. The maximum descent latency was established at 180 s. Catalepsy tests were performed in triplicate.

Akinesia test. This test estimates the delay taken for the animal to initiate a movement, also giving information regarding the upper limb motor function. Akinesia test was carried out on days 16, 25, 35, and 44 by estimating the latency in seconds required for the animals to move all four limbs. When latency surpassed 180 s the test was terminated. Before initiating the experiments, animals were adapted to the procedure by placing them for 5 min on an elevated (100 cm) platform (100 × 150 cm). Akinesia tests were carried out in triplicate.

Swim-test. Swimming scores were obtained on days 16, 25, 35, and 44 of the study. The procedure used is that of Haobam et al. [27] with minor modifications. For this, animals were placed in warm water tubs (27 ± 2 °C). The following swim-scores were used: score 0 (hind part sinks with head floating), score 1 (occasional swimming using hind limbs while floating on one side), score 2 (occasional swimming/floating), and score 3 (continuous swimming). Tests were carried out in triplicate.

2.5.4. Histochemical Assessments

Brain processing. At the end of the study (44 days), animals were decapitated using a guillotine. Brains were removed, frozen on dry ice, and stored at −80 °C until analysis. Coronal brain sections (30 μm thick) at the level of striatum and substantia nigra were obtained by means of a cryostat (Leica CM1850, Leica Biosystems Nussloch GmbH, Nußloch, Germany). All brain slices were thaw-mounted onto Superfrost Plus slides (Thermo Fisher Scientific, Dreieich, Germany), dried at 36 °C on a hot plate, and then kept frozen at −80 °C.

Nissl-staining. For this test, brain samples were fixed with 4% formaldehyde prepared in PBS at pH 7.4. Samples were washed twice with phosphate buffer and submerged in 0.5% cresyl violet acid solution for 30 min. Samples were then washed with distilled water and dehydrated in graded ethanol solutions (70%, 95%, and 100%). Finally, all samples were cleared in xylene (twice, 5 min each) and coverslipped with DPX mounting medium (dibutyl phthalate in xylene) (Sigma-Aldrich, Madrid, Spain). Images of the substantia nigra were obtained by means of a DFC425 digital camera (Leica Biosystems Nussloch GmbH, Nußloch, Germany) coupled to a light microscope (Leitz Laborlux S microscope, Leica Biosystems Nussloch GmbH, Nußloch, Germany).

TH immunohistochemistry. A 1:500 dilution of the TH (tyrosine hydroxylase) antibody (Sigma-Aldrich, Madrid, Spain) was added to the samples once fixed, permeabilized with 0.1% Tween 20 in TBS (tris buffered saline), washed, and blocked. After overnight incubation at 4 °C, all slides were washed with TBS/0.1% Tween 20 (3 × 5 min at RT), and then the corresponding secondary FITC (fluorescein isothiocyanate)-labeled antibody (dilution 1:500; Sigma-Aldrich, Madrid, Spain) was added. Thereafter, samples were incubated for 2 h at RT, washed, and mounted with Mowiol aqueous medium. Images were obtained by means of a fluorescence microscope (Leica DM 2000LED, Leica Biosystems Nussloch GmbH, Nußloch, Germany). Digital images were captured using the FITC filter (Leica DFC 3000G, Leica Biosystems Nussloch GmbH, Nußloch, Germany).

GFAP immunohistochemistry. Glial fibrillary acidic protein (GFAP) immunohistochemistry was carried out as reported by Garcia-Garcia et al. (Garcia-Garcia et al., 2015). For this, samples were fixed with 4% formaldehyde, washed, permeabilized in TBS/0.1% Tween 20, and blocked in 5% albumin dissolved in TBS. Overnight incubation was carried out at 4 °C with a fluorescent anti-GFAP antibody conjugated with a 1:500 dilution of the Cy3 cyanine dye (Sigma-Aldrich, Madrid, Spain). With this procedure, there is no need for a secondary antibody. The unbound antibody was eliminated by washing the samples. Finally, brain slices were coverslipped with Mowiol mounting medium. Images were observed using a fluorescence digital camera (Leica DFC 3000G, Leica Biosystems Nussloch GmbH, Nußloch, Germany) coupled to a microscope (Leica DM 2000LED, Leica Biosystems Nussloch GmbH, Nußloch, Germany) using the tetramethylrhodamine isothiocyanate (TRITC) filter.

2.6. Statistical Analysis

One-way ANOVA was used for analysis, with statistical significance defined as $p < 0.05$ with data obtained from the experiments expressed as mean ± standard error of the mean. All statistical analyses were performed with the Statgraphics® *Plus* v.5.1 software (Statistical Graphics Corporation, Warrenton, VA, USA). Results from the animal behavioral tests were analyzed by means of non-parametric analyses (multifactorial Kruskal–Wallis one-way ANOVA).

3. Results and Discussion

Controlled drug delivery systems are very interesting approaches when dealing with active compounds exhibiting short elimination plasma half-lives, non-specific biodistribution, and off-site toxicities as they can facilitate the access of drugs to their specific target sites. When targeting to the CNS, there is a growing interest in the development of micro- and nano-based systems for improving the pharmacological and therapeutic properties of conventional drugs, increasing dosage intervals and reducing adverse peripheral side-effects.

In this work, we have developed two new controlled release systems (microparticles and nanoparticles) for tolcapone (TC) using PLGA 502 as a polymer. PLGA, a copolymer of poly lactic acid (PLA) and poly glycolic acid (PGA), is approved by the FDA [28] and the EMA [8] for its use in pharmaceutical products administered to humans via conventional oral and parenteral routes as well as suspension formulations for implantation without surgical procedures [29], due to its biocompatibility and biodegradability, long clinical experience, favorable degradation characteristics, and possibilities for sustained drug delivery. After administration, PLGA yields to glycolic and lactic acids, which are rapidly cleared from the body after entering the Krebs' cycle to be degraded into CO_2 and H_2O [30,31].

Several TC-loaded PLGA formulations of microparticles (MPs) have been prepared with different amounts of TC ranging from 70 mg to 120 mg (Table 1, formulations MP-TC1 to MP-TC4). Mean values of process yield for all TC-loaded PLGA MPs ranged from 62.33 ± 15.10% to 87.69 ± 7.04%. Encapsulation efficiency (EE) increased with the amount of TC used (70 to 120 mg), with the highest value obtained for the formulation prepared with 120 mg of TC (85.13 ± 2.08%) (Table 1). A successful microparticle system should have a high drug-loading capacity in order to reduce the number of MPs administered, thereby reducing the amount of polymer given.

Mean particle sizes ranged from 16.35 ± 0.10 µm to 27.73 ± 2.59 µm, being in all cases lower than 35 µm (Table 1). From the results obtained, formulation MP-TC4 was selected to perform further studies. This formulation was prepared with 120 mg of TC and presents an EE of 85.13% and mean particle size of 17.00 µm. Figure 1a shows microphotographs of formulation MP-TC4 and its particle size distribution (DLS image).

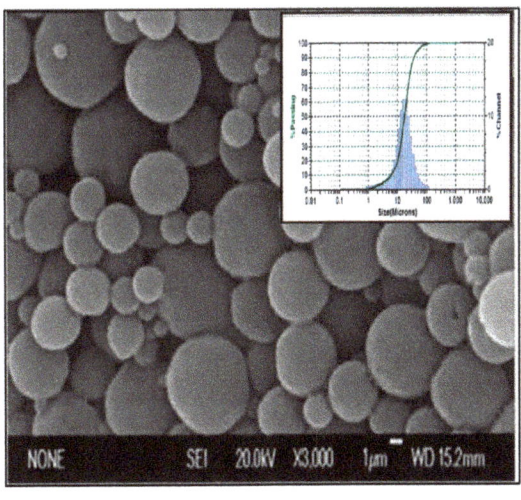
(a)

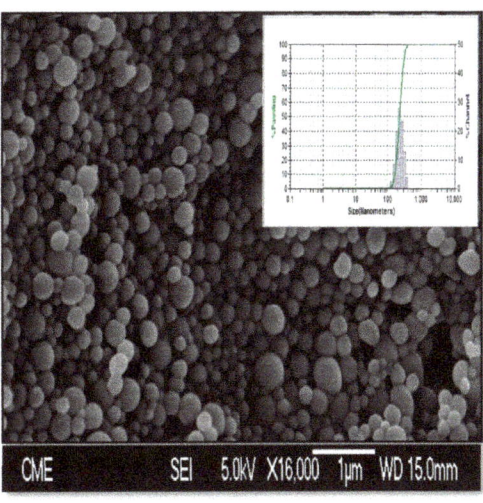
(b)

Figure 1. SEM microphotograph of TC-loaded PLGA MPs (formulation MP-TC4) and particle size distribution (**a**). SEM microphotograph of TC-loaded PLGA NPs (formulation NP-TC3) and particle size distribution (**b**). TC (tolcapone).

In our work, we have also developed several TC-loaded PLGA formulations of NPs using different amounts of the drug (Table 1, formulations NP-TC1 to NP-TC4). Taking into consideration the importance of particle size and size distribution regarding drug loading capacity, drug release, and stability of NPs as well as regarding their biological fate within the body, toxicity, and targeting ability, we have determined mean particle sizes of NPs by means of dynamic light scattering (DLS) (Table 1). For all formulations prepared, the mean particle size was around 200 nm, which is suitable for improving the access of TC to the brain. Several studies have demonstrated that NPs prepared with polymers such as PLGA and particle sizes of 250 nm are able to reach the CNS [32,33]. Figure 1b shows microphotographs of formulation NP-TC3 with its particle size distribution. The mean values of process yield for all TC-loaded PLGA NPs ranged from 55.78 ± 16.87% to 75.28 ± 5.73% (Table 1). Mean EE of TC within the NPs ranged from 46.16 ± 5.99% to 56.16 ± 4.65%. Loading efficiency increased as the amount of TC increased from 6 to 10 mg, but not when 12 mg was used. In this case, loading efficiency was similar to that obtained with 10 mg (0.88 mg TC/10 mg of NPs vs. 0.89 mg TC/10 mg of NPs). Higher values of loading efficiency are desirable in order to minimize the number of NPs administered. From the results obtained, formulation NP-TC3 was selected to continue the study.

Figure 2a shows the cumulative in vitro release profiles of TC obtained for the microparticle formulation selected, MP-TC4. For PLGA MPs, the release of drugs occurs via diffusion and/or homogeneous bulk erosion of the biopolymer, with the diffusion rate dependent upon drug diffusivity and partition coefficient [34]. Moreover, burst release occurs because of the formation of surface cracks in the MPs, which facilitates their erosion [35]. In our case, the initial burst release of TC from formulation MP-TC4 was low (around 15% within the first hour). High burst release is usually regarded as a negative effect when considering the long-term performance of a drug delivery system. Moreover, this burst release effect leads to undesirable consequences such as more frequent dosing intervals and local toxicity due to the release of high drug concentrations at short times. Burst release has been associated with different chemical, physical, and processing parameters when preparing MPs [36]. For instance, the migration of the drug during the drying process leads to heterogeneous drug distribution, thereby facilitating this burst release.

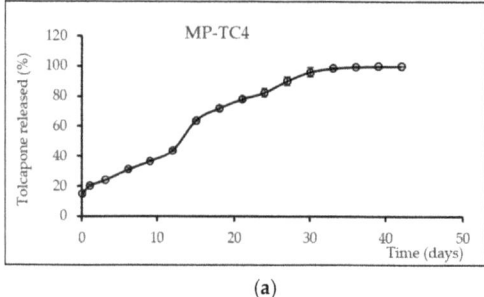
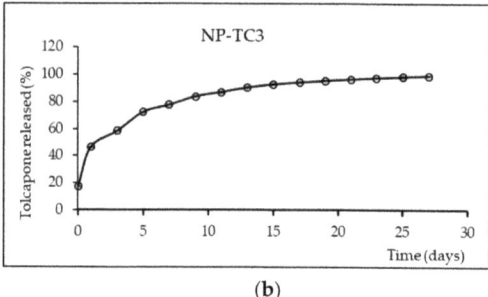

(a)   (b)

Figure 2. Mean release profiles (±SEM, n = 3) of TC from formulations MP-TC4 (**a**) and NP-TC3 (**b**). TC (tolcapone).

For formulation MP-TC4, the burst release was followed by zero-order release kinetics for around 30 days. The mean zero-order release rate constant was 2.13 µg/h. After 30 days, the percentage of TC released was around 95%. This slow release could be explained by the hydrophobic nature of TC, which hinters water diffusion into the MPs, thereby reducing the rate of polymer degradation [37].

Figure 2b shows the in vitro cumulative TC release profiles obtained for the nanoparticle formulation selected (NP-TC3). A burst release of around 18% was obtained within the first hour. At 24 h, 46% of TC was released followed by a slower release for 8 days with mean zero-order release rate constant of 1.77 µg/h/10 mg NPs. Drug release can be affected by particle size. Small particles such as NPs have large surface area-to-volume ratios, being therefore most of the drug associated with small particles that would be at or near the particle surface, thereby leading to faster drug release.

Zeta potential is a key parameter regarding the surface charge properties of NPs. It reflects the electrical potential of the particles being influenced by their composition and that of the medium in which they are dispersed. It has been demonstrated that NPs with zeta potential values above ±30 mV are stable in suspension as this surface charge prevents the particles from aggregation [38]. Additionally, zeta potential has an influence on the passage of NPs across the BBB. It has been described that, at low concentrations, negatively charged NPS do no influence the BBB passage, but if positively charged interaction with the cell surfaces can occur, thereby facilitating their passage, a stronger immune response can also occur [39]. In our case, the value of zeta potential for the formulation selected (NP-TC3) was -26.32 ± 0.48 mV, being adequate for crossing the BBB. This value can be due to the ionization of the PLGA carboxylic groups, which lead to a negative charge in the surface of the particles. In fact, it has been indicated that NPs prepared with PLGA 502 exhibit a negative zeta potential of around -33 mV [40]. The zeta potential value increased when loading the NPs with TC as a consequence of the modification of the surface due to the incorporation of the drug.

Moreover, previous research studies have demonstrated that nanoparticles prepared with PLGA of sizes around 250 nm were able to cross the BBB [32,33,41]. In our case, NPs presented mean particle sizes of around 200 nm.

To determine the efficacy of the two new controlled delivery systems developed for TC, the selected formulations (MP-TC4 and NP-TC3) were evaluated in an experimental rotenone-model of PD, which was induced in male Wistar rats. Several studies have demonstrated that, in animal models, RT can induce several PD-like abnormalities including Lewy body formation in the nigral neurons due to systematic inhibition of mitochondrial complex I, oxidative stress, alpha-synuclein phosphorylation and DJ-1 acidification and translocation, proteasomal dysfunction, and nigral iron accumulation [26,42,43].

In our study, behavioral, histological, and immunochemistry tests were carried out in order to determine the efficacy of the formulations developed for TC.

Regarding mortality in our study, RT was given at a low dose (2 mg/kg/day), which resulted in a mortality rate of 12.3% in group G2 (animals treated only with RT), without any deaths occurring in control animals. This value is similar to that reported by Cannon et al. [44] when using RT (2.75–3 mg/kg/day) and for which 10% mortality occurred shortly after administration of the neurotoxin. In another study, RT was assayed at two dose levels (2 and 2.5 mg/kg), resulting in mortality rates of 6.7% and 46.7%, respectively [30].

Figure 3a shows the evolution of body weight with time. Control groups (G1A and G1B) corresponding to animals receiving the vehicles (sunflower oil or saline) experienced a gradual and steady weight gain throughout the study, with non-significant differences ($p > 0.05$) observed between both subgroups. Animals treated with RT showed a slight weight increase for the first 10 days, with no gain in weight thereafter. Animals treated with TC-containing formulations showed a steady weight gain throughout the study.

The mean results obtained in the catalepsy test (bar and grid) are depicted in Figure 3b,c, with non-statistically significant differences found between both control subgroups (G1A and G1B), indicating that the vehicles used did not have any influence on the test. The neurotoxin RT induced an increase in latency, both in the bar and grid test (group G2) as compared to control animals that was reverted by the active compound (groups G3, G4, and G5). Among these groups, the best results correspond to animals receiving the NP formulation (group G4), for which non-statistically significant differences were found when compared to group G1 at the end of the study period ($p > 0.05$).

Akinesia results demonstrated non-statistically significant differences within control subgroups G1A and G1B (Figure 3d). Latency was clearly prolonged with RT (group G2), resulting in a latency value of around 7 times higher in group G2 with respect to G1 at the end of the study period (44 days).

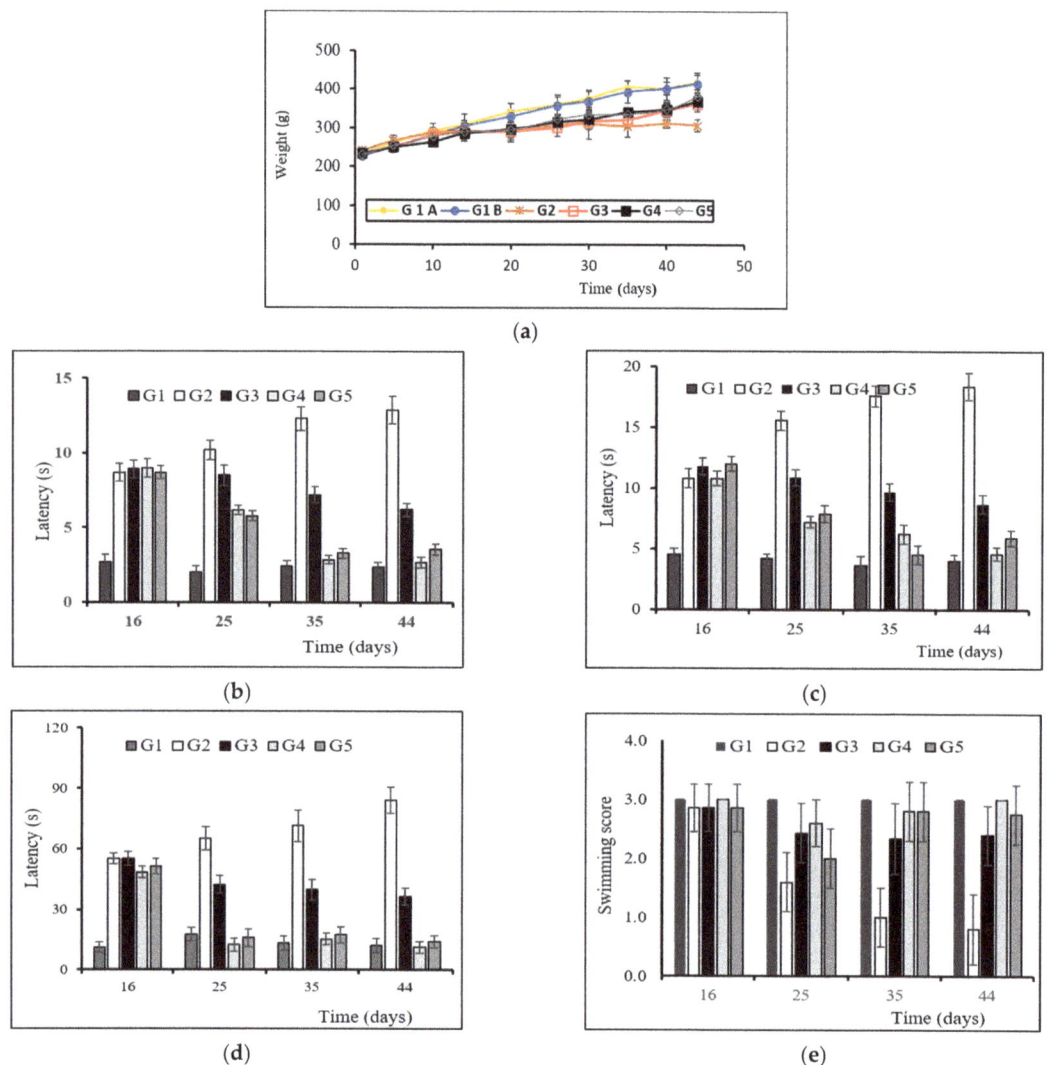

Figure 3. Evolution of rat-body weight throughout the study (44 days) (**a**). Results of the behavioral tests: catalepsy test on bar (**b**) and grid (**c**), akinesia test (**d**), and swim-test (**e**). Animal groups: control subgroups (G1A and G1B); RT-treated control group (G2); RT-treated animals also receiving formulation MP-TC4 (G3), formulation NP-TC3 (G4), and TC in saline (G5). RT (rotenone), TC (tolcapone).

Reversion of akinesia was observed in groups G3, G4, and G5 at times 25, 35, and 44 days. After 44 days, the latency values obtained for groups G4 and G5 were similar to that of the control group, without any statistically significant differences ($p > 0.05$) found between both groups (G4 and G5). In the case of group G5, this could be attributed to the fact that TC was given once daily in solution, indicating that the formulation exhibited a very rapid effect on the brain. Regarding formulation G4, which corresponds TC-loaded PLGA NPs, the results obtained confirm the ability of NPs to deliver TC to the brain and maintain TC levels in the CNS between dosing intervals.

Swim-tests were performed to evaluate the animals' overall motor capacity/deficit. The results obtained are depicted in Figure 3e. At all times, assayed animals corresponding to the control group (G1) obtained the highest values (score = 3). The swimming ability of the animals treated with RT (group G2) markedly decreased when compared to the control group ($p < 0.05$). At the end of the study, all animal groups receiving TC (G3, G4 and G5) showed high swimming scores (score > 2), but only group G4 resulted in swim scores equal to control animals.

The histological method of Nissl staining is widely used to study the morphology and pathology of neurons, as the stain used binds to DNA from nuclei and RNA from cytoplasm of cells, allowing study of the cytoarchitectony of the brain [45]. To determine the effects of the neurotoxin RT and the different formulations on neuronal loss in the SNpc, Nissl staining was performed, with the images obtained shown in Figure 4. Rotenone is a highly lipophilic compound that readily crosses the BBB, thereby allowing for the development of PD-like symptoms in animals. After systemic administration, RT induces progressive degeneration of the nigrostriatal pathway, resembling that occurring in PD patients [44,46]. The results obtained in our study confirm that i.p. injection of RT reproduced the characteristic behavioral and histopathological features of PD, including loss of neuronal cells in the SNpc [47–49]. The administration of TC in solution (group G5), or encapsulated within PLGA MPs (group G3) or PLGA NPs (group G4), prevented the cell death induced by RT in SNpc. This effect was more marked when TC was given encapsulated within PLGA NPs, indicating an improved access to the brain.

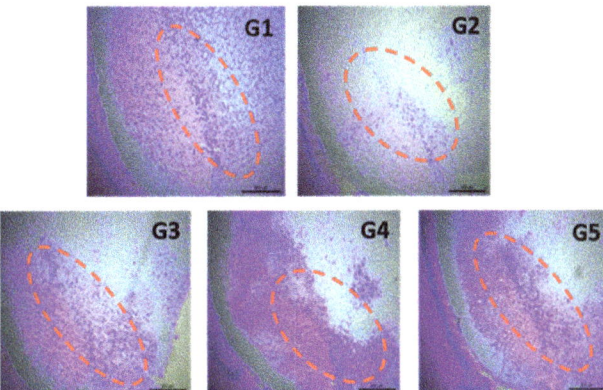

Figure 4. Representative Nissl-staining (cresyl violet) of nigral neurons from brain sections (substantia nigra, 30 μm) corresponding to all animal groups. Control group (G1); RT-treated control group (G2); RT-treated animals also receiving formulation MP-TC4 (G3), formulation NP-TC3 (G4), and TC in saline (G5). RT (rotenone), TC (tolcapone).

The glial fibrillary acidic protein (GFAP) is one of the fibrous proteins forming the intermediate filaments of the intracellular cytoskeleton. This glial response is a source of trophic factors and can protect against the formation of reactive oxygen species (ROS) and glutamate [50], taking into consideration that PD is associated with a glial response mainly composed of activated microglial cells and, to a lesser extent, reactive astrocytes. Moreover, when a brain insult occurs, a slow astrocytic response maintains microglia activation, eventually leading to a chronic brain lesion [51].

For this reason, and in order to determine whether there is a possible astrocytic activation associated with the neurodegeneration caused by RT, non-quantitative immunohistochemical studies of GFAP were performed (Figure 5). The administration of RT at a dose of 2 mg/kg/day for 43 days (group G2) produced intense gliosis. These results are in agreement with those obtained by other authors that described an intense astrocytic activation caused by RT, both in vitro [49] and in vivo [47]. This astrocytic response includes hypertrophy and thickened cell bodies, as occurred in group G2, features which are typical of reactive astrogliosis [52]. Activation of astrocytes causes brain damage due to an increase in the production of ROS [53] and the release of pro-inflammatory cytokines [54,55].

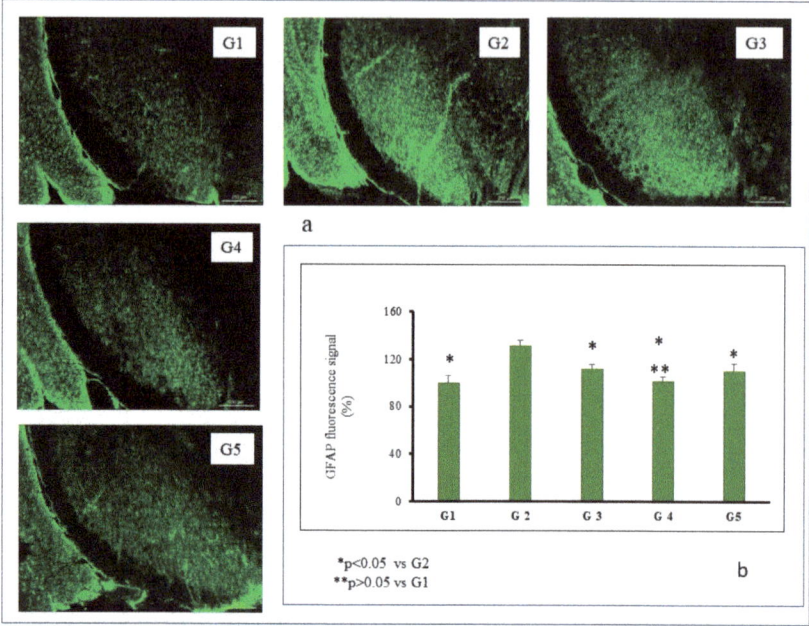

Figure 5. Representative GFAP fluorescence (**a**) and GFAP fluorescence signal (**b**) in coronal brain slices at the level of the substantia nigra for all animal groups. Control group (G1); RT-treated control group (G2); RT-treated animals also receiving: formulation MP-TC4 (G3), formulation NP-TC3 (G4), and TC in saline (G5). GFAP (glial fibrillary acidic protein), RT (rotenone), TC (tolcapone).

As seen in Figure 5b, intense gliosis occurred in the SNpc after 43 days of RT administration (group G2). This astrocytic response was almost reverted in all animal groups receiving TC either encapsulated (groups G3 and G4) or in solution (group G5). However, the response was completely reverted only when TC-loaded PLGA NPs were given to the animals. For this group, non-statistically significant differences were found when compared with control animals ($p > 0.05$).

A significant alteration occurring in PD is the degeneration of dopaminergic neurons, which leads to a reduction of striatal dopamine levels. Dopamine is synthesized in dopaminergic neurons of the SNpc area, stored in synaptic vesicles and released in the striatum to exert its physiological function [41]. Taking into consideration that tyrosine hydroxylase (TH) catalyzes the formation of levodopa, which is a rate-limiting step for the biosynthesis of dopamine, PD can be considered as a TH-deficiency syndrome of the striatum. For this, the TH immunohistochemical test is useful as it allows quantifying the degree of loss of dopaminergic cells in postmortem brains of individuals diagnosed with PD. Moreover, the use of RT as a neurotoxin has been associated with an observable reduction of TH-immunoreactive neurons in the SNpc [56–58].

Figure 6 depicts the results of fluorescence intensity obtained in our study for the different animal groups. It can be seen that TH immunoreactivity in SNpc was decreased in group G2, which corresponds to animals treated with daily doses of RT. This reduction was partially reversed in animals receiving TC-containing formulations, with the strongest reversion obtained with TC-loaded PLGA NPs (group G4). For this formulation, non-statistically significant differences were found when compared to the control group

($p > 0.05$), thereby demonstrating the potential interest of this new drug delivery system developed for TC.

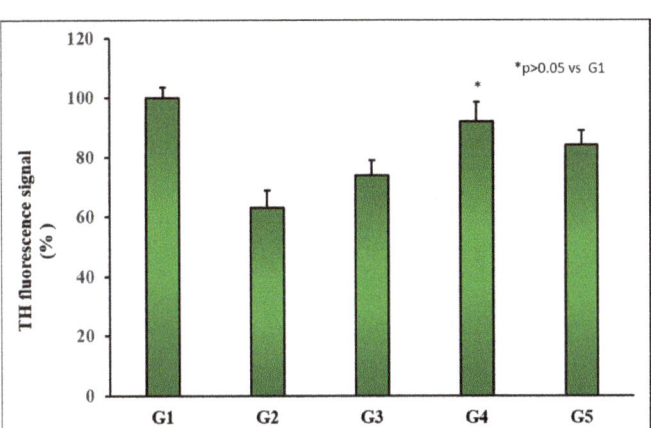

Figure 6. Representative TH fluorescence signal in coronal brain slices at the level of the substantia nigra for all animal groups. Control group (G1); RT-treated control group (G2); RT-treated animals also receiving formulation MP-TC4 (G3), formulation NP-TC3 (G4), and TC in saline (G5). TH (tyrosine hydroxylase), RT (rotenone), TC (tolcapone).

4. Conclusions

In vivo evaluation of both controlled delivery systems developed for TC consisting of biodegradable PLGA 502 microparticles (formulation MP-TC4) and nanoparticles (formulation NP-TC3) resulted in satisfactory results, with the nanoparticulate system being able to almost completely reverse the rotenone-induced neurodegeneration in the animal model assayed. With both formulations, extending the dosage intervals could be achieved.

Author Contributions: Conceptualization, E.B. and S.N.; methodology, E.B., S.N. and A.F.-C.; formal analysis, S.N., E.B., Y.C. and L.G.-G.; investigation, Y.C., K.S. and L.G.-G.; data curation, S.N. and E.B.; writing—original draft preparation, S.N. and E.B.; writing—review and editing, E.B., S.N. and M.R.; funding acquisition, E.B., S.N. and A.F.-C. All authors have read and agreed to the published version of the manuscript.

Funding: This work was partially supported by Complutense University of Madrid (UCM) research group "Formulation and Bioavailability of New Drugs" (funder UCM, funding number 910939).

Institutional Review Board Statement: Not applicable.

Informed Consent Statement: Not applicable.

Data Availability Statement: Not applicable.

Conflicts of Interest: The authors declare no conflict of interest.

References

1. Kouli, A.; Torsney, K.M.; Kuan, W.L. Parkinson's Disease: Etiology, Neuropathology, and Pathogenesis. In *Parkinson's Disease: Pathogenesis and Clinical Aspects*; Stoker, T.B., Greenland, J.C., Eds.; Codon Publications: Brisbane, Australia, 2018; Chapter 1. [CrossRef]
2. GBD 2015 Neurological Disorders Collaborator Group. Global, regional, and national burden of neurological disorders during 1990–2015: A systematic analysis for the Global Burden of Disease Study 2015. *Lancet Neurol.* **2017**, *16*, 877–897. [CrossRef]
3. Schapira, A.H.V. Treatment Options in the Modern Management of Parkinson Disease. *Arch. Neurol.* **2007**, *64*, 1083–1088. [CrossRef] [PubMed]
4. Leegwater-Kim, J.; Waters, C. Role of tolcapone in the treatment of Parkinson's disease. *Expert Rev. Neurother.* **2007**, *7*, 1649–1657. [CrossRef] [PubMed]

5. Zhang, P.-L.; Wang, Y.-X.; Chen, Y.; Zhang, C.-H.; Li, C.-H. The efficacy of homemade tolcapone in the treatment of patients with Parkinson's disease. *Exp. Ther. Med.* **2018**, *15*, 127–130. [CrossRef] [PubMed]
6. Olanow, C.W. Tolcapone and Hepatotoxic Effects. *Arch. Neurol.* **2000**, *57*, 263–267. [CrossRef] [PubMed]
7. Suchowersky, O.; Bailey, P.; Pourcher, E.; Bulger, L.; Facciponte, G. Comparison of Two Dosages of Tolcapone Added to Levodopa in Nonfluctuating Patients with PD. *Clin. Neuropharmacol.* **2001**, *24*, 214–220. [CrossRef] [PubMed]
8. Tolcapone and Hepatotoxic Effects. Tasmar Advisory Panel. Available online: https://www.ema.europa.eu/en/medicines/human/EPAR/tasmar (accessed on 3 March 2022).
9. Keating, G.M.; Lyseng-Williamson, K.A. Tolcapone: A review of its use in the management of Parkinson's disease. *CNS Drugs* **2005**, *19*, 165–184. [CrossRef]
10. Truong, D.D. Tolcapone: Review of its pharmacology and use as adjunctive therapy in patients with Parkinson's disease. *Clin. Interv. Aging* **2009**, *4*, 109–113. [CrossRef]
11. Dingemanse, J.; Jorga, K.M.; Schmitt, M.; Gieschke, R.; Fotteler, B.; Zürcher, G.; Prada, M.; Van Brummelen, P. Integrated pharmacokinetics and pharmacodynamics of the novel catechol-O-methyltransferase inhibitor tolcapone during first administration to humans. *Clin. Pharmacol. Ther.* **1995**, *57*, 508–517. [CrossRef]
12. Dankyi, B.O.; Amponsah, S.K.; Allotey-Babington, G.L.; Adams, I.; Goode, N.A.; Nettey, H. Chitosan-Coated Hydroxypropylmethyl Cellulose Microparticles of Levodopa (and Carbidopa): In Vitro and Rat Model Kinetic Characteristics. *Curr. Ther. Res.* **2020**, *93*, 100612. [CrossRef]
13. Arisoy, S.; Sayiner, O.; Comoglu, T.; Onal, D.; Atalay, O.; Pehlivanoglu, B. In vitro and in vivo evaluation of levodopa-loaded nanoparticles for nose to brain delivery. *Pharm. Dev. Technol.* **2020**, *25*, 735–747. [CrossRef] [PubMed]
14. Bali, N.R.; Salve, P.S. Impact of rasagiline nanoparticles on brain targeting efficiency via gellan gum based transdermal patch: A nanotheranostic perspective for Parkinsonism. *Int. J. Biol. Macromol.* **2020**, *164*, 1006–1024. [CrossRef] [PubMed]
15. Jiang, Y.; Zhang, X.; Mu, H.; Hua, H.; Duan, D.; Yan, X.; Wang, Y.; Meng, Q.; Lu, X.; Wang, A.; et al. Preparation and evaluation of injectable Rasagiline mesylate dual-controlled drug delivery system for the treatment of Parkinson's disease. *Drug Deliv.* **2018**, *25*, 143–152. [CrossRef] [PubMed]
16. Chen, T.; Liu, W.; Xiong, S.; Li, D.; Fang, S.; Wu, Z.; Wang, Q.; Chen, X. Nanoparticles Mediating the Sustained Puerarin Release Facilitate Improved Brain Delivery to Treat Parkinson's Disease. *ACS Appl. Mater. Interfaces* **2019**, *11*, 45276–45289. [CrossRef] [PubMed]
17. Sa, F.; Zhang, L.Q.; Chong, C.M.; Guo, B.J.; Li, S.; Zhang, Z.J.; Zheng, Y.; Hoi, P.M.; Lee, S.M.Y. Discovery of novel anti-parkinsonian effect of schisantherin A in in vitro and in vivo. *Neurosci. Lett.* **2015**, *593*, 7–12. [CrossRef]
18. Lu, C.-T.; Jin, R.-R.; Jiang, Y.-N.; Lin, Q.; Yu, W.-Z.; Mao, K.-L.; Tian, F.-R.; Zhao, Y.-P.; Zhao, Y.-Z. Gelatin nanoparticle-mediated intranasal delivery of substance P protects against 6-hydroxydopamine-induced apoptosis: An in vitro and in vivo study. *Drug Des. Dev. Ther.* **2015**, *9*, 1955–1962. [CrossRef]
19. Negro, S.; Boeva, L.; Slowing, K.; Fernandez-Carballido, A.; García-García, L.; Barcia, E. Efficacy of Ropinirole-Loaded PLGA Microspheres for the Reversion of Rotenone-Induced Parkinsonism. *Curr. Pharm. Des.* **2017**, *23*, 3423–3431. [CrossRef]
20. Regnier-Delplace, C.; du Boullay, O.T.; Siepmann, F.; Martin-Vaca, B.; Degrave, N.; Demonchaux, P.; Jentzer, O.; Bourissou, D.; Siepmann, J. PLGA microparticles with zero-order release of the labile anti-Parkinson drug apomorphine. *Int. J. Pharm.* **2013**, *443*, 68–79. [CrossRef]
21. Linazasoro, G. Potential applications of nanotechnologies to Parkinson's disease therapy. *Park. Relat. Disord.* **2008**, *14*, 383–392. [CrossRef]
22. Spuch, C.; Saida, O.; Navarro, C. Advances in the Treatment of Neurodegenerative Disorders Employing Nanoparticles. *Recent Pat. Drug Deliv. Formul.* **2012**, *6*, 2–18. [CrossRef]
23. Marcianes, P.; Negro, S.; Garcia-Garcia, L.; Montejo, C.; Barcia, E.; Fernandez-Carballido, A. Surface-modified gatifloxacin nanoparticles with potential for treating central nervous system tuberculosis. *Int. J. Nanomed.* **2017**, *12*, 1959–1968. [CrossRef] [PubMed]
24. Barcia, E.; Boeva, L.; García-García, L.; Slowing, K.; Fernández-Carballido, A.; Casanova, Y.; Negro, S. Nanotechnology-based drug delivery of ropinirole for Parkinson's disease. *Drug Deliv.* **2017**, *24*, 1112–1123. [CrossRef] [PubMed]
25. Katiyar, S.S.; Muntimadugu, E.; Rafeeqi, T.A.; Domb, A.J.; Khan, W. Co-delivery of rapamycin- and piperine-loaded polymeric nanoparticles for breast cancer treatment. *Drug Deliv.* **2016**, *23*, 2608–2616. [CrossRef] [PubMed]
26. Fernández, M.; Barcia, E.; Fernández-Carballido, A.; Garcia, L.; Slowing, K.; Negro, S. Controlled release of rasagiline mesylate promotes neuroprotection in a rotenone-induced advanced model of Parkinson's disease. *Int. J. Pharm.* **2012**, *438*, 266–278. [CrossRef]
27. Haobam, R.; Sindhu, K.M.; Chandra, G.; Mohanakumar, K.P. Swim-test as a function of motor impairment in MPTP model of Parkinson's disease: A comparative study in two mouse strains. *Behav. Brain Res.* **2005**, *163*, 159–167. [CrossRef]
28. Makadia, H.K.; Siegel, S.J. Poly lactic-co-glycolic acid (PLGA) As biodegradable controlled drug delivery carrier. *Polymers* **2011**, *3*, 1377–1397. [CrossRef]
29. Freiberg, S.; Zhu, X.X. Polymer microspheres for controlled drug release. *Int. J. Pharm.* **2004**, *282*, 1–18. [CrossRef]
30. Vert, M.; Schwach, G.; Engel, R.; Coudane, J. Something new in the field of PLA/GA bioresorbable polymers? *J. Control. Release* **1998**, *53*, 85–92. [CrossRef]

31. Anderson, J.M.; Shive, M.S. Biodegradation and biocompatibility of PLA and PLGA microspheres. *Adv. Drug Deliv. Rev.* **1997**, *28*, 5–24. [CrossRef]
32. Hillaireau, H.; Couvreur, P. Nanocarriers' entry into the cell: Relevance to drug delivery. *Cell. Mol. Life Sci.* **2009**, *66*, 2873–2896. [CrossRef]
33. Wohlfart, S.; Gelperina, S.; Kreuter, J. Transport of drugs across the blood–brain barrier by nanoparticles. *J. Control. Release* **2012**, *161*, 264–273. [CrossRef] [PubMed]
34. Kamaly, N.; Yameen, B.; Wu, J.; Farokhzad, O.C. Degradable Controlled-Release Polymers and Polymeric Nanoparticles: Mechanisms of Controlling Drug Release. *Chem. Rev.* **2016**, *116*, 2602–2663. [CrossRef] [PubMed]
35. Park, T.G.; Cohen, S.; Langer, R. Poly(L-lactic acid)/Pluronic blends: Characterization of phase separation behavior, degradation, and morphology and use as protein-releasing matrixes. *Macromolecules* **1992**, *25*, 116–122. [CrossRef]
36. Huang, X.; Brazel, C.S. On the importance and mechanisms of burst release in matrix-controlled drug delivery systems. *J. Control. Release* **2001**, *73*, 121–136. [CrossRef]
37. Klose, D.; Siepmann, F.; Elkharraz, K.; Krenzlin, S.; Siepmann, J. How porosity and size affect the drug release mechanisms from PLGA-based microparticles. *Int. J. Pharm.* **2006**, *314*, 198–206. [CrossRef]
38. Singh, R.; Lillard, J.W., Jr. Nanoparticle-based targeted drug delivery. *Exp. Mol. Pathol.* **2009**, *86*, 215–223. [CrossRef]
39. Lockman, P.; Koziara, J.M.; Mumper, R.J.; Allen, D.D. Nanoparticle Surface Charges Alter Blood–Brain Barrier Integrity and Permeability. *J. Drug Target.* **2004**, *12*, 635–641. [CrossRef]
40. Fonseca, C.; Simões, S.; Gaspar, R. Paclitaxel-loaded PLGA nanoparticles: Preparation, physicochemical characterization and in vitro anti-tumoral activity. *J. Control. Release* **2002**, *83*, 273–286. [CrossRef]
41. Kreuter, J. Mechanism of polymeric nanoparticle-based drug transport across the blood-brain barrier (BBB). *J. Microencapsul.* **2013**, *30*, 49–54. [CrossRef]
42. Betarbet, R.; Canet-Aviles, R.M.; Sherer, T.; Mastroberardino, P.G.; McLendon, C.; Kim, J.-H.; Lund, S.; Na, H.-M.; Taylor, G.; Bence, N.F.; et al. Intersecting pathways to neurodegeneration in Parkinson's disease: Effects of the pesticide rotenone on DJ-1, α-synuclein, and the ubiquitin–proteasome system. *Neurobiol. Dis.* **2006**, *22*, 404–420. [CrossRef]
43. Sindhu, K.M.; Saravanan, K.S.; Mohanakumar, K.P. Behavioral differences in a rotenone-induced hemiparkinsonian rat model developed following intranigral or median forebrain bundle infusion. *Brain Res.* **2005**, *1051*, 25–34. [CrossRef] [PubMed]
44. Cannon, J.R.; Tapias, V.; Na, H.M.; Honick, A.S.; Drolet, R.E.; Greenamyre, J.T. A highly reproducible rotenone model of Parkinson's disease. *Neurobiol. Dis.* **2009**, *34*, 279–290. [CrossRef] [PubMed]
45. Pilati, N.; Barker, M.; Panteleimonitis, S.; Donga, R.; Hamann, M. A Rapid Method Combining Golgi and Nissl Staining to Study Neuronal Morphology and Cytoarchitecture. *J. Histochem. Cytochem.* **2008**, *56*, 539–550. [CrossRef] [PubMed]
46. Zhang, Z.-N.; Zhang, J.-S.; Xiang, J.; Yu, Z.-H.; Zhang, W.; Cai, M.; Li, X.-T.; Wu, T.; Li, W.-W.; Cai, D.-F. Subcutaneous rotenone rat model of Parkinson's disease: Dose exploration study. *Brain Res.* **2017**, *1655*, 104–113. [CrossRef] [PubMed]
47. Tapias, V.; Greenamyre, J.T.; Watkins, S.C. Automated imaging system for fast quantitation of neurons, cell morphology and neurite morphometry in vivo and in vitro. *Neurobiol. Dis.* **2013**, *54*, 158–168. [CrossRef] [PubMed]
48. Zhang, Y.; Guo, H.; Guo, X.; Ge, D.; Shi, Y.; Lu, X.; Lu, J.; Chen, J.; Ding, F.; Zhang, Q. Involvement of Akt/mTOR in the Neurotoxicity of Rotenone-Induced Parkinson's Disease Models. *Int. J. Environ. Res. Public Health* **2019**, *16*, 3811. [CrossRef]
49. Swarnkar, S.; Singh, S.; Goswami, P.; Mathur, R.; Patro, I.K.; Nath, C. Astrocyte Activation: A Key Step in Rotenone Induced Cytotoxicity and DNA Damage. *Neurochem. Res.* **2012**, *37*, 2178–2189. [CrossRef]
50. Vila, M.; Jackson-Lewis, V.; Guégan, C.; Wu, D.C.; Teismann, P.; Choi, D.-K.; Tieu, K.; Przedborski, S. The role of glial cells in Parkinson's disease. *Curr. Opin. Neurol.* **2001**, *14*, 483–489. [CrossRef]
51. Gao, Z.; Zhu, Q.; Zhang, Y.; Zhao, Y.; Cai, L.; Shields, C.B.; Cai, J. Reciprocal Modulation Between Microglia and Astrocyte in Reactive Gliosis Following the CNS Injury. *Mol. Neurobiol.* **2013**, *48*, 690–701. [CrossRef]
52. Sofroniew, M.V.; Vinters, H.V. Astrocytes: Biology and pathology. *Acta Neuropathol.* **2010**, *119*, 7–35. [CrossRef]
53. Thomas, D.M.; Walker, P.D.; Benjamins, J.A.; Geddes, T.J.; Kuhn, D.M. Methamphetamine Neurotoxicity in Dopamine Nerve Endings of the Striatum Is Associated with Microglial Activation. *J. Pharmacol. Exp. Ther.* **2004**, *311*, 1–7. [CrossRef] [PubMed]
54. Choi, W.-S.; Kim, H.-W.; Xia, Z. JNK inhibition of VMAT2 contributes to rotenone-induced oxidative stress and dopamine neuron death. *Toxicology* **2015**, *328*, 75–81. [CrossRef] [PubMed]
55. Gomez, C.; Bandez, M.J.; Navarro, A. Pesticides and impairment of mitochondrial function in relation with the parkinsonian syndrome. *Front. Biosci.* **2007**, *12*, 1079–1093. [CrossRef]
56. Bassani, T.B.; Gradowski, R.W.; Zaminelli, T.; Barbiero, J.K.; Santiago, R.M.; Boschen, S.L.; da Cunha, C.; Lima, M.M.S.; Andreatini, R.; Vital, M.A. Neuroprotective and antidepressant-like effects of melatonin in a rotenone-induced Parkinson's disease model in rats. *Brain Res.* **2014**, *1593*, 95–105. [CrossRef] [PubMed]
57. Betarbet, R.; Sherer, T.B.; MacKenzie, G.; Garcia-Osuna, M.; Panov, A.V.; Greenamyre, J.T. Chronic systemic pesticide exposure reproduces features of Parkinson's disease. *Nat. Neurosci.* **2000**, *3*, 1301–1306. [CrossRef]
58. Sherer, T.; Betarbet, R.; Kim, J.-H.; Greenamyre, J. Selective microglial activation in the rat rotenone model of Parkinson's disease. *Neurosci. Lett.* **2003**, *341*, 87–90. [CrossRef]

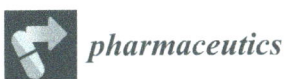

Article

High-Dose Acetaminophen Alters the Integrity of the Blood–Brain Barrier and Leads to Increased CNS Uptake of Codeine in Rats

Junzhi Yang [1], Robert D. Betterton [2], Erica I. Williams [2], Joshua A. Stanton [2], Elizabeth S. Reddell [2], Chidinma E. Ogbonnaya [2], Emma Dorn [2], Thomas P. Davis [1,2], Jeffrey J. Lochhead [2,*] and Patrick T. Ronaldson [1,2,*]

[1] Department of Pharmacology and Toxicology, College of Pharmacy, University of Arizona, Tucson, AZ 85721, USA; jzyang345@email.arizona.edu (J.Y.); davistp@email.arizona.edu (T.P.D.)

[2] Department of Pharmacology, College of Medicine, University of Arizona, Tucson, AZ 85724, USA; rdbetter@email.arizona.edu (R.D.B.); eiwilliams@email.arizona.edu (E.I.W.); joshuastanton@email.arizona.edu (J.A.S.); ekurilko@email.arizona.edu (E.S.R.); ceogbonn@email.arizona.edu (C.E.O.); emmadorn@email.arizona.edu (E.D.)

* Correspondence: lochhead@email.arizona.edu (J.J.L.); pronald@email.arizona.edu (P.T.R.)

Abstract: The consumption of acetaminophen (APAP) can induce neurological changes in human subjects; however, effects of APAP on blood–brain barrier (BBB) integrity are unknown. BBB changes by APAP can have profound consequences for brain delivery of co-administered drugs. To study APAP effects, female Sprague–Dawley rats (12–16 weeks old) were administered vehicle (i.e., 100% dimethyl sulfoxide (DMSO), intraperitoneally (i.p.)) or APAP (80 mg/kg or 500 mg/kg in DMSO, i.p.; equivalent to a 900 mg or 5600 mg daily dose for a 70 kg human subject). BBB permeability was measured via in situ brain perfusion using [^{14}C]sucrose and [^{3}H]codeine, an opioid analgesic drug that is co-administered with APAP (i.e., Tylenol #3). Localization and protein expression of tight junction proteins (i.e., claudin-5, occludin, ZO-1) were studied in rat brain microvessels using Western blot analysis and confocal microscopy, respectively. Paracellular [^{14}C]sucrose "leak" and brain [^{3}H]codeine accumulation were significantly enhanced in rats treated with 500 mg/kg APAP only. Additionally, claudin-5 localization and protein expression were altered in brain microvessels isolated from rats administered 500 mg/kg APAP. Our novel and translational data show that BBB integrity is altered following a single high APAP dose, results that are relevant to patients abusing or misusing APAP and/or APAP/opioid combination products.

Keywords: acetaminophen; blood–brain barrier; claudin-5; CNS drug delivery; opioids; tight junction

Citation: Yang, J.; Betterton, R.D.; Williams, E.I.; Stanton, J.A.; Reddell, E.S.; Ogbonnaya, C.E.; Dorn, E.; Davis, T.P.; Lochhead, J.J.; Ronaldson, P.T. High-Dose Acetaminophen Alters the Integrity of the Blood–Brain Barrier and Leads to Increased CNS Uptake of Codeine in Rats. *Pharmaceutics* **2022**, *14*, 949. https://doi.org/10.3390/pharmaceutics14050949

Academic Editors: Flávia Sousa and Xavier Declèves

Received: 18 March 2022
Accepted: 25 April 2022
Published: 27 April 2022

Publisher's Note: MDPI stays neutral with regard to jurisdictional claims in published maps and institutional affiliations.

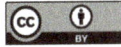

Copyright: © 2022 by the authors. Licensee MDPI, Basel, Switzerland. This article is an open access article distributed under the terms and conditions of the Creative Commons Attribution (CC BY) license (https://creativecommons.org/licenses/by/4.0/).

1. Introduction

The blood–brain barrier (BBB) is essential for maintenance and regulation of brain homeostasis. The BBB selectively and dynamically regulates solute exchange between the central nervous system (CNS) and systemic circulation and simultaneously restricts entry of harmful substances into the brain. The BBB is susceptible to disruption or modulation by stress factors including disease states (e.g., ischemic stroke [1–3], inflammatory pain [4–6], and Alzheimer's disease [7–10]), as well as the presence of circulating intrinsic regulators (e.g., hormones [11,12]) and xenobiotics including environmental toxins [13–15] and drugs [16,17]). For example, morphine is an inducer of ATP-binding cassette transporters at the BBB including P-glycoprotein and breast cancer resistance protein [18–20], which reduces blood-to-brain permeability of many drugs and is suggested to be an underlying mechanism for development of opioid tolerance following chronic use. Besides opioid analgesics, other common psychoactive substances including cocaine [21,22], nicotine [23,24], alcohol [25,26], methamphetamine [27–30] and methylenedioxymethamphetamine (MDMA,

"Ecstasy") [31,32] have been shown to modulate or damage the BBB in varying capacities by changing expression levels and/or post-translational modification status of endothelial transporters or tight junction proteins, or by disruption of functioning tight junction BBB protein assemblies. Indeed, modifications to BBB function by drugs of abuse and polypharmacy can have serious consequences leading to dysregulation of brain homeostasis [33,34], neuronal degeneration [9,10], and concomitant drug–drug interactions [35–37]. In contrast, investigations on the potential of therapeutics that are not classified as drugs of abuse to alter the BBB is lacking.

Acetaminophen (i.e., paracetamol, APAP) is a potent antipyretic and analgesic agent and one of the most commonly used and abused medications, both in the United States and worldwide. According to the Consumer Healthcare Products Association (CHPA), 23% of adults in the United States use an APAP-containing medication on a weekly basis [38]. Although APAP is generally regarded as safe when taken as directed, it is often consumed in excessive amounts. A five-year national survey over the period of 2011–2016 indicated an overall 6.3% rate of overuse of APAP-containing products among participants that significantly exceeded the 4000 mg recommended daily dose [39]. In line with this survey, Blieden and colleagues reported that approximately 6% of their recruited chronic pain patients each year in the United States were prescribed by their physician with an over-4000 mg daily dosage of APAP [40]. Similarly, an Australian study, which recruited chronic non-cancer pain patients, described that 6.1% of participants used considerably more than 4000 mg of APAP per day during the week-long study, and 8.0% of participants consumed quantities of APAP higher than 4000 mg, up to 9540 mg, in a given day [41].

According to StatPearls in 2021, approximately 50% of all APAP-related hospital visits were related to unintentional overdose [42]. Indeed, overuse of APAP is strongly associated with the use of concomitant medications [43]. This is not surprising given that a substantial portion of the over-six-hundred APAP-containing medications are combination drugs, a classic example of polypharmacy. Notably, opioids including hydrocodone (i.e., Vicodin®), oxycodone (i.e., Percocet®), and codeine (i.e., Tylenol #3®) are commonly co-administered with APAP. A cohort study in 1998–2003 in the United States found that opioid-containing products were involved in 63% of unintentional APAP overdoses [44]. In fact, the hydrocodone–APAP combination was the most frequently prescribed medication between the years of 2006–2011 [45], and a medical surveillance in 2004–2005 study identified hydrocodone–APAP and oxycodone–APAP combination medications as some of the most commonly implicated drugs in medication-related adverse events for emergency visits [46]. Both hydrocodone–APAP and oxycodone–APAP combinations are now classified as Schedule II controlled substances by the United States Drug Enforcement Administration (DEA), leaving the codeine–APAP combination as the only Schedule III opioid-containing analgesics on market [47]. The Schedule III classification allows for less stringent prescription regulations (i.e., written, verbal, or electronic prescriptions), and is currently a cause for concern in pediatric medicine [48]. According to analysis of death-certificate data of 2010, opioids were involved in 75.2% of all pharmaceutical overdose deaths of the year, and high-dose APAP was implicated in 2.4% of deaths due to opioid overdose [49]. It is important to note that complete toxicology analyses were not performed in all patients in this study, suggesting that high APAP levels may be involved in a greater percentage of patient deaths.

Considering the prevalence of APAP use and the fact that opioids are frequently co-administered with APAP, it is of critical importance to understand its effects on the BBB. Hepatotoxicity of APAP has been extensively studied, and the consumption of APAP has been linked to neurological alterations without achieving acute liver injury [50,51]; however, there is a marked gap in knowledge regarding effects of APAP directly at the BBB. Furthermore, the current opioid epidemic indicates an urgent need to expand our knowledge on effects of APAP at the BBB in order to understand how it impacts the delivery of concomitantly administered drugs (i.e., opioids) into the CNS. In this study, we hypothesized that APAP modulates paracellular permeability of the BBB by disrupting tight junction barrier proteins at the brain microvascular endothelium, thereby exacerbating CNS opioid exposure through the "leak" of codeine into the brain. To test this hypothesis, we studied, in vivo, paracellular solute "leak" and localization/expression of critical tight junction proteins at the BBB (i.e., claudin-5, occludin and ZO-1) following APAP administration. Our work demonstrated, for the first time, that an acute high dosage (500 mg/kg) of APAP increases paracellular leak of the BBB to both sucrose (i.e., a vascular marker) and codeine, a commonly prescribed opioid that is concomitantly administered with APAP. Of particular significance, low-dose APAP (80 mg/kg) did not have significant effects on BBB permeability to sucrose or codeine. In addition to BBB permeability changes in response to high-dose APAP, we showed that tight junction protein complex disruption by acute APAP exposure is characterized by altered expression of claudin-5 in rat brain microvessels.

2. Materials and Methods

2.1. Animals and Treatments

Animal protocols were approved by the University of Arizona Institutional Animal Care and Use Committee (Protocol #18-377; Approval Date: 25 February 2021) and were conducted in compliance with both National Institutes of Health and Animal Research: Reporting In Vivo Experiments (ARRIVE) guidelines. Female Sprague–Dawley rats were purchased from Envigo (Madison, WI, USA). At the time of experimentation, rats were 3–4 months old with body weights of 200–250 g. We purposely focused our study on female experimental animals to enable robust comparison with our previous study on APAP effects at the BBB [52]. Animals were housed under controlled conditions (22.2–22.4 °C; 50% relative humidity; 12 h light/dark cycle) with free access to food and water for a minimum of seven days. For low- and high-dose drug treatments groups, APAP (Millipore-Sigma, St. Louis, MO, USA) was dissolved in vehicle (100% dimethyl sulfoxide; DMSO) to achieve doses of 80 mg/mL and 500 mg/mL, respectively. Animals received a single intraperitoneal (i.p.) injection of either APAP or vehicle (1 mL/kg). Three hours after treatment and prior to further experimentation, animals were anesthetized with 100 mg/mL ketamine with 10 mg/mL xylazine (i.p.).

2.2. In Situ Brain Perfusion

In situ brain perfusion was performed as described previously by our laboratory [53,54]. Briefly, after anesthesia, experimental animals (n = 6) were given an i.p. dose of heparin (10,000 U/kg) to prevent coagulation. Common carotid arteries were exposed and bilaterally canulated to connect to the perfusion circuit. Both jugular veins were severed to provide drainage. The perfusion buffer (117 mM NaCl, 4.7 mM KCl, 0.8 mM $MgSO_4$, 1.2 mM KH_2PO_4, 2.5 mM $CaCl_2$, 10 mM d-glucose, 3.9% dextran (75,000 g/mol), and 1.0 g/L bovine serum albumin; pH 7.4) was warmed to 37 °C and oxygenated with 95% O_2 and 5% CO_2. Evan's blue dye was added to the perfusion buffer as a visual indicator for tight junction intactness. Rat brains were perfused for 10 min at a total flow rate of 3.6 mL per min under a perfusion pressure of 95 to 105 mmHg. In control experiments, we monitored EKG and respiratory waveforms in animals subjected to in situ brain perfusion for up to 30 min. In all animals, these physiological parameters remained within normal limits, which implies that our in situ brain perfusion method allows for evaluation of BBB integrity and permeability in a stable, well-controlled environment for the entire duration of the perfusion. For measurement of the BBB paracellular leak, [^{14}C]sucrose (Specific Activity = 0.5000 mCi/mL; PerkinElmer Life and Analytical Sciences, Boston, MA, USA) was used as a vascular marker and infused into the perfusate at 0.5 mL per min using a slow-drive syringe pump (Harvard Apparatus, Cambridge, MA, USA). For the measurement of cerebral exposure to opioids, [^{3}H]codeine (Specific Activity = 2.0000 mCi/mL; Research Triangle Institute, Research Triangle, NC, USA) was infused into the perfusion circuit with identical settings to the sucrose experiments. Immediately after perfusion, rat brains were extracted and processed by removing cerebellum, meninges and choroid plexus. The processed brains were divided into three parts and solubilized for two days using

1 mL TS2 tissue solubilizer. At this time, a 2 mL Optiphase SuperMix liquid scintillation cocktail (PerkinElmer Life and Analytical Sciences) was added to each tube to enable the measurement of radioactivity and 100 µL 30% (v/v) glacial acetic acid was added to quench background counts. Radioactivity was measured with a 1450 Liquid Scintillation and Luminescence Counter (PerkinElmer Life and Analytical Sciences) and reported as brain-to-perfusate radioactivity ratios (Rbr %; pmol/mg brain tissue) by dividing the measured amount of radioisotope in brain per brain weight by the known amount of radioisotope in the perfusate:

$$\text{RBr (\%; pmol/mg brain tissue)} = C_{Brain}/C_{Perfusate} \times 100\% \qquad (1)$$

The brain vascular volume in rats has been previously shown to range between 6 and 9 µL/g of brain tissue in perfusion studies utilizing a saline-based bicarbonate buffer [55]. Since brain tissue was processed immediately after perfusion with radiolabeled substrate, all uptake values obtained for [^{14}C]sucrose or [^{3}H]codeine required correction for brain vascular volume (i.e., 8.0 µL/g brain tissue as calculated from data reported by Takasato and colleagues [55]).

2.3. Microvessel Isolation

Rat brain microvessels were isolated according to a protocol developed and published by our laboratory [56]. Briefly, animals ($n = 9$) were euthanized with ketamine/xylazine and decapitated. Brains were removed, processed (i.e., removal of cerebellum, meninges and choroid plexus), and homogenized in ice-cold brain microvessel buffer (pH 7.4) with 0.1% protease inhibitor cocktail (Millipore-Sigma, St. Louis, MO, USA). After thoroughly mixing the brain homogenate with 26% dextran (75,000 g/mol), samples were centrifuged at 6500× g at 4 °C for 30 min. Following centrifugation, the supernatant was aspirated, and pellets were resuspended in the same buffer, mixed with 26% dextran, and were once again centrifuged for 30 min under the same conditions. The microvessel-enriched pellets from the second centrifugation were resuspended in Pierce™ IP Lysis Buffer (Thermo Fisher Scientific, Waltham, MA, USA) with cOmplete™ Mini Protease Inhibitor Cocktail (Roche, Basel, Switzerland), and Phosphatase Inhibitor Cocktail II and III (Research Products International) and stored at −80 °C until further analysis.

2.4. Western Blotting

The total protein concentration of the samples was measured with the Pierce™ BCA Protein Assay Kit (Thermo Fisher Scientific, Waltham, MA, USA). Western blots were performed using the Criterion™ XT Bis-Tris electrophoresis and blotting system (Bio-Rad Laboratories, Hercules, CA, USA). After electrophoresis and protein transfer, the blotting membranes were blocked with SuperBlock™ Blocking Buffer (ThermoFisher Scientific, Waltham, MA, USA) and incubated with appropriate primary antibodies overnight at 4 °C. Primary antibodies that were used in these experiments were designed to detect claudin-5 (4C3C2; Cat #35-2500; 0.5 mg/mL; 1:2000 dilution), occludin (Cat #40-6100; 0.25 mg/mL; 1:500 dilution), and ZO-1 (Cat #40-2200; 0.25 mg/mL; 1:1000 dilution) and were purchased from Thermo Fisher Scientific (Waltham, MA, USA). As a loading control, α-tubulin was detected using a commercially available primary antibody (DM1A; Cat #ab7291; 1.0 mg/ml; 1:1000 dilution) from Abcam, Inc. (Cambridge, MA, USA). After overnight incubation, membranes were washed and incubated with horseradish peroxidase (HRP)-conjugated AffiniPure Goat Anti-Rabbit secondary IgG antibody (Cat #111-035-144; 1:5000 dilution) or HRP-conjugated AffiniPure Goat Anti-Mouse secondary IgG antibody (Cat #115-035-166; 1:5000 dilution) from Jackson ImmunoResearch Laboratories. Inc. (West Grove, PA, USA). The specificity of claudin-5, ZO-1, and occludin primary antibodies has been confirmed for Western blotting experiments by demonstrating the enrichment of specific protein bands corresponding to each tight junction protein in rat brain microvessel samples as compared to rat skeletal muscle homogenate (Figure S1A). Protein signals were detected with SuperSignal™ West Pico PLUS Chemiluminescent Substrate (Thermo Fisher Scientific,

Waltham, MA, USA) and imaged using the ChemiDoc™ Touch Imaging System from Bio-Rad Laboratories. Densitometry analysis of protein bands was performed using ImageJ (Wayne Rasband, Research Services Branch, National Institute of Mental Health, Bethesda, MD, USA). Band intensities of tight junction proteins (i.e., claudin-5, occludin, ZO-1) were normalized to those of the loading control (i.e., α-tubulin) for statistical analysis.

2.5. Immunofluorescence Staining

Three hours after treatment with vehicle or APAP, rats were anesthetized with ketamine/xylazine and decapitated. The brain was immediately removed and snap-frozen at −75 °C in isopentane on dry ice. Cryosections (20 µm) were mounted onto glass slides and stored at −80 °C until needed for staining. Sections were fixed in methanol at −20 °C, blocked in PBS with 0.3% Triton X-100 + 5% goat serum and then incubated in primary antibody overnight at 4 °C. Primary antibodies used for immunofluorescence were rabbit anti-ZO-1 (Cat #40-2200; 1:750 dilution; Thermo Fisher Scientific, Waltham, MA, USA), mouse anti-claudin-5 (Cat #35-2500; 1:500 dilution; Thermo Fisher Scientific, Waltham, MA, USA), and mouse anti-occludin (OC-3F10; Cat #33-1500; 0.5 mg/mL; 1:500 dilution; Thermo Fisher Scientific, Waltham, MA, USA). These antibodies were detected with Alexa 488 goat anti-rabbit (Cat #A11008; 1:500 dilution; Thermo Fisher Scientific, Waltham, MA, USA) and Alexa 568 goat anti-mouse (Cat #A11004; 1:500 dilution; Thermo Fisher Scientific, Waltham, MA, USA). DyLight 649-tomato lectin (Cat #DL-1178-1; Vector Laboratories, Burlingame, CA, USA) was used to label and visualize the cerebral vasculature. Control experiments were conducted by incubating sections in the presence of secondary antibody only (i.e., no primary antibody controls). Data for these control experiments are presented in Figure S1B.

2.6. Confocal Microscopy

Confocal microscopy was performed on a Leica SP8 confocal microscope (Leica Biosystems, Wetzlar, Germany) with 488 and 552 nm excitation lasers. Emitted light was detected with a Leica hybrid detector (HyD). Images were acquired from randomly chosen areas of the somatosensory cortex between 2 mm rostral to 1 mm caudal relative to Bregma. Images from control and treated animals were acquired using matching laser power and gain settings with emission windows set to prevent bleed-through between fluorophores. Adjustments for brightness and contrast levels were performed with ImageJ software (NIH) in an identical manner for both control and treated images.

2.7. Statistical Analysis

In situ brain perfusion brain-to-perfusate radioactivity ratios (RBr %) and Western blot densitometric analysis data (normalized to loading control) were reported as mean ± S.D. Statistically significant differences between control and treatment groups were determined with one-way analysis of variance (ANOVA) followed by post hoc two-tailed unpaired homoscedastic Student's t-test to examine differences between groups. A value of $p < 0.05$ was considered to be statistically significant.

3. Results

3.1. Increased BBB Paracellular "Leak" in Response to High-Dose APAP Treatment

To investigate whether there is a change in BBB paracellular permeability (i.e., "leak") in the presence of APAP, radiolabeled sucrose (i.e., [^{14}C]sucrose) was used. We administered 80 mg/kg of APAP, a low dose emulating approximately 900 mg for an average-weight human adult (i.e., 70 kg), and 500 mg/kg of APAP, an acute dosage equivalent to approximately 5600 mg for an average-weight human adult (i.e., 70 kg), for the low- and high-dose treatments, respectively, 3 h prior to in situ brain perfusion with [^{14}C]sucrose. As shown in Figure 1A, only the high-dose APAP treatment resulted in significantly elevated codeine and sucrose radioactivity in perfused rat brains, which indicates disruption of BBB functional integrity leading to paracellular leak.

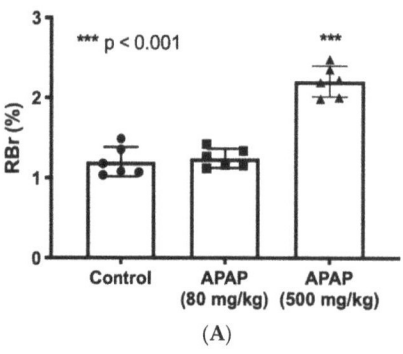 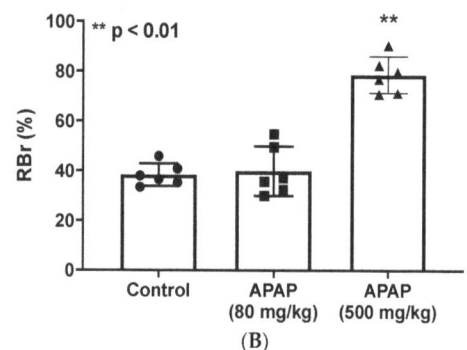

Figure 1. BBB paracellular permeability to sucrose and codeine is increased at three hours following high-dose APAP administration. (**A**): In situ brain perfusion with [^{14}C]sucrose as a vascular paracellular permeability marker shows significantly elevated radioactivity level represented in brain-to-perfusate radioactivity ratios (RBr %) in brains of high-dose APAP-treated rats ($n = 6$) in comparison to vehicle or low-dose APAP-treated rats. No significant change radioactivity level was measured in the low-dose APAP (80 mg/kg) treated rats. (**B**): In situ perfusion with [^{3}H]codeine following APAP injection shows significantly higher radioactivity represented in brain-to-perfusate radioactivity ratios (RBr %) in brains of APAP (500 mg/kg)-treated rats ($n = 6$) in comparison to vehicle. Data are expressed as mean ± S.D. (** $p < 0.01$; *** $p < 0.001$).

3.2. Elevated CNS Exposure to Codeine after APAP Treatment

To investigate whether the increase in BBB paracellular permeability due to APAP stress contributes to elevated CNS exposure to drugs, we utilized in situ brain perfusion to measure [^{3}H]codeine uptake into brain tissue 3 h following APAP injection (80 mg/kg or 500 mg/kg; i.p.). Codeine was purposely selected for these experiments since it is commonly co-administered with APAP in combination products including, but not limited to, Tylenol #3®. It is also an opioid analgesic drug that accesses the CNS primarily by passive diffusion and not by facilitated transport processes [54,57], which renders it an ideal drug to use in the evaluation of altered BBB functional integrity by APAP. Codeine radioactivity levels measured in brain tissue of high-dose APAP (500 mg/kg)-treated rats were significantly increased as compared to those of low-dose APAP (80 mg/kg) or vehicle controls (Figure 1B). This indicates that concomitantly administered medications such as high-dose APAP and codeine can interact at the BBB, thereby causing a serious risk of adverse effects associated with the codeine due to the elevated brain penetration of this opioid analgesic drug in the presence of a high dose of APAP.

3.3. Increased Claudin-5 Expression in Brain Microvessel after High-Dose APAP Treatment

Since claudin-5 is considered to be the primary determinant of BBB tight junction integrity [17], we measured changes in claudin-5 content in rat brain microvessels 3 h after an acute low dose (80 mg/kg; i.p.) or high dose (500 mg/kg; i.p.) of APAP in accordance with our in situ brain perfusion experiment. Western blot analysis of microvessel samples indicated a significant elevation in claudin-5 expression in response to high-dose APAP treatment as compared to low-dose APAP ($p < 0.0001$) or vehicle-treated rats ($p < 0.0001$) (Figure 2A). Both a cross-section (Figure 2B) and longitudinal section (Figure 2C) of a rat brain microvessel show localization of claudin-5 at endothelial cell margins, evidence for its role as a critical constituent of tight junction protein complexes. Confocal imaging of microvessels in rat brain cryosections corroborated with our Western blot data, demonstrating an overall increase in claudin-5 staining throughout cortices of rats three hours after high-dose APAP treatment as compared to vehicle (Figure 2D).

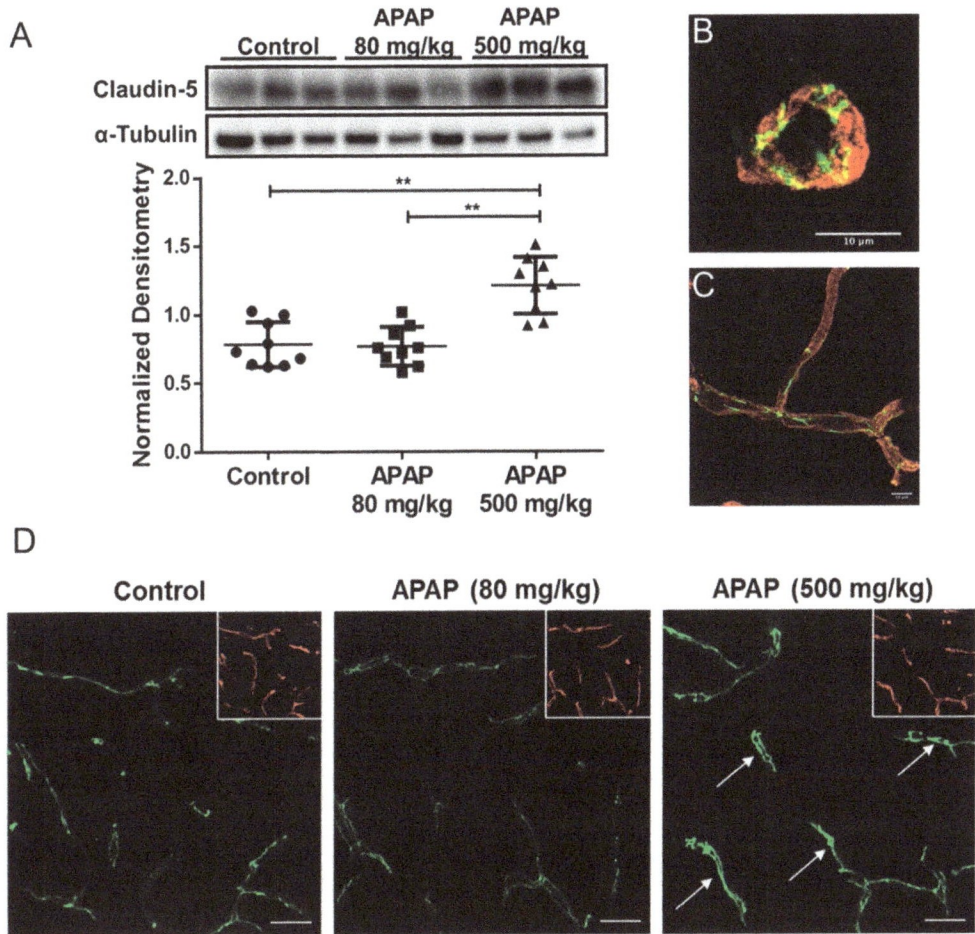

Figure 2. Claudin-5 level increases in BBB microvessel endothelial cells three hours after high-dose APAP treatment. (**A**) Western blot (**top**) and densitometric analysis (**bottom**) of claudin-5 levels in isolated brain microvessel of rats ($n = 9$) treated with low-dose APAP (80 mg/kg) and high-dose APAP (500 mg/kg) shows statistical significance between the three groups ($p = 0.000012$), as well as between vehicle and the high-dose groups ($p = 0.00018$; Student's t-test) and between low-dose and high-dose groups ($p = 0.000074$). No statistical significance was detected between the vehicle and the low-dose APAP group ($p = 0.84$). Densitometric data are expressed as mean ± S.D. (** $p < 0.0001$). High magnification confocal microscopy images of a cross-section (**B**) and a longitudinal section (**C**) of a cortical microvessel showing claudin-5 localization (green) within the microvessel labeled with the vascular marker tomato lectin (red). (**D**) confocal microscopy images indicate higher overall claudin-5 expression in cortical microvessel of rats treated with high-dose APAP (500 mg/kg) than vehicle, but not in those treated with low-dose APAP (80 mg/kg). Arrows show sites of claudin-5 upregulation. Microvessels were stained with lectin (red) and are shown in the inset to demonstrate vascular localization of claudin-5. Scale bar = 20 μm.

We also evaluated APAP effects on other tight junction proteins including the transmembrane protein occludin and the intracellular accessory protein zonula occludens-1 (ZO-1). In contrast to our results with claudin-5, Western blot analysis and confocal microscopy of occludin (Figure 3A,C) and ZO-1 (Figure 3B,D) in cortical microvessels showed no detectable change in either APAP-treated or untreated rats at the three-hour timepoint. Taken together, these observations suggest that the changes in claudin-5 is likely involved in the process leading up to the observed BBB paracellular "leak" in response to high-dose APAP treatment, while occludin and ZO-1 are likely not responsible for the disruption of BBB tight junctions in the acute phase of the high-dose APAP stress response.

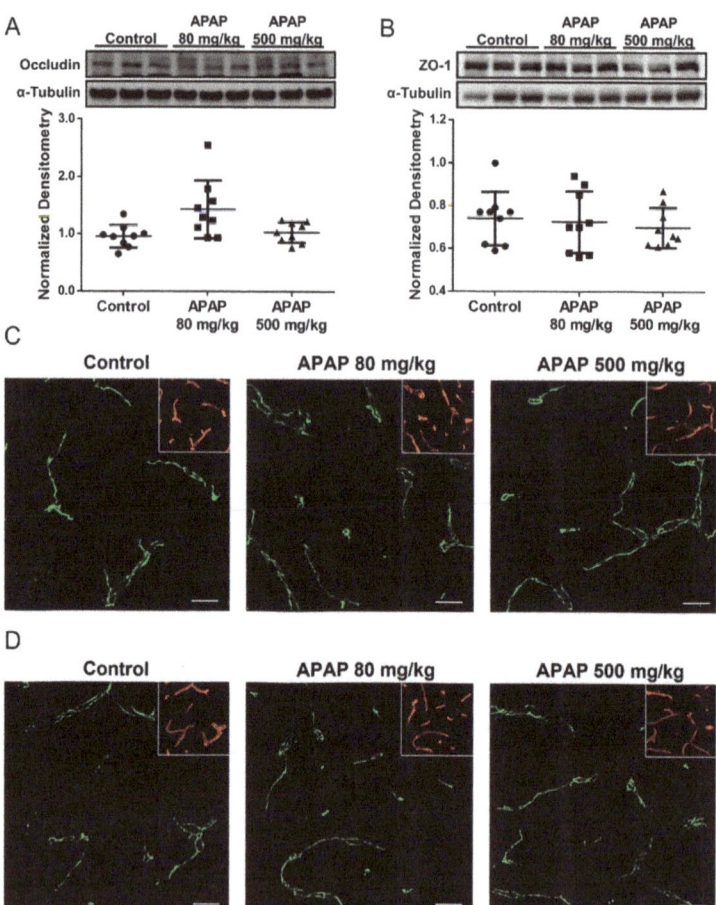

Figure 3. Occludin and ZO-1 levels remain unchanged three hours following APAP treatment. (**A**) Western blot (**top**) and densitometric analysis (**bottom**) shows comparable occludin levels in isolated brain microvessel of APAP (500 mg/mL)-treated and control rats ($n = 9$). Densitometric data are expressed as mean ± S.D. (**B**) Western blot (**top**) and densitometric analysis (**bottom**) shows comparable ZO-1 levels in isolated brain microvessel of APAP (500 mg/mL)-treated and control rats ($n = 9$). Densitometric data are expressed as mean ± S.D. (**C**) Confocal microscopy shows similar overall occludin expression in cortical microvessel of rats treated with APAP (80 or 500 mg/kg) as vehicle. Microvessels were stained with lectin (red) and are shown in the inset to demonstrate vascular localization of occludin. Scale bar = 20 μm. (**D**) Confocal microscopy shows similar overall ZO-1 expression in cortical microvessel of rats treated with APAP (80 or 500 mg/kg) as vehicle. Microvessels were stained with lectin (red) and are shown in the inset to demonstrate vascular localization of ZO-1. Scale bar = 20 μm.

4. Discussion

The BBB plays an essential role in regulation of brain homeostasis and preservation of the optimal microenvironment for proper neuronal function. Dysregulation of BBB permeability is associated with many pathologies [17] and can lead to increased vulnerability (i.e., leak) of the brain to harmful substances in the systemic circulation [52,54,57–62]. For example, peripheral inflammatory pain can cause BBB dysfunction that is manifested by increased paracellular "leak" to circulating small molecule solutes including drugs [54]. Such enhancement in paracellular permeability was shown to result from modulation of tight junction protein complexes at the brain microvascular endothelium. Claudins, as well as occludin, are critical transmembrane tight junction proteins at the BBB that form protein complexes responsible for physically sealing paracellular gaps between adjacent endothelial cells [17,63]. Changes to protein expression levels of claudins and occludin are frequently observed in modulation of stress responses by tight junctions at the BBB [17]. ZO-1 is an important intracellular accessory protein at the tight junction that links transmembrane proteins to the actin cytoskeleton, thus forming complex networks essential for the dynamic regulation of the BBB [17]. In the present study, we are the first to demonstrate that acute treatment of APAP disrupts tight junction protein complexes in the cerebral microvasculature, as evidenced by an increase in paracellular permeability at the BBB and an upregulation of claudin-5. We believe these changes are due specifically to APAP administration rather than the DMSO solvent. Our previous work has shown that BBB permeability to sucrose or small molecule drugs in control (i.e., untreated animals) is not altered in vivo following acute (i.e., up to 3 h) administration of DMSO vehicle [53,64]. Preliminary time-point experiments showed that this increase in claudin-5 levels was sustained until 6 h after APAP treatment and returned to baseline by 12 h (data not shown). Additionally, as increased levels of claudin-5 in the systemic circulation have been implicated in BBB breakdown [65,66], we conducted an ELISA analysis of rat plasma that detected a slight but statistically significant ($p = 0.03$) increase in plasma claudin-5 protein levels at 3 h following APAP administration (data not shown). In contrast, occludin and ZO-1 were not affected by APAP treatment, indicating that claudin-5 is likely the primary tight junction protein that controls the response to high-dose APAP-induced stress and, by extension, enhanced paracellular "leak" associated with APAP administration.

Although a simultaneous increase in both claudin-5 expression and BBB permeability may seem paradoxical, it is essential to note that many publications in the scientific literature have reported that claudin-5 upregulation is associated with an increase in barrier permeability or neuronal injury due to pathophysiological stressors. For example, studies in the kainic acid model of temporal lobe epilepsy demonstrated a significant increase in claudin-5 levels 24–72 h after kainic acid injection in correspondence with neuronal injury [67]. Our laboratory's studies in a rat model of peripheral inflammatory pain showed a 6-fold increase in microvessel claudin-5 levels with BBB paracellular "leak" but no detectable change in claudin-5 localization [6]. Further investigation into the underlying mechanism revealed that transforming growth factor (TGF)-β-signaling mediated this disruption of the BBB that was manifested by sucrose extravasation and claudin-5 upregulation at the brain microvascular endothelium [53]. Claudin-5 is also elevated in epithelial tight junctions in lung tissue isolated from alcoholic rats with diminished barrier functions, likely a result of disrupted protein-protein interactions between claudins [68]. Interestingly, overexpression of claudins 1 and 3 in stably transfected NIH/3T3 or IB3.1 cells leads to a decrease in permeability to dextrans but overexpression of claudin-5 in these same cells results in an increase in permeability to dextrans [69]. Additionally, it is essential to consider that changes in monomeric tight junction protein expression following exposure to a pathological or pharmacological stressor may reflect altered tight junction integrity via collapse of oligomeric structures. Indeed, claudin-5 has been shown to form oligomers in HEK293 cells transfected with native claudin-5 [70] or chimeric claudin-5 proteins [71]. The ability of claudin-5 to assemble into higher order structures was proposed to be required for the formation of tight junction strands and, subsequently, the sealing function of tight junction protein complexes in endothelial cells [70–72]. These findings highlight the fact that elevated claudin-5 protein expression in brain microvascular endothelial cells is not necessarily indicative of improved neurovascular integrity. Rather, any change in claudin-5 expression, regardless of directionality, can be reflective of tight junction dysregulation and paracellular leak, depending on the specific pathological or mechanistic processes involved and the resulted state of functional intact nature of tight junction assembly. Future work by our group will elucidate the mechanism of action pertaining to the upregulation of claudin-5 in response to APAP treatment.

APAP may also affect BBB permeability through interactions with phospholipids in the plasma membrane. APAP directly binds to phospholipids and significantly increases membrane fluidity in a dose-dependent manner [73]. Alterations in physicochemical properties of the plasma membrane are likely to alter the function of the tight junction protein complex by dynamically affecting the organization, oligomerization, and structure of the proteins comprising the tight junction at the BBB [74–76]. These changes may affect paracellular permeability at the BBB independent of changes in expression levels of individual proteins comprising the TJ complex.

In pharmacological studies, BBB disruption is frequently studied as a clinical goal for optimization of drug delivery into the CNS, while its role as an adverse effect of pharmaceutical agents, polypharmacy, and risk factor for brain microenvironment dysregulation is frequently overlooked. APAP is an extraordinarily effective and useful substance used in hundreds of combination medications and consumed by millions of individuals each day in the United States alone [38]. Contrary to APAP popularity, there is limited knowledge on effects of APAP and its potential for drug–drug interactions at the BBB. Previous studies indicate that, while APAP has been shown to preserve brain endothelial cell survival and reduce the neurovascular inflammatory response under oxidative stress in vitro and at low doses in vivo [77,78], APAP at a higher dose (>200 mg/kg) induces cortical oxidative stress and produces reactive astrocytosis without achieving acute liver injury [50,78]. As another example, one prominent site for potential drug interactions at the BBB is P-glycoprotein, a critical efflux transporter at the BBB responsible for restricting entrance of a wide range of substances into the CNS. Our laboratory has previously shown that APAP at 500 mg/kg significantly increases the expression level of P-glycoprotein in brain microvessels and thereby reduces morphine uptake and antinociception [52]. Of particular significance, we demonstrated that APAP activated endothelial signaling pathways such as the constitutive androstane receptor, a nuclear receptor known to be involved in the induction of drug metabolizing enzymes and transporters [52]. In the present study, we further demonstrate that a high dose of APAP elicits drug–drug interactions at the BBB by increasing paracellular permeability and, as a result, can also increase CNS exposure to concomitantly administered drugs that are not transport substrates for P-glycoprotein (i.e., codeine). Importantly, we found that APAP administered at a dose considered safe and effective for analgesia did not alter BBB integrity. Taken together with our previous work, these data imply that an acute, high dose of APAP can have profound effects on cerebral microvascular homeostasis and contribute to unexpected changes in CNS drug disposition.

In addition to drug exposures, the BBB is susceptible to modulation by various physiological stress stimuli. As APAP is the most prevalent and most used analgesic on the market, it is important to note that inflammatory pain by itself could damage tight junction integrity at the BBB. We have previously shown that the induction of inflammatory pain in the hind paw with several different agents (i.e., λ-carrageenan, complete Freund's adjuvant, formalin) also increases paracellular "leak" of the BBB to sucrose and codeine. Associated with these changes in the λ-carrageenan model are alterations to the tight junction proteins claudin-5, occludin, and ZO-1 as well as the cytoskeletal scaffolding protein, actin [4–6]. Studies with the λ-carrageenan model further illustrated prolonged BBB tight junction injury, most prominently at the 3 and 48 h timepoints, which correlated with increased CNS codeine uptake and enhanced codeine analgesia [57]. Given that APAP is commonly used in the presence of pain, it is of our interest to further investigate the effect of APAP in inflammatory pain models and understand their concurrent effects on the function of the BBB.

In conclusion, our novel data show that high-dose APAP increases paracellular permeability of the BBB, an effect that is correlated with increased protein expression of claudin-5 in brain microvessels, an effect that indicates dysregulation of tight junction assembly. The APAP-induced paracellular "leak" contributes to higher CNS exposure to codeine. As noted, many human subjects regularly consume excessive amounts of APAP, including doses greater than or equal to those used in this study on rats, on a daily basis in order to manage acute or chronic pain [43]. Our data suggest that further investigation into effects of APAP on BBB integrity at both the molecular and functional level is warranted. Such studies are likely to yield paradigm-shifting findings that will lead to safer prescribing of APAP and improved formulation of APAP-containing combination products to lower occurrence of accidental overdose of concomitantly administered drugs such as opioids.

Supplementary Materials: The following supporting information can be downloaded at: https://www.mdpi.com/article/10.3390/pharmaceutics14050949/s1, Figure S1: Western blot and confocal microscopy demonstrate antibody specificity.

Author Contributions: J.Y., J.J.L. and P.T.R. designed and carried out the experiments with assistance from R.D.B., E.I.W., J.A.S., E.S.R., C.E.O., E.D. and T.P.D. The writing and editing of the manuscript were conducted by J.Y., J.J.L., T.P.D. and P.T.R. All authors have read and agreed to the published version of the manuscript.

Funding: This work was supported by a grant from the National Institute on Drug Abuse (NIDA), National Institutes of Health (R01-DA051812) to PTR and TPD.

Institutional Review Board Statement: Animal protocols were approved by the University of Arizona Institutional Animal Care and Use Committee (IACUC; Protocol #18-377; Date of approval: 25 February 2021) and were conducted in compliance with both National Institutes of Health and Animal Research: Reporting In Vivo Experiments (ARRIVE) guidelines.

Informed Consent Statement: Not applicable.

Data Availability Statement: If reasonably requested or needed, data and samples/models will be made available for sharing to qualified parties provided that such a request does not compromise intellectual property interests, interfere with publication, or betray confidentiality. Data that are shared will include standards and notations required to accurately interpret the data, following commonly accepted practices in the field. Data and samples/materials will be available for access and sharing as soon as reasonably possible and no longer than two years after acquisition of the data.

Conflicts of Interest: The authors have no competing interests to declare.

References

1. Bernardo-Castro, S.; Sousa, J.A.; Bras, A.; Cecilia, C.; Rodrigues, B.; Almendra, L.; Machado, C.; Santo, G.; Silva, F.; Ferreira, L.; et al. Pathophysiology of Blood-Brain Barrier Permeability Throughout the Different Stages of Ischemic Stroke and Its Implication on Hemorrhagic Transformation and Recovery. *Front. Neurol.* **2020**, *11*, 594672. [CrossRef] [PubMed]
2. Abdullahi, W.; Tripathi, D.; Ronaldson, P.T. Blood-brain barrier dysfunction in ischemic stroke: Targeting tight junctions and transporters for vascular protection. *Am. J. Physiol. Cell Physiol.* **2018**, *315*, C343–C356. [CrossRef] [PubMed]
3. Nadareishvili, Z.; Simpkins, A.N.; Hitomi, E.; Reyes, D.; Leigh, R. Post-Stroke Blood-Brain Barrier Disruption and Poor Functional Outcome in Patients Receiving Thrombolytic Therapy. *Cerebrovasc. Dis.* **2019**, *47*, 135–142. [CrossRef] [PubMed]
4. Huber, J.D.; Witt, K.A.; Hom, S.; Egleton, R.D.; Mark, K.S.; Davis, T.P. Inflammatory pain alters blood-brain barrier permeability and tight junctional protein expression. *Am. J. Physiol. Heart Circ. Physiol.* **2001**, *280*, H1241–H1248. [CrossRef] [PubMed]
5. Huber, J.D.; Hau, V.S.; Borg, L.; Campos, C.R.; Egleton, R.D.; Davis, T.P. Blood-brain barrier tight junctions are altered during a 72-h exposure to lambda-carrageenan-induced inflammatory pain. *Am. J. Physiol. Heart Circ. Physiol.* **2002**, *283*, H1531–H1537. [CrossRef]
6. Brooks, T.A.; Hawkins, B.T.; Huber, J.D.; Egleton, R.D.; Davis, T.P. Chronic inflammatory pain leads to increased blood-brain barrier permeability and tight junction protein alterations. *Am. J. Physiol. Heart Circ. Physiol.* **2005**, *289*, H738–H743. [CrossRef]
7. Cai, Z.; Qiao, P.F.; Wan, C.Q.; Cai, M.; Zhou, N.K.; Li, Q. Role of Blood-Brain Barrier in Alzheimer's Disease. *J. Alzheimers Dis.* **2018**, *63*, 1223–1234. [CrossRef]
8. Ishii, M.; Iadecola, C. Risk factor for Alzheimer's disease breaks the blood-brain barrier. *Nature* **2020**, *581*, 31–32. [CrossRef]

9. Sweeney, M.D.; Sagare, A.P.; Zlokovic, B.V. Blood-brain barrier breakdown in Alzheimer disease and other neurodegenerative disorders. *Nat. Rev. Neurol.* **2018**, *14*, 133–150. [CrossRef]
10. Palmer, A.M. The role of the blood brain barrier in neurodegenerative disorders and their treatment. *J. Alzheimers Dis.* **2011**, *24*, 643–656. [CrossRef]
11. Wilson, A.C.; Clemente, L.; Liu, T.; Bowen, R.L.; Meethal, S.V.; Atwood, C.S. Reproductive hormones regulate the selective permeability of the blood-brain barrier. *Biochim. Biophys. Acta* **2008**, *1782*, 401–407. [CrossRef] [PubMed]
12. Mahringer, A.; Fricker, G. BCRP at the blood-brain barrier: Genomic regulation by 17beta-estradiol. *Mol. Pharm.* **2010**, *7*, 1835–1847. [CrossRef] [PubMed]
13. Tobwala, S.; Wang, H.-J.; Carey, J.; Banks, W.; Ercal, N. Effects of Lead and Cadmium on Brain Endothelial Cell Survival, Monolayer Permeability, and Crucial Oxidative Stress Markers in an in Vitro Model of the Blood-Brain Barrier. *Toxics* **2014**, *2*, 258–275. [CrossRef]
14. Calderon-Garciduenas, L.; Solt, A.C.; Henriquez-Roldan, C.; Torres-Jardon, R.; Nuse, B.; Herritt, L.; Villarreal-Calderon, R.; Osnaya, N.; Stone, I.; Garcia, R.; et al. Long-term air pollution exposure is associated with neuroinflammation, an altered innate immune response, disruption of the blood-brain barrier, ultrafine particulate deposition, and accumulation of amyloid beta-42 and alpha-synuclein in children and young adults. *Toxicol. Pathol.* **2008**, *36*, 289–310. [PubMed]
15. Oppenheim, H.A.; Lucero, J.; Guyot, A.C.; Herbert, L.M.; McDonald, J.D.; Mabondzo, A.; Lund, A.K. Exposure to vehicle emissions results in altered blood brain barrier permeability and expression of matrix metalloproteinases and tight junction proteins in mice. *Part. Fibre Toxicol.* **2013**, *10*, 62. [CrossRef] [PubMed]
16. Pimentel, E.; Sivalingam, K.; Doke, M.; Samikkannu, T. Effects of Drugs of Abuse on the Blood-Brain Barrier: A Brief Overview. *Front. Neurosci.* **2020**, *14*, 513. [CrossRef]
17. Lochhead, J.J.; Yang, J.; Ronaldson, P.T.; Davis, T.P. Structure, Function, and Regulation of the Blood-Brain Barrier Tight Junction in Central Nervous System Disorders. *Front. Physiol.* **2020**, *11*, 914. [CrossRef]
18. Yousif, S.; Saubamea, B.; Cisternino, S.; Marie-Claire, C.; Dauchy, S.; Scherrmann, J.M.; Decleves, X. Effect of chronic exposure to morphine on the rat blood-brain barrier: Focus on the P-glycoprotein. *J. Neurochem.* **2008**, *107*, 647–657. [CrossRef]
19. Yousif, S.; Chaves, C.; Potin, S.; Margaill, I.; Scherrmann, J.M.; Decleves, X. Induction of P-glycoprotein and Bcrp at the rat blood-brain barrier following a subchronic morphine treatment is mediated through NMDA/COX-2 activation. *J. Neurochem.* **2012**, *123*, 491–503. [CrossRef]
20. Chaves, C.; Gomez-Zepeda, D.; Auvity, S.; Menet, M.C.; Crete, D.; Labat, L.; Remiao, F.; Cisternino, S.; Decleves, X. Effect of Subchronic Intravenous Morphine Infusion and Naloxone-Precipitated Morphine Withdrawal on P-gp and Bcrp at the Rat Blood-Brain Barrier. *J. Pharm. Sci.* **2016**, *105*, 350–358. [CrossRef]
21. Fiala, M.; Eshleman, A.J.; Cashman, J.; Lin, J.; Lossinsky, A.S.; Suarez, V.; Yang, W.; Zhang, J.; Popik, W.; Singer, E.; et al. Cocaine increases human immunodeficiency virus type 1 neuroinvasion through remodeling brain microvascular endothelial cells. *J. Neurovirol.* **2005**, *11*, 281–291. [CrossRef] [PubMed]
22. Dhillon, N.K.; Peng, F.; Bokhari, S.; Callen, S.; Shin, S.H.; Zhu, X.; Kim, K.J.; Buch, S.J. Cocaine-mediated alteration in tight junction protein expression and modulation of CCL2/CCR2 axis across the blood-brain barrier: Implications for HIV-dementia. *J. Neuroimmune Pharmacol.* **2008**, *3*, 52–56. [CrossRef] [PubMed]
23. Hawkins, B.T.; Abbruscato, T.J.; Egleton, R.D.; Brown, R.C.; Huber, J.D.; Campos, C.R.; Davis, T.P. Nicotine increases in vivo blood-brain barrier permeability and alters cerebral microvascular tight junction protein distribution. *Brain Res.* **2004**, *1027*, 48–58. [CrossRef] [PubMed]
24. Manda, V.K.; Mittapalli, R.K.; Bohn, K.A.; Adkins, C.E.; Lockman, P.R. Nicotine and cotinine increases the brain penetration of saquinavir in rat. *J. Neurochem.* **2010**, *115*, 1495–1507. [CrossRef] [PubMed]
25. Haorah, J.; Knipe, B.; Gorantla, S.; Zheng, J.; Persidsky, Y. Alcohol-induced blood-brain barrier dysfunction is mediated via inositol 1,4,5-triphosphate receptor (IP3R)-gated intracellular calcium release. *J. Neurochem.* **2007**, *100*, 324–336. [CrossRef] [PubMed]
26. Abdul Muneer, P.M.; Alikunju, S.; Szlachetka, A.M.; Haorah, J. The mechanisms of cerebral vascular dysfunction and neuroinflammation by MMP-mediated degradation of VEGFR-2 in alcohol ingestion. *Arterioscler. Thromb. Vasc. Biol.* **2012**, *32*, 1167–1177. [CrossRef] [PubMed]
27. Mahajan, S.D.; Aalinkeel, R.; Sykes, D.E.; Reynolds, J.L.; Bindukumar, B.; Adal, A.; Qi, M.; Toh, J.; Xu, G.; Prasad, P.N.; et al. Methamphetamine alters blood brain barrier permeability via the modulation of tight junction expression: Implication for HIV-1 neuropathogenesis in the context of drug abuse. *Brain Res.* **2008**, *1203*, 133–148. [CrossRef]
28. Ramirez, S.H.; Potula, R.; Fan, S.; Eidem, T.; Papugani, A.; Reichenbach, N.; Dykstra, H.; Weksler, B.B.; Romero, I.A.; Couraud, P.O.; et al. Methamphetamine disrupts blood-brain barrier function by induction of oxidative stress in brain endothelial cells. *J. Cereb. Blood Flow Metab.* **2009**, *29*, 1933–1945. [CrossRef]
29. Abdul Muneer, P.M.; Alikunju, S.; Szlachetka, A.M.; Murrin, L.C.; Haorah, J. Impairment of brain endothelial glucose transporter by methamphetamine causes blood-brain barrier dysfunction. *Mol. Neurodegener.* **2011**, *6*, 23. [CrossRef]
30. Xue, Y.; He, J.T.; Zhang, K.K.; Chen, L.J.; Wang, Q.; Xie, X.L. Methamphetamine reduces expressions of tight junction proteins, rearranges F-actin cytoskeleton and increases the blood brain barrier permeability via the RhoA/ROCK-dependent pathway. *Biochem. Biophys. Res. Commun.* **2019**, *509*, 395–401. [CrossRef]

31. Torres, E.; Gutierrez-Lopez, M.D.; Mayado, A.; Rubio, A.; O'Shea, E.; Colado, M.I. Changes in interleukin-1 signal modulators induced by 3,4-methylenedioxymethamphetamine (MDMA): Regulation by CB2 receptors and implications for neurotoxicity. *J. Neuroinflamm.* **2011**, *8*, 53. [CrossRef]
32. Rubio-Araiz, A.; Perez-Hernandez, M.; Urrutia, A.; Porcu, F.; Borcel, E.; Gutierrez-Lopez, M.D.; O'Shea, E.; Colado, M.I. 3,4-Methylenedioxymethamphetamine (MDMA, ecstasy) disrupts blood-brain barrier integrity through a mechanism involving P2X7 receptors. *Int. J. Neuropsychopharmacol.* **2014**, *17*, 1243–1255. [CrossRef]
33. Weiss, N.; Miller, F.; Cazaubon, S.; Couraud, P.O. The blood-brain barrier in brain homeostasis and neurological diseases. *Biochim. Biophys. Acta* **2009**, *1788*, 842–857. [CrossRef]
34. Xiao, M.; Xiao, Z.J.; Yang, B.; Lan, Z.; Fang, F. Blood-Brain Barrier: More Contributor to Disruption of Central Nervous System Homeostasis Than Victim in Neurological Disorders. *Front. Neurosci.* **2020**, *14*, 764. [CrossRef]
35. Sun, J.J.; Xie, L.; Liu, X.D. Transport of carbamazepine and drug interactions at blood-brain barrier. *Acta Pharmacol. Sin.* **2006**, *27*, 249–253. [CrossRef]
36. Wanek, T.; Romermann, K.; Mairinger, S.; Stanek, J.; Sauberer, M.; Filip, T.; Traxl, A.; Kuntner, C.; Pahnke, J.; Bauer, F.; et al. Factors Governing P-Glycoprotein-Mediated Drug-Drug Interactions at the Blood-Brain Barrier Measured with Positron Emission Tomography. *Mol. Pharm.* **2015**, *12*, 3214–3225. [CrossRef]
37. Karbownik, A.; Stanislawiak-Rudowicz, J.; Stachowiak, A.; Romanski, M.; Grzeskowiak, E.; Szalek, E. The Influence of Paracetamol on the Penetration of Sorafenib and Sorafenib N-Oxide through the Blood-Brain Barrier in Rats. *Eur. J. Drug Metab. Pharmacokinet.* **2020**, *45*, 801–808. [CrossRef]
38. Safe Use of Acetaminophen. Available online: https://www.chpa.org/about-consumer-healthcare/activities-initiatives/safe-use-acetaminophen (accessed on 27 September 2021).
39. Kaufman, D.W.; Kelly, J.P.; Battista, D.R.; Malone, M.K.; Weinstein, R.B.; Shiffman, S. Five-year trends in acetaminophen use exceeding the recommended daily maximum dose. *Br. J. Clin. Pharmacol.* **2019**, *85*, 1028–1034. [CrossRef]
40. Blieden, M.; Paramore, L.C.; Shah, D.; Ben-Joseph, R. A perspective on the epidemiology of acetaminophen exposure and toxicity in the United States. *Expert Rev. Clin. Pharmacol.* **2014**, *7*, 341–348. [CrossRef]
41. Hoban, B.; Larance, B.; Gisev, N.; Nielsen, S.; Cohen, M.; Bruno, R.; Shand, F.; Lintzeris, N.; Hall, W.; Farrell, M.; et al. The use of paracetamol (acetaminophen) among a community sample of people with chronic non-cancer pain prescribed opioids. *Int. J. Clin. Pract.* **2015**, *69*, 1366–1376. [CrossRef]
42. Agrawal, S.; Khazaeni, B. Acetaminophen Toxicity. In *StatPearls*; StatPearls Publishing: Treasure Island, FL, USA, 2021.
43. Shiffman, S.; Rohay, J.M.; Battista, D.; Kelly, J.P.; Malone, M.K.; Weinstein, R.B.; Kaufman, D.W. Patterns of acetaminophen medication use associated with exceeding the recommended maximum daily dose. *Pharmacoepidemiol. Drug Saf.* **2015**, *24*, 915–921. [CrossRef] [PubMed]
44. Larson, A.M.; Polson, J.; Fontana, R.J.; Davern, T.J.; Lalani, E.; Hynan, L.S.; Reisch, J.S.; Schiodt, F.V.; Ostapowicz, G.; Shakil, A.O.; et al. Acetaminophen-induced acute liver failure: Results of a United States multicenter, prospective study. *Hepatology* **2005**, *42*, 1364–1372. [CrossRef] [PubMed]
45. Manchikanti, L.; Helm, S., 2nd; Fellows, B.; Janata, J.W.; Pampati, V.; Grider, J.S.; Boswell, M.V. Opioid epidemic in the United States. *Pain Physician* **2012**, *15* (Suppl. 3), ES9–ES38. [CrossRef] [PubMed]
46. Budnitz, D.S.; Pollock, D.A.; Weidenbach, K.N.; Mendelsohn, A.B.; Schroeder, T.J.; Annest, J.L. National surveillance of emergency department visits for outpatient adverse drug events. *JAMA* **2006**, *296*, 1858–1866. [CrossRef]
47. Drug Enforcement Administration, US Department of Justice. *Lists of: Scheduling Actions Controlled Substances Regulated Chemicals*; 2022. Available online: https://www.deadiversion.usdoj.gov/schedules/orangebook/orangebook.pdf (accessed on 18 April 2022).
48. Prows, C.A.; Zhang, X.; Huth, M.M.; Zhang, K.; Saldana, S.N.; Daraiseh, N.M.; Esslinger, H.R.; Freeman, E.; Greinwald, J.H.; Martin, L.J.; et al. Codeine-related adverse drug reactions in children following tonsillectomy: A prospective study. *Laryngoscope* **2014**, *124*, 1242–1250. [CrossRef]
49. Jones, C.M.; Mack, K.A.; Paulozzi, L.J. Pharmaceutical overdose deaths, United States, 2010. *JAMA* **2013**, *309*, 657–659. [CrossRef]
50. Vigo, M.B.; Perez, M.J.; De Fino, F.; Gomez, G.; Martinez, S.A.; Bisagno, V.; Di Carlo, M.B.; Scazziota, A.; Manautou, J.E.; Ghanem, C.I. Acute acetaminophen intoxication induces direct neurotoxicity in rats manifested as astrogliosis and decreased dopaminergic markers in brain areas associated with locomotor regulation. *Biochem. Pharmacol.* **2019**, *170*, 113662. [CrossRef]
51. Ghanem, C.I.; Perez, M.J.; Manautou, J.E.; Mottino, A.D. Acetaminophen from liver to brain: New insights into drug pharmacological action and toxicity. *Pharmacol. Res.* **2016**, *109*, 119–131. [CrossRef]
52. Slosky, L.M.; Thompson, B.J.; Sanchez-Covarrubias, L.; Zhang, Y.; Laracuente, M.L.; Vanderah, T.W.; Ronaldson, P.T.; Davis, T.P. Acetaminophen modulates P-glycoprotein functional expression at the blood-brain barrier by a constitutive androstane receptor-dependent mechanism. *Mol. Pharmacol.* **2013**, *84*, 774–786. [CrossRef]
53. Ronaldson, P.T.; Demarco, K.M.; Sanchez-Covarrubias, L.; Solinsky, C.M.; Davis, T.P. Transforming growth factor-beta signaling alters substrate permeability and tight junction protein expression at the blood-brain barrier during inflammatory pain. *J. Cereb. Blood Flow Metab.* **2009**, *29*, 1084–1098. [CrossRef]
54. Lochhead, J.J.; McCaffrey, G.; Sanchez-Covarrubias, L.; Finch, J.D.; Demarco, K.M.; Quigley, C.E.; Davis, T.P.; Ronaldson, P.T. Tempol modulates changes in xenobiotic permeability and occludin oligomeric assemblies at the blood-brain barrier during inflammatory pain. *Am. J. Physiol. Heart Circ. Physiol.* **2012**, *302*, H582–H593. [CrossRef] [PubMed]

55. Takasato, Y.; Rapoport, S.I.; Smith, Q.R. An in situ brain perfusion technique to study cerebrovascular transport in the rat. *Am. J. Physiol.* **1984**, *247 Pt 2*, H484–H493. [CrossRef] [PubMed]
56. Brzica, H.; Abdullahi, W.; Reilly, B.G.; Ronaldson, P.T. A Simple and Reproducible Method to Prepare Membrane Samples from Freshly Isolated Rat Brain Microvessels. *J. Vis. Exp.* **2018**, *135*, e57698. [CrossRef] [PubMed]
57. Hau, V.S.; Huber, J.D.; Campos, C.R.; Davis, R.T.; Davis, T.P. Effect of lambda-carrageenan-induced inflammatory pain on brain uptake of codeine and antinociception. *Brain Res.* **2004**, *1018*, 257–264. [CrossRef]
58. Raabe, A.; Schmitz, A.K.; Pernhorst, K.; Grote, A.; von der Brelie, C.; Urbach, H.; Friedman, A.; Becker, A.J.; Elger, C.E.; Niehusmann, P. Cliniconeuropathologic correlations show astroglial albumin storage as a common factor in epileptogenic vascular lesions. *Epilepsia* **2012**, *53*, 539–548. [CrossRef]
59. Salimi, H.; Klein, R.S. Disruption of the Blood-Brain Barrier during Neuroinflammatory and Neuroinfectious Diseases. In *Neuroimmune Diseases*; Springer: Berlin/Heidelberg, Germany, 2019; pp. 195–234.
60. Al-Obaidi, M.M.J.; Desa, M.N.M. Mechanisms of Blood Brain Barrier Disruption by Different Types of Bacteria, and Bacterial-Host Interactions Facilitate the Bacterial Pathogen Invading the Brain. *Cell. Mol. Neurobiol.* **2018**, *38*, 1349–1368. [CrossRef]
61. Chen, Z.; Li, G. Immune response and blood-brain barrier dysfunction during viral neuroinvasion. *Innate Immun.* **2021**, *27*, 109–117. [CrossRef]
62. Zhang, L.; Zhou, L.; Bao, L.; Liu, J.; Zhu, H.; Lv, Q.; Liu, R.; Chen, W.; Tong, W.; Wei, Q.; et al. SARS-CoV-2 crosses the blood-brain barrier accompanied with basement membrane disruption without tight junctions alteration. *Signal Transduct. Target. Ther.* **2021**, *6*, 337. [CrossRef]
63. Suzuki, H.; Nishizawa, T.; Tani, K.; Yamazaki, Y.; Tamura, A.; Ishitani, R.; Dohmae, N.; Tsukita, S.; Nureki, O.; Fujiyoshi, Y. Crystal structure of a claudin provides insight into the architecture of tight junctions. *Science* **2014**, *344*, 304–307. [CrossRef]
64. Thompson, B.J.; Sanchez-Covarrubias, L.; Slosky, L.M.; Zhang, Y.; Laracuente, M.L.; Ronaldson, P.T. Hypoxia/reoxygenation stress signals an increase in organic anion transporting polypeptide 1a4 (Oatp1a4) at the blood-brain barrier: Relevance to CNS drug delivery. *J. Cereb. Blood Flow Metab.* **2014**, *34*, 699–707. [CrossRef]
65. Andersson, E.A.; Mallard, C.; Ek, C.J. Circulating tight-junction proteins are potential biomarkers for blood-brain barrier function in a model of neonatal hypoxic/ischemic brain injury. *Fluids Barriers CNS* **2021**, *18*, 7. [CrossRef] [PubMed]
66. Kazmierski, R.; Michalak, S.; Wencel-Warot, A.; Nowinski, W.L. Serum tight-junction proteins predict hemorrhagic transformation in ischemic stroke patients. *Neurology* **2012**, *79*, 1677–1685. [CrossRef] [PubMed]
67. Yan, B.C.; Xu, P.; Gao, M.; Wang, J.; Jiang, D.; Zhu, X.; Won, M.H.; Su, P.Q. Changes in the Blood-Brain Barrier Function Are Associated With Hippocampal Neuron Death in a Kainic Acid Mouse Model of Epilepsy. *Front. Neurol.* **2018**, *9*, 775. [CrossRef] [PubMed]
68. Schlingmann, B.; Overgaard, C.E.; Molina, S.A.; Lynn, K.S.; Mitchell, L.A.; Dorsainvil White, S.; Mattheyses, A.L.; Guidot, D.M.; Capaldo, C.T.; Koval, M. Regulation of claudin/zonula occludens-1 complexes by hetero-claudin interactions. *Nat. Commun.* **2016**, *7*, 12276. [CrossRef]
69. Coyne, C.B.; Gambling, T.M.; Boucher, R.C.; Carson, J.L.; Johnson, L.G. Role of claudin interactions in airway tight junctional permeability. *Am. J. Physiol. Lung Cell. Mol. Physiol.* **2003**, *285*, L1166–L1178. [CrossRef]
70. Rossa, J.; Lorenz, D.; Ringling, M.; Veshnyakova, A.; Piontek, J. Overexpression of claudin-5 but not claudin-3 induces formation of trans-interaction-dependent multilamellar bodies. *Ann. N. Y. Acad. Sci.* **2012**, *1257*, 59–66. [CrossRef]
71. Rossa, J.; Ploeger, C.; Vorreiter, F.; Saleh, T.; Protze, J.; Gunzel, D.; Wolburg, H.; Krause, G.; Piontek, J. Claudin-3 and claudin-5 protein folding and assembly into the tight junction are controlled by non-conserved residues in the transmembrane 3 (TM3) and extracellular loop 2 (ECL2) segments. *J. Biol. Chem.* **2014**, *289*, 7641–7653. [CrossRef]
72. Krause, G.; Protze, J.; Piontek, J. Assembly and function of claudins: Structure-function relationships based on homology models and crystal structures. *Semin. Cell Dev. Biol.* **2015**, *42*, 3–12. [CrossRef]
73. De Mel, J.U.; Gupta, S.; Harmon, S.; Stingaciu, L.; Roth, E.W.; Siebenbuerger, M.; Bleuel, M.; Schneider, G.J. Acetaminophen Interactions with Phospholipid Vesicles Induced Changes in Morphology and Lipid Dynamics. *Langmuir* **2021**, *37*, 9560–9570. [CrossRef]
74. Ikenouchi, J. Roles of membrane lipids in the organization of epithelial cells: Old and new problems. *Tissue Barriers* **2018**, *6*, 1–8. [CrossRef]
75. Otani, T.; Furuse, M. Tight Junction Structure and Function Revisited. *Trends Cell Biol.* **2020**, *30*, 805–817. [CrossRef] [PubMed]
76. Vu, D.D.; Tuchweber, B.; Raymond, P.; Yousef, I.M. Tight junction permeability and liver plasma membrane fluidity in lithocholate-induced cholestasis. *Exp. Mol. Pathol.* **1992**, *57*, 47–61. [PubMed]
77. Tripathy, D.; Grammas, P. Acetaminophen protects brain endothelial cells against oxidative stress. *Microvasc. Res.* **2009**, *77*, 289–296. [CrossRef] [PubMed]
78. Naziroglu, M.; Uguz, A.C.; Kocak, A.; Bal, R. Acetaminophen at different doses protects brain microsomal Ca^{2+}-ATPase and the antioxidant redox system in rats. *J. Membr. Biol.* **2009**, *231*, 57–64. [CrossRef] [PubMed]

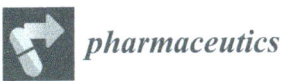

Review

Drug Delivery Systems in the Development of Novel Strategies for Glioblastoma Treatment

Wiam El Kheir [1,2], Bernard Marcos [3], Nick Virgilio [4], Benoit Paquette [5,6], Nathalie Faucheux [2,6] and Marc-Antoine Lauzon [1,7,*]

1. Advanced Dynamic Cell Culture Systems Laboratory, Department of Chemical Engineering and Biotechnology Engineering, Faculty of Engineering, Université de Sherbrooke, 2500 Boul. Université, Sherbrooke, QC J1K 2R1, Canada; wiam.el.kheir@usherbrooke.ca
2. Laboratory of Cell-Biomaterial Biohybrid Systems, Department of Chemical Engineering and Biotechnology Engineering, Faculty of Engineering, Université de Sherbrooke, 2500 Boul. Université, Sherbrooke, QC J1K 2R1, Canada; nathalie.faucheux@usherbrooke.ca
3. Department of Chemical Engineering and Biotechnology Engineering, Faculty of Engineering, Université de Sherbrooke, 2500 Boul. Université, Sherbrooke, QC J1K 2R1, Canada; bernard.marcos@usherbrooke.ca
4. Department of Chemical Engineering, Polytechnique Montréal, 2500 Chemin de Polytechnique, Montréal, QC H3T 1J4, Canada; nick.virgilio@polymtl.ca
5. Department of Nuclear Medicine and Radiobiology, Faculty of Medicine and Health Sciences, Université de Sherbrooke, 12e Avenue Nord, Sherbrooke, QC J1H 5N4, Canada; benoit.paquette@usherbrooke.ca
6. Clinical Research Center of the Centre Hospitalier Universitaire de l'Université de Sherbrooke, 12e Avenue Nord, Sherbrooke, QC J1H 5N4, Canada
7. Research Center on Aging, 1036 Rue Belvédère Sud, Sherbrooke, QC J1H 4C4, Canada
* Correspondence: marc-antoine.lauzon@usherbrooke.ca; Tel.: +1-819-821-8000 (ext. 66457)

Abstract: Glioblastoma multiforme (GBM) is a grade IV glioma considered the most fatal cancer of the central nervous system (CNS), with less than a 5% survival rate after five years. The tumor heterogeneity, the high infiltrative behavior of its cells, and the blood–brain barrier (BBB) that limits the access of therapeutic drugs to the brain are the main reasons hampering the current standard treatment efficiency. Following the tumor resection, the infiltrative remaining GBM cells, which are resistant to chemotherapy and radiotherapy, can further invade the surrounding brain parenchyma. Consequently, the development of new strategies to treat parenchyma-infiltrating GBM cells, such as vaccines, nanotherapies, and tumor cells traps including drug delivery systems, is required. For example, the chemoattractant CXCL12, by binding to its CXCR4 receptor, activates signaling pathways that play a critical role in tumor progression and invasion, making it an interesting therapeutic target to properly control the direction of GBM cell migration for treatment proposes. Moreover, the interstitial fluid flow (IFF) is also implicated in increasing the GBM cell migration through the activation of the CXCL12-CXCR4 signaling pathway. However, due to its complex and variable nature, the influence of the IFF on the efficiency of drug delivery systems is not well understood yet. Therefore, this review discusses novel drug delivery strategies to overcome the GBM treatment limitations, focusing on chemokines such as CXCL12 as an innovative approach to reverse the migration of infiltrated GBM. Furthermore, recent developments regarding in vitro 3D culture systems aiming to mimic the dynamic peritumoral environment for the optimization of new drug delivery technologies are highlighted.

Keywords: brain cancer; chemoattractant; CXCL; CXCR; glioblastoma multiforme; 3D cell culture systems

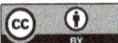

1. Introduction

Malignant tumors of the central nervous system (CNS) are a widely heterogeneous and polygenic disease that constitutes 1.6% of all cancer cases worldwide [1]. The GLOBOCAN cancer tomorrow prediction tool at the Global Cancer Observatory (GCO) (gco.iarc.fr) expects the incidence and mortality rates to increase by more than 41.3% and 46.6%, respectively, by 2040 [2]. In the US, more than 13,000 new patients are diagnosed with Glioblastoma (GBM) every year, 50% of them die within one year, and 90% within three years post-diagnosis [3].

The 2021 WHO fifth edition classified the CNS neoplasms into twelve categories. Within the category of "gliomas, glioneuronal and neuronal tumors", six large groups of diffuse gliomas are defined: (1) Adults diffuse gliomas, including three types (Grade 2, 3 or 4 Isocitrate Dehydrogenase (IDH)-mutated diffuse astrocytomas, grade 2 or 3 IDH-mutated diffuse astrocytomas, and grade 4 IDH-mutated astrocytoma or Glioblastomas), (2) Pediatric-type diffuse low-grade gliomas, (3) Pediatric-type diffuse high-grade gliomas, (4) Circumscribed astrocytic gliomas, (5) Glioneuronal and neuronal tumors, and (6) Ependymal tumors [4]. Based on the level of the tumor malignancy, grade 1 gliomas can usually be cured by surgical resection, chemotherapy, and radiotherapy. Whereas grade 2 gliomas are highly malignant and can progress to grades 3 and 4, which are more aggressive, invasive, and resistant to the actual standard treatments [5].

GBM accounts for more than 82% of all malignant gliomas [6]. GBM is considered the most aggressive and fatal primary brain tumor, with a worldwide incidence rate of less than 10 per 100,000 [7] and a survival rate of less than 5% after five years post-diagnosis [6]. The incidence of GBM is 1.6 times higher in males compared to females and diagnosed at an older age with a median age of 64 at diagnosis [7,8]. GBM incidence is twice higher in Caucasians compared to Africans and Afro-Americans, and lower in Asians and American Indians [9]. GBM includes "Primary GBM (or de novo)" progressing from low-grade astrocytomas or oligodendrocytomas, which occurs mostly in elderly patients (usually over 60 years old), and accounts for 90% of the GBM cases. On the other hand, "Secondary GBM" accounts for the remaining 10%, generally observed in younger patients (45 years old), and arises from already existing grade I or II gliomas.

GBM is characterized by considerable mitotic activity, high vascular proliferation, abundant necrosis, recurrent mutation in IDH in most of its cells, and a high resistance of GBM cells to radio- and chemotherapy. These are the critical factors that make GBM extremely complicated to eradicate. Furthermore, GBM cells have a highly invasive nature and can modulate their microenvironment to disperse and invade the brain parenchyma using the blood vessels and the white matter (Figure 1).

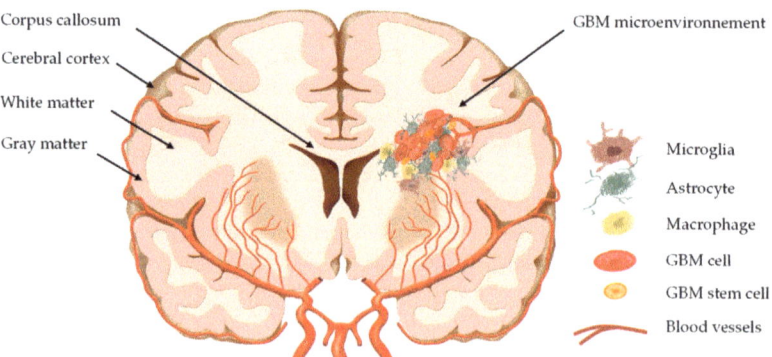

Figure 1. Schematic illustration of GBM.

These cells make GBM a disseminated tumor that is impossible to completely resect or cure by the standard treatments that consist of a primary resection surgery, followed by chemotherapy and radiotherapy. Surgery is often powerless due to the depth of the lesion and its location, whereas the radiation tolerance of the brain limits the radiotherapy efficacy. Furthermore, the systemic delivery of chemotherapeutic drugs into the tumor site is limited due to the blood–brain barrier (BBB). Despite its high local aggressiveness, GBM rarely leaves the brain. The estimated incidence of metastasis is seldom up to 0.5% [10], but when it occurs, metastatic cells target mostly the lungs, lymph nodes, liver, bones, and pancreas [10–14]. All these data illustrate the urgent need for novel and innovative alternative treatments for GBM. Here, we first review some of the actual treatments used for GBM. Then, we discuss the roles of chemokines and the interstitial fluid flow in GBM cell invasion (particularly the chemokine CXCL12 and its receptor CXCR4). Finally, we review the recent innovations in drug delivery technology for GBM treatment. We focus on drug delivery devices in GBM and their systemic or local administration, and we finally discuss the strategy we are developing, which is a gliotrap based on the controlled delivery of a chemoattractant. The gliotrap consists of chemoattracting GBM cells with the aim to inverse their migration direction towards being well-confined meaning they can be more efficiently irradiated.

2. GBM Traditional Treatments

The high mobility of invading cells, the cellular heterogeneity within GBM clusters, and the ability of GBM cells to transit between proliferative and non-proliferative phases are the main factors responsible for the failure of GBM standard treatment [15–18].

2.1. Surgical Resection

Surgical resection is considered the most important component in the treatment of GBM. Surgery is mainly used for reducing tumor burden, reversing neurological deficits, and the local introduction of therapeutic agents [19]. The feasibility of surgery depends basically on the localization and the size of the tumor. Tumors located in sites such as the eloquent cortex, brainstem, or basal ganglia do not allow surgery, and patients generally have the worst prognosis [20]. However, a successful identification of the tumor margins and its location are still the major challenges that face a total excision. Imaging is the key tool for GBM resection to guide biopsies and identify the tumor margins [19,21,22]. Imaging techniques such as functional magnetic resonance imaging (MRI), computed tomography (CT), and ultrasound now make it possible to process a more aggressive surgical resection with fewer side effects in patients [23]. Even if the surgical resection can remove most of the tumor bulk, the main problem remaining is that a subset of GBM cells at the time of treatment will have already migrated and spread beyond the visible boundary of the main mass [24]. Due to this, radiotherapy postsurgical treatment is usually necessary to prevent recurrence.

2.2. Radiotherapy

In the late 1970s, radiation therapy after surgery was shown to improve survival in patients with GBM and has since become progressively optimized for focused applications [25]. After the resection of the tumor, the total radiotherapy dose administrated is typically 60 Gy delivered through 30 fractions of 2 Gy per day (5/7 days) for 6 weeks with intervals [26,27]. In addition to the tumor, a 20–25 mm margin is irradiated in order to kill the infiltrated GBM cells [28,29]. The use of radiotherapy has revealed several limitations and different side effects including cognitive impairment, radiological necrosis, radiation-induced neuronal damage, radio-resistance of some tumors, and reduced proliferation of normal cells caused by DNA damage [30]. However, the other potential radiotherapies-based strategies that have been explored, such as treatments with conformal radiation therapy, stereotactic radiosurgery [31], intensity-modulated radiation therapy [26], and boron neutron capture therapy [32], have shown less toxicity and less exposure in comparison with normal tissues [33]. Conformal radiation therapy, for example, is designed to target the residual GBM cells while maintaining the healthy brain tissue and minimizing the cognitive side effects [25]. Stereotaxic radiosurgery (SRS) consists of delivering X-ray energy in a few sessions (<5) over 6 to 8 weeks [34,35]. Although, clinical neurological complications such as motor deficit, visual deficit, cognitive deficit, sensory deficit, headache, and others are often reported [34]. Nevertheless, the best results for GBM treatment are obtained when radiotherapy (60 Gy) is usually combined with concurrent daily temozolomide (TMZ) chemotherapy [27].

2.3. Chemotherapy

Chemotherapy was found to be beneficial for improving patient survival, but the systemic administration of drugs is known to be very limited due to the presence of the BBB [36]. The BBB is the boundary between the circulatory system and the brain extracellular space and is mainly composed of endothelial cells that make tight junctions along the wall of blood vessels [37]. After surgery, the standard treatment regimen includes 6 weeks of concomitant TMZ (75 mg/m^2 of body-surface area per day for each week) and radiation followed by the administration of adjuvant TMZ (150–200 mg/m^2) for 5 days every 28 days on six cycles [38]. TMZ, which is a small alkylating agent that methylates the purine bases of the DNA, was first approved by the Food and Drugs Administration (FDA) and used to treat brain tumors in 1993 [39]. So far, its use has shown a significantly better overall survival in treated patients [40]. TMZ reduces the activity of the DNA repair enzyme O 6 methylguanine-DNA methyltransferase (MGMT) to promote GBM tumor cells death. MGMT gene methylation is correlated with a positive prognostic of TMZ [41]. Generally, the major side effect of TMZ is hematologic toxicity [42]. Several agents which alkylate DNA base pairs have been explored in the context of GBM treatments [43]. Carmustine (BCMU), for example, induces a crosslink between the guanine and cytosine. It has been approved by the FDA to treat high grade gliomas (3 and 4) [44]. In addition, in 2014, the FDA approved the use of Lomustine (CCNU) in patients with GBM, following surgery and radiotherapy [45]. Lomustine is a small lipophobic alkylating anti-tumor reagent able to cross the BBB [38].

However, several studies have shown that combining therapies were more effective than using a single approach [46,47]. In 2005, a phase 3 clinical trial conducted by the European Organization for Research and Treatment of Cancer (EORTC) and the Clinical Trials Group of the National Cancer Institute of Canada (NCIC CTG) showed that patient survival significantly increases when treated with TMZ in combination with radiotherapy and complete surgical resection [48]. Unfortunately, due to its various genetic–epigenetic alterations and its high heterogeneity, the standard treatments for GBM remain mostly ineffective to completely heal patients. Therefore, understanding the pathways used by GBM cells to migrate, the molecules that regulate it, and the different mechanisms responsible for the cancer cells extensive invasiveness and migration is critical to develop therapeutic approaches to treat GBM patients.

3. CXCL12–CXCR4 in Glioblastoma Invasion
3.1. The Pathways of GBM Cell Invasion

Despite several studies and current therapies, GBM treatment remains a challenging task in clinical oncology because of its highly invasive properties, GBM cells being capable of invading local and distant brain tissues. In 1938, Dr. Scherer described the migration of GBM cells following four pathways (Figure 2): (a) within the brain parenchyma while interacting with cells and neuronal extensions; (b) along the blood vessels; (c) following the fibrous pathways of the white matter tracts (in the corpus callosum); and (d) along the subarachnoid space in continuity with the ventricles [17].

The invasion of the parenchyma by the GBM cells is a complex process based on different interactions between the tumor cells and their microenvironment [49–51]. The GBM cells have the ability to adapt their microenvironment by modifying the brain extracellular matrix (ECM), which is a complex mixture of molecules such as glycoproteins—fibronectin, laminins, tenascins (TN) as well as glycosaminoglycans (hyaluronic acid, HA), and proteoglycans that contribute to GBM angiogenesis, invasion, and therapeutic resistance [52]. GBM cells synthesize some ECM components such as HA, TN-C, and fibronectin, and express their cell receptors, such as specific integrins [53] and CD44 (receptor of hyaluronic acid (HA)), which leads to cell adhesion and migration [54].

Proteases, such as plasminogen/plasmin system, and cathepsins, that are divided into six groups including gelatinases, collagenases, stromelysins, matrilysins, and metalloproteinases (MMP), are other essential components of the ECM playing an important role in its remodeling during tumor cell migration [53]. For example, the ECM changes its conformation through the action of MMPs, which can be expressed by brain cells and favor GBM cell migration [55]. Through signals mediated by integrins, the ECM also allows GBM cells to develop protrusions and eventually remodel their cytoskeleton to create new connections and influence their migration [53].

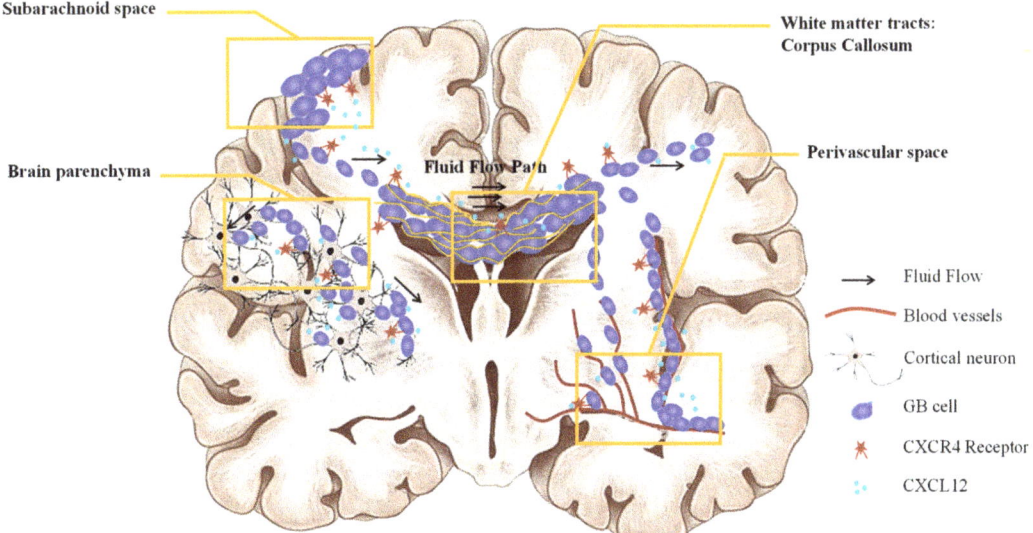

Figure 2. Routes of GBM cells to metastasize in the brain (Adapted from deGooijer et al., 2018 [56]).

The name "integrin" was first proposed by the research group of Hynes in 1986 for a protein complex linking the ECM to the actin-based cytoskeleton [57]. Integrins are the major receptors of the ECM proteins [58], composed of α and β transmembrane heterodimer subunits combined to make 24 different integrins [59]. Currently, 18 α subunits and 8 β subunits have been identified, and each combination determines the functional specificity of the receptors [60]. Based on affinities to ligands, integrins can be classified into four groups: the (a) Collagen receptors group, (b) Laminin receptors group, (c) Leukocyte-specific receptors group, and (d) the group of receptors that recognizes the sequence of three amino-acids RGD (Arginine–Glycine–Aspartate) [61].

Integrins play different roles, such as cell adhesion, intracellular transduction, and the regulation of several signaling pathways (Figure 3) [62]. They are also involved in the survival, proliferation, and migration of cancer cells [63]. The integrin-mediated signaling pathway maintains homeostasis, but is dysregulated in tumors and generally associated with the invasive phenotype of GBM cells [64]. For example, RGD-binding integrins include a series of αv dimers, such as αvβ3 and αvβ5, highly expressed in GBM cells in which ligands are ECM proteins, such as fibrinogen (one of the markers of inflammation in brain injury [65]), fibronectin, and TN [66,67]. Types of TN, such as TN-C, can promote cell migration, angiogenesis, and proliferation. TN-C is highly associated with blood vessels which enable glioma cells to invade into other regions of the brain either by binding to integrins to affect the cell directly or by binding to ECM molecules and affecting the cell indirectly [54].

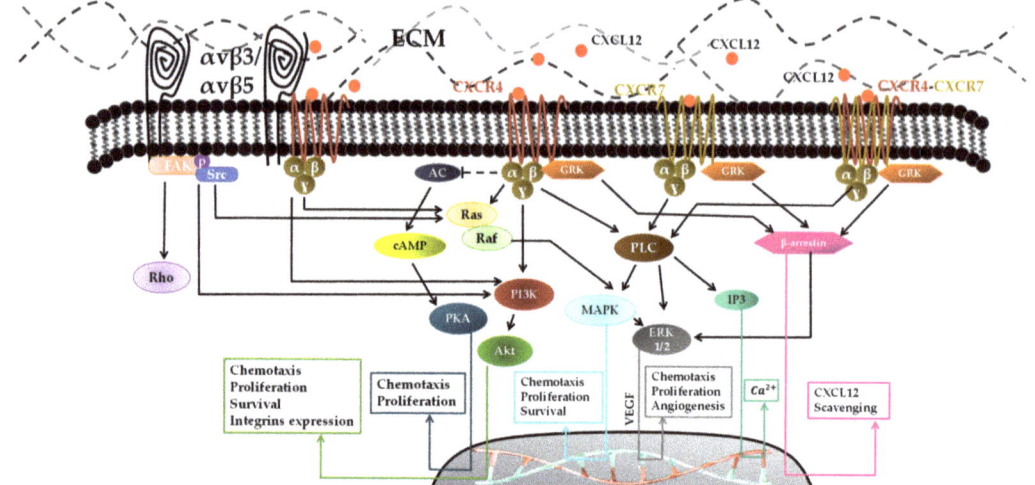

Figure 3. Schematic representation of different signaling pathways activated by CXCL12/CXCR4/CXCR7 axis and integrins. FAK: focal adhesion kinase; p: phosphorylation; Src: proto-oncogene tyrosine-protein kinase; cAMP: cyclic AMP, adenosine 3′,5′-cyclic monophosphate; AC: adenylate cyclase; PKA: protein kinase A; PI3K: phosphoinositide 3 kinase; Akt: protein kinase B; MAPK: mitogen-activated protein kinase; PLC: phospholipase C; ERK: extracellular signal-regulated kinase; IP3: inositol trisphosphate; GRK: G-protein coupled receptor kinase; ECM: extracellular matrix; Ca^{2+}: Calcium; CXCL12: CXC chemokine ligand 12; CXCR4: receptor CXC type 4; CXCR7: receptor CXC type 7; αβγ : G protein complex; αvβ3: integrin alpha V and integrin beta 3; αvβ5: integrin alpha V and integrin beta 5; VEGF: vascular endothelial growth factor.

3.2. CXCL12–CXCR4 Axis in GBM Cell Migration

Different studies have shown that integrins such as αvβ3, αvβ5, α3β1, α5β1, α6β1, and α9β1 are associated with the invasive phenotype of GBM cells [68–71]. Blandin et al. demonstrated that αv integrin allows the dissemination of GBM cells in the presence of a rich microenvironment of fibronectin, while its absence reinforces cells adhesion [72]. The stimulation of αv integrins subunits by ECM proteins leads to the activation of different signaling pathways such as phosphatidylinositol-3-kinase (PI3K) and protein kinase B (AKT) pathways, for which several studies have proven their induction of GBM cell migration [64,72,73]. Rat sarcoma virus (RAS) and extracellular signal-regulated kinase (ERK) pathways are also activated via the increased activity of MMP-2 and MMP-9 [74,75]. In conclusion: (a) Integrins' activation via ECM proteins leads to changes in the GBM cell cytoskeleton and the activation of gene transcription for cell adhesion, migration, and invasion [76–79]. (b) The ECM has become a target for many researchers due to the important role it plays in GBM progression. For more information about the emerging therapeutic approaches for GBM that target ECM, see Mohiuddin et al., 2021 [54].

However, in addition to the ECM, the GBM microenvironment is constituted from several other components, such as fluids, molecules such as chemokines that play a crucial role in the migration of GBM cells, and others, such as neurons, astrocytes, and immune cells [55].

3.3. Chemokines Implicated in GBM Cell Invasion

Chemokines are a family of small (8–10 kDa) secretory proteins whose name comes from their ability to be "chemoattractant cytokines" [80]. Chemokines are known to allow the migration of various cell types such as leukocytes, fibroblasts, and both normal and malignant epithelial cells [80]. Chemokines are divided into four subfamilies based on the positioning of their cysteine residues from the amino-terminus side: CXC, CC, C, and

CX3C [81]. By binding to their receptors, chemokines activate various intracellular signaling pathways and play a crucial role in the regulation of many biological processes such as angiogenesis, immune response, hematopoiesis, chemotaxis, as well as cell proliferation, migration, apoptosis, and others [82].

Forty-seven chemokines and twenty chemokine receptors have been identified in humans so far [83]. Chemokine receptors such as CXCR are G-protein-coupled receptors (GPCR) that include a central common core made of seven transmembrane helices (TM-1 to -7). Helices are connected by three intracellular and three extracellular loops, also an N-terminal extracellular domain and C-terminal intracellular domain that is specific to every protein receptor [84]. A GPCR can bind to its ligand either by homodimerization (one receptor for one G-protein) or by heterodimerization [84]. Once stimulated, GPCR modifies its three-dimensional conformation; guanosine triphosphate (GTP) and guanosine diphosphate (GDP) exchange is activated, which leads to the dissociation of the GTP-bound α-subunit and βγ-dimer [85]. Gαi induces the inhibition of adenylate cyclase, which prevents cyclic adenosine monophosphate (cAMP) production and activates Src-like tyrosine kinases, while Gαq activates phospholipase C (PLC). This enzyme hydrolyzes the phosphatidylinositol 4,5-bisphosphate into diacylglycerol and inositol 1,4,5 trisphosphate (IP3), allowing the release of intracellular Ca^{2+} from the endoplasmic reticulum (Figure 3) [86,87]. On the other side, the Gβγ dimer activates numerous signaling pathways involved in the migration of GBM cells, in particular, PI3K, Akt, ERK1/2, mitogen-activated protein kinase (MAPK), and serine/threonine-specific kinases (Raf) pathways [88–90]. CXCL12 can also induce the phosphorylation of CXCR4 by GPCR kinase (GRK), leading to its subsequent interaction with β-arrestin. Certainly, for its formation and progression, GBM cells engage different chemokines such as CXCL8, CXCL16, CX3CL, CCL5, CXCL12, and their receptors CXCR1-2, CXCR6, CX3CR1, CCR5, CXCR4-7, respectively, for a chemokine network communication mechanism to maintain and increase the tumor malignancy (Table 1).

Table 1. Some activated axes in GBM and their actions.

Axis	Actions in GBM			Ref
	Migration and Invasiveness	Proliferation	Growth, Survival, and Apoptosis	
CXCL12–CXCR4	Chemotaxis	Activation of Ras, Raf kinase	Ca^{2+} mobilization via inhibition of cAMP (survival)	[91]
		ERK1/2 phosphorylation		
CXCL12–CXCR7	Activation of β-arrestin by heterodimerization with CXCR4		Activation of ERK1/2 via GRK	[92,93]
	Activation of ERK1/2			
CXCL8–CXCR1-2	Overexpression of MMP-9 and MMP-2	High density of macrophage promotes a high degree of microvascular proliferation	Activation of IL-6	[94]
			Activation of JAK pathway	
	EMT transition		Increase of anti-apoptotic protein secretion	
CXCL16–CXCR6	Overexpression of anti-inflammatory genes and modulating microglia polarization		Establishing a pro-tumoral microenvironment in the brain	[95]
	Increase of MMP-9 and MMP-2 expression			
CCL5–CCR5	Activation of Akt kinase		Stimulation of AKT pathway	[94,96]
CX3CL1–CX3CR1	Modulation of the activation of TGF-beta1	Not clear	CX3CR1 polymorphism through isoleucine V249I (survival)	[97,98]

Ca^{2+}: Calcium; CXCR7: receptor C-X-C type 7; GRK: G protein-coupled receptor kinases; CXCL8: C-X-C motif chemokine ligand 8; CXCR1-2: C-X-C chemokine receptor 1 and C-X-C chemokine receptor 2; CXCL16: C-X-C motif chemokine ligand 16; CXCR6: C-X-C motif chemokine receptor 6; CX3CL1: chemokine [C-X3-C motif] ligand 1; CX3CR1: C-X3-C motif chemokine receptor 1; CCL5: C-C motif chemokine ligand 5; CCR5: C-C chemokine receptor type 5; IL-6: Interleukin 6; TGF-beta1: transforming growth factor beta 1; EMT: epithelial–mesenchymal transition.

Among several chemokines and their receptors, CXC chemokine ligand 12 (CXCL12) and its two GPCR receptors, CXC type 4 (CXCR4) and type 7 (CXCR7), are mainly involved in the migration and the spreading of GBM cells into distant tissues.

CXCL12 plays an important role in the regulation of different processes such as neuronal development and stem cell motility [91]. CXCL12 has been found in the white matter tracts, blood vessels, and subpial regions, suggesting chemotactic direction cues for GBM cell invasion [99]. Its high expression in some areas, such as white matter tracts, can also attract the spread of the cells toward those areas, causing invasion [14]. CXCR7 has been recently identified as a second receptor for CXCL12, and its expression has been shown to be increased in many tumor cell lines, including gliomas cells [100]. It has a 10-fold higher affinity to CXCL12 than CXCR4 [101]. Nonetheless, CXCR4 plays a crucial role in GBM invasion [100] by mediating chemotaxis in the brain. Being widely expressed within the human body, the CXCR4 upregulated state has been reported in over 20 types of human malignant tumors such as breast, prostate, lung, ovarian, and brain cancer [102–104]. The receptor is also overexpressed in GBM and is considered as a hallmark of the tumor aggressiveness [105,106]. The CXCL12/CXCR4 axis has gained increased focus during the recent decade [107] and has been extensively studied in brain tumors (GBM, astrocytoma, medulloblastoma, oligodendroglioma, and oligodendroastrocytoma) [108] due to its key role in the communication of tumor cells with their microenvironment [109]. The axis is implicated in GBM immunosuppression, chemotherapy and radiotherapy resistance [107,110], cellular reprogramming, and ECM remodeling [107]. CXCL12 acts primarily via two mechanisms in cancer: (a) through an autocrine effect that promotes cancer cell growth, invasion, and angiogenesis, and (b) indirectly by recruiting cancer cells expressing CXCR4 into regions or organs containing CXCL12 to initiate metastasis [111].

Both in vitro and in vivo studies proved that CXCL12 promotes GBM growth and cell migration, and inhibits apoptosis through the activation of various signal transductions [112]. The CXCL12–CXCR4–CXCR7 axis has been extensively studied over recent years [91]. It acts via three mechanisms (Figure 3):

(a) Through CXCR7, which has been known for decades and has an inability to activate the G-protein complex [113]. Lately, it has been proved in vitro that CXCR7 activation by CXCL12 is mediated via G-protein and β-arrestin and increases the intracellular calcium concentration. β-arrestin has four isoforms and plays a key role in GPCR signal transduction [114]. It activates numerous intracellular signaling pathways such as MAPK-ERK1/2 pathways for cell proliferation and migration [115]. An in vivo study demonstrated that the inhibition of CXCR7 after irradiation prolonged survival and blocked tumor recurrence of intracranial U251 GBM in nude mice [116]. Yang Liu et al. showed that knocking down CXCR7 in GBM cells (U251MG and U373MG) using siRNA to block ERK1/2 in response to CXCL12 decreases cell proliferation, invasion, and migration [93].

(b) CXCR7 can heterodimerize with CXCR4 in response to CXCL12, which modulates CXCR4-mediated G-protein and β-arrestin signaling pathways such as MAPK-ERK1/2 inducing cell migration [92].

(c) One CXCL12 binds to its receptor CXCR4 [117,118], the tertiary structure of CXCR4 changes to activate the G-protein through its intracellular component. Multiple signals are activated via GRK, such as phospholipase C (PLC), PI3K, and MAPK/ERK, for vascular endothelial growth factor (VEGF) production, which is mainly responsible for recruiting new vessels for GBM neovascularizations [119]. The activation of the PI3K pathway followed by the activation of Akt contributes to the CXCL12/CXCR4-induced survival, invasion and proliferation. CXCL12–CXCR4-mediated migration is reported to be regulated by the PI3K and MAPK/ERK pathways [119].

Overall, targeting the CXCL12–CXCR4–CXCR7 axis to develop new therapeutic approaches in GBM treatment is required. AMD3100, Peptide R, CPZ1344, and AMD3465 are inhibitors for CXCR4 that reduce tumor growth and inhibit GBM cell invasiveness and migration [120]. The most extensively studied, AMD3100, also known as plerixafor (Mozobil®), is an FDA-licensed CXCR4 antagonist that was approved in 2008 [121]. In addition, AMD3100 reduces the chemotaxis, survival, and proliferation of glioma cell lines [120]. For instance, Cornelison et al. proved that AMD3100 can inhibit CXCR4-dependant GBM invasion induced by convective flow forces within the tumor tissue [106].

Furthermore, it has been also demonstrated that CXCL12 and CXCR4 induce the activation of integrins which suggests a cooperation between the CXCL12–CXCR4 axis and the integrins in mediating cancer cell behavior, such as adhesion and survival [122]. For example, the adhesion of prostate tumor cells to the endothelium or proteins of the ECM is transmitted via CXCL12-induced signals depending on CXCR4. The binding of CXCL12 to its receptor leads to an upregulated expression of α5 and β3 integrin subunits. In contrast, the level of α2, β1, β4, and αv integrin subunits remains unchanged in CXCL12-treated cells. This provides evidence of existing links between CXCR4 expression, CXCL12, and α5 and β3 integrin subunits [118,123,124]. As the CXCL12–CXCR4 axis is the potent driver for GBM invasion under static conditions, studies have shown that cell invasion and migration may be enhanced by another factor, interstitial fluid flow [99,106,125].

4. Interstitial Fluid Flow in Glioblastoma

4.1. Cerebral Fluids

Within the brain, many processes occur to regulate different mechanisms with the aim of maintaining homeostasis. Cell communication, environment interactions, and chemical gradients are necessary to ensure the brain function. On another scale, biophysical forces such as fluid flow act by ensuring the creation of the chemokine gradient in neonatal and adult development, and by recruiting immune cells into target sites [69]. Brain tissues are composed of three compartments: neural cells, the vascular system, and the interstitial space (IS) [126]. The latter occupies 15% to 20% of the total brain volume and is composed mainly of interstitial fluid (IF) and the extracellular matrix (ECM) [126]. IF is one of the most important axes studied because of its behavioral changes in pathological diseases such as CNS cancers and Alzheimer's disease [127]. IF surrounds every cell in the brain, allowing it to be the carrier for proteins and different molecules to and from cells [128]. The interstitial fluid flow (IFF) can be defined as the movement of fluid between cells in the interstitial space. It is mainly composed of water, ions, and gaseous and organic molecules (O_2, CO_2, hormones) [128]. Chary and Jain measured the interstitial flow velocity using fluorescence intensity after bleaching on a rabbit ear, which was found to be 6×10^{-5} cm/s. In GBM, the IFF develops due to the high interstitial pressure between the tumor and the healthy tissue [129]. Besides the hypotheses that the ECM and cytokines increase GBM cells' invasion, the IFF has been proved to enhance GBM cells' migration as well.

4.2. Interstitial Fluid Flow and CXCL12 in the Migration of GBM

The IFF plays a critical role in the GBM cell invasion of the brain parenchyma [99,106,125] by enhancing CXCL12 secretion along white matter tracts, blood vessels, and subpial regions [130]. The fluid flow in the brain also follows the same pathways, providing the information that the fluid flow, CXCL12 gradients, and white matter tracts may be interrelated. The IFF stimulates GBM cell migration mainly by mediating two mechanisms: (a) Autologous chemotaxis, in which the GBM cell stimulates its migration via a self-secreted chemokines mechanism. The secreted chemokine allows the cell to be transported following the direction of the flow, creating a gradient around individual cells [106]. (b) Mechanotransduction, which occurs when a cell detects mechanical changes in its environment, leading to the activation of different signaling pathways mediating the migration [131].

For example, the fluid flow was found to enhance glioma cell migration via a CXCL12–CXCR4 signaling-dependent mechanism in both 3D in vitro models using invasive cells (RT2, rat astrocytoma; U87MG, human glioblastoma; C6, rat astrocytoma) in a HA/collagen I matrix and in vivo models such as rats [99]. The response of these invasive cells to the fluid flow (velocity of 0.7 μm/s) was prevented by blocking CXCR4, either by adding its inhibitor AMD3100 (Mozobil®, Plerixafor) or CXCL12 at 100 nM (uniform CXCL12 treatment) to abrogate any chemoattractant gradient [99]. Nonetheless, blocking CXCR4 did not stop the GBM cell invasion entirely under static or flow conditions, suggesting that the cells are capable of producing their CXCL12 to migrate [99]. Cornelison et al. used an in vitro 3D tissue culture insert model to show that GL261 cells can migrate under static conditions, which can be significantly enhanced after flow application. Furthermore, they used convection enhanced delivery (CED), a technique known to enhance the local perfusion of chemotherapeutic agents in the treatment of GBM, to highlight the invasion effects of convective forces on glioma cell invasion into the surrounding brain parenchyma in an in vivo mice model [106]. The flow effect can be mitigated by blocking the CXCL12 gradient or its receptor using uniform CXCL12 and AMD3100, respectively, [106].

However, Kingsmore et al., using G2, G34, G62, and G528 GBM stem cell lines, proved that the response to the fluid flow is heterogenous and can vary from one cell line to another, both in vitro and in vivo [125]. The invasion of G34, G62, and G528 GBM stem cell lines increased in response to the interstitial fluid flow as compared to the static conditions, unlike the G2 invasion that was not increased, which was in accordance with their in vivo results. Using antibodies against CXCR4 and CXCL12, the authors also found that G34 and G528 cells respond to the flow through CXCR4/CXCL12 chemotaxis. Uniform CXCL12 also decreased the flow-stimulated invasion in both G34 and G528 GBM stem cells, confirming the crucial role played by the chemoattractant for flow-responsive invasion in these cells [125]. Interestingly, flow-stimulated invasion in G34 cells also depended on CD44, a receptor of HA mediating mechanotransduction [125].

In contrast, Qazi et al., by culturing U87 human glioma, rat CNS-1 glioma, and U251 human glioma cell lines in 3D modified Boyden chambers containing collagen type I in a dynamic microenvironment with various flow velocities (0.8–3 μm/s), found that the migration rate of the cells diminished after exposure to the flow. This decrease of migratory activity by flow was dependent on MMP-1 and MMP-2 for U87 and CNS-1 cells, respectively. In contrast, the migration of U251 cells was not affected by the shear stress. However, adding chemoattractant TGF-α with the flow enhanced the U87, CNS-1, as well as U251 cell migratory activity by 89%, 566%, and 101%, respectively, compared to controls [132]. All this indicates that CXCR4/CXCL12 mechanisms can have different impacts on the GBM cell population depending on their heterogeneity, which may contribute to different invasion behavioral responses to fluid flow. However, since studying GBM cell migration in vivo is currently limited, bioengineers focus on the development of in vitro models that mimic different elements of the in vivo microenvironment.

5. Models to Study Glioblastoma Cells Migration

5.1. Two-Dimensional Models for Glioblastoma Studies

Several studies performed in two/three-dimensional in vitro and in vivo models have proved that GBM cells invade either by an amoeboid or mesenchymal manner [133,134]. Two-dimensional models are simple to use, but have proved to have several limitations in terms of mimicking the natural microenvironment of the parenchyma. Scratch assays are the commonly used technique. They allow the study of migration in favor of invasion, but do not allow the distinction between the proliferative and invasive behavior of the cells. Transwell assays, on the other hand, give more information but produce a wider range of results [135]. However, these kinds of tests fail to recapitulate the real microenvironment of the brain [136] (Table 2).

Table 2. Advantages and disadvantages of different models used in the study of GBM.

		GBM Study Models	Advantages	Disadvantages	Applications	Ref
2D	In vitro	Scratch assays	• Easily implemented • Low cost • Real-time cell tracking	• Low physiological relevance • Migration and invasion are not distinguished	Migration Matrix remodeling Drug screening	[137]
		Transwell assays	• Technically easy • Low cost • A matrix can be added to study ECM	• Lacks tumor complexity • Lack of 3D environment without matrix • Difficult to distinguish between migration and invasion		
3D		3D bioscaffolds (Spheroids)	• Simple • Control of spheroids size • Control of growth parameters • High throughput • Allow ECM interactions study • Allow pathways signaling study	• Long-term culture difficulties • Lack tumors complexity • Lack vascularization	Migration/Invasion Cell biology (proliferation, apoptosis, etc.) Drug Screening	[138]
		Microfluidic co-culture	• Real-time cell tracking • Allow ECM interactions study • Allow pathways signaling study • Cell–Cell interactions study	• High cost • Lack of native microenvironment • Lack of tumor complexity	Migration/Invasion Cell adhesion	[139]
	Ex vivo	Organotypic brain slices cultures	• Native ECM composition • Real-time cells tracking • Maintain tumor heterogeneity • Allow ECM interactions study • Allow cell signaling study	• Ethical issues associated with animal studies • Lacks blood • Flow • Lack of tumor complexity	Migration/Invasion Tumor growth Study of drugs delivery	[140]
	In vivo	Orthotopic xenograft	• Native microenvironment • Studies under the effect of the flow • Cell–Cell interactions study • Allow pathway's signaling study	• Ethical issues associated with animal studies • High cost • Less experimental control • Time consuming	Migration/Invasion Signaling Study of drugs delivery Tumor growth	[141]

5.2. Three-Dimensional Models for Glioblastoma Studies

Three-dimensional assays are a step forward to investigate cell invasion as they mimic the cellular microenvironment more closely. Boyden chambers are the most used. They consist in evaluating the cell invasion through a porous insert that can be coated with different matrices, such as the mouse sarcoma-derived matrigel or collagen-based matrices [56]. The matrices are static, so the addition of chemo-attractants in the lower compartment is usually required in most cases [142]. Microfluidic co-culture platforms are 3D in vitro models made of a gel scaffold bound by two channels in which cells can be seeded. This allows the study of the impact of intracellular interactions on GBM invasion (see Table 2) [56,143]. Cerebral organoids on another side have been recently developed to culture tumor cells retaining part of the original brain morphology [144]. Models such as organotypic brain slice cultures are ex vivo models that have emerged at the beginning of this century to mimic in vivo orthotopic xenograft invasion models [56]. These models allow GBM cells to express their invasive characteristics in a physiological microenvironment as well as their interactions with the ECM [52,145].

6. Innovative Treatments for Glioblastoma

Despite the advanced clinical therapeutic approaches, the combination of classical treatments yet fails to cure GBM due to tumor recurrence and metastasis. Therefore, varied applications of biotechnology and many innovative approaches such as immunotherapies, gene therapies, and drug delivery-based therapies have been explored (Figure 4) and will be briefly discussed. In this review, we will focus mainly on describing the different drug delivery therapies used in the development of new GBM treatments.

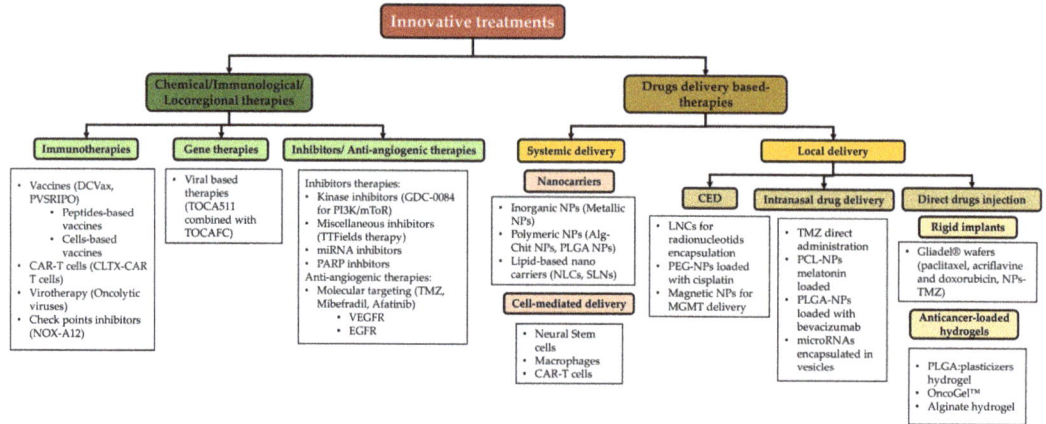

Figure 4. Summary of some different innovative treatments for GBM. DCVax: dendritic cells vaccine; PVSPIRO: recombinant nonpathogenic polio-rhinovirus chimera; CAR-T: chimeric antigen receptor T cell; CLTX-CAR T: chlorotoxin-chimeric antigen receptor T cell; NOX-A12: olaptesed pegol; TOCA511: vocimagene amiretrorepvec; TOCAFC: toca 511 (vocimagene amiretrorepvec) + FC (5-fluorouracil); GDC-0084: paxalisib; TTFields: tumor-treating fields; PARP: poly (ADP-ribose) polymerase; Alg: alginate; Chit: chitosan; PLGA: poly D,L-lactic-co-glycolic acid; NLCs: nanostructured Lipid Carriers; SLNs: solid lipid nanoparticles; LNCs: lipid nanocapsules; PEG: polyethylene glycol; PCL: polycaprolactone.

6.1. Some Innovative Treatments in Glioblastoma

6.1.1. Gene Therapies

Gene therapy consists of integrating a functional version of a gene instead of the defective one. There is no gene therapy clinically approved at the moment, but various clinical trials with encouraging results are ongoing [146,147]. Many strategies have been used in the context of gene delivery, such as antiangiogenic gene therapy and nano-technology-based gene therapy in the past twenty years [148].

Some of the antiangiogenic gene therapies have been successful to suppress tumor angiogenesis and growth [148]. Angiogenic gene therapy strategies consist mostly in disrupting the normal function of VEGF [149]. For example, ofranergene obadenovec (VB-111) is a genetically modified non-replicating adenovirus type 5 containing a specific promoter and a transgene encoding for a chimeric death receptor (proapoptotic Fas-TNFR1 chimeric protein) [150,151]. Cloughesy et al. have performed a phase III clinical trial (256 patients at 57 sites) studying the effect of VB-111 administration with and without bevacizumab, a humanized monoclonal antibody for VEGF-A, approved for use in recurrent GBM in 2009 [152,153]. The patients treated with VB-111 showed apoptotic cell areas in the tumor with an increase in the number of infiltrated CD8 and CD4 lymphocytes. However, the administration of VB-111 and bevacizumab did not improve the outcomes in recurrent GBM [152]. Some other studies hypothesized that combining TMZ chemotherapy with gene therapy may be beneficial for a synergistic effect against GBM and that the decrease of the MGMT level with gene therapy can overcome TMZ resistance and enhance GBM cell death [154–156]. For example, Przystal et al. introduced a unique prokaryotic viral-based approach combined to TMZ to target tumors [155]. Using a M13 bacteriophage that specifically infects bacterial cells, the single-stranded genome of human adeno-associated virus (AAV) was inserted in and the phage capsid was engineered to display the CDCRGDCFC (RGD4C) ligand that binds to $\alpha v \beta 3$ integrins [155]. Once bonded to these integrins, the RGD4C/AAV-Phage (AAVP) viral particles penetrate the GBM cells, releasing the AAV genome that expresses a tumor-specific gene from the *Grp78* promoter. Przystal et al. first verified that TMZ increases the expression of the endogenous Grp78 protein in human GBM cells (LN229, U87, and SNB19 cells) in a dose-dependent manner. They also showed that RGD4C/AAVP-*Grp78* gene expression is strongly increased by TMZ. Interestingly, the combination of the TMZ with the RGD4C/AAVP-Grp78-HSVtk mutant SR39 encoding the Herpes simplex virus type I thymidine kinase in the presence of ganciclovir (GCV) induced strong tumor cell killing both in vitro and in vivo (mice with established intracranial U87 tumors) [155].

mRNA and siRNA in GBM Gene Therapy:

mRNA-based gene therapy is an efficient gene transfection tool that emerged to adapt with the high heterogeneity and diffusing invasiveness nature of the GBM. Xiangjun et al. explored a new therapeutic strategy using an in vitro synthesized mRNA encoding for (a) a phosphatase and tensin homolog on chromosome ten (PTEN) that can induce apoptosis or (b) a tumor-necrosis-factor-related apoptosis-inducing ligand (TRAIL)- in tumor cells derived from -*PTEN*-deletion patients [157]. They confirmed that a low survival rate is observed in GBM patients who have a high frequency mutation of PTEN. Using patient-derived primary GBM stem cells with *PTEN* alteration and a Denver Brain Tumor Research Group (DBTRG)-cell-derived xenograft to detect the cytotoxicity of mRNA in vitro and tumor suppression in vivo, they showed that the combined treatment of PTEN-mRNA and TRAIL-mRNA significantly reduced the growth of both the GBM cells and tumor. The tumor growth is suppressed after two months compared with the control PBS (96.4%) and single mRNA group (PTEN-mRNA (89.7%) or TRAIL-mRNA (84.5%)) [157]. mRNAs can also be encapsulated into nanocarriers such as liposomes and nanoparticles (NP) to overcome the natural barriers and protect them from degradation [158]. The delivery routes and the carrier forms of mRNA depend on the patients glioma grade, stage, surgery, and chemotherapy history [158]. To our knowledge, no clinical trial of mRNA-based GBM therapy has been completed, and has not been widely adopted in treating GBM yet.

On another side, small interfering RNA (siRNA) are known by their ability to silence the genes responsible for cancer progression by targeting tumor-promoting factors, such as VEGF and EGFR [159,160]. Since GBM cells are resistant to anti-tumor drugs, the use of siRNA in combination with chemotherapy could be beneficial to enhancing the treatment efficiency [161]. For example, the combination of resveratrol (RES) and heat shock protein 27-knockdown using siRNA (Hsp27) was tested to treat the disease [162]. Hsp27 is a tumor-promoting factor in GBM implicated in ECM remodeling and cell survival. RES at 15 µM decreases the Hsp27 protein level in a similar way than quercetin, a well-known Hsp27 inhibitor (47% and 41%, respectively). However, combining RES at 15 µM with Hsp27 siRNA induces a decrease in the level of Hsp27 by 93.4% in transfected human U87 MG cells [162]. This combined treatment increases the caspase-3 activity by 101% and induces GBM cell apoptosis. [162]. This study proves that the use of Hsp27-siRNA combined with an anti-tumor agent could be beneficial to induce apoptosis in GBM cells. However, the BBB, the degradation by RNAse enzymes, and reaching the tumor site are the main challenges preventing the efficiency of siRNA therapy [163]. Under these conditions, nanocarriers can promote a targeted delivery of siRNA and protect them against degradation at the same time. A wide range of siRNA-loaded nanocarriers have been tested in GBM therapy [164]. For instance, loaded MGMT-siRNA liposomes have been tested in GBM treatment resulting in MGMT downregulation, DNA repair induction, and decreased drug efflux capacities responsible for increasing GBM cell sensitivity to TMZ [164]. In another study, RGD-functionalized pH-responsive polyamidoamine (PAMAM) dendrimers were investigated for delivery of both c-myc siRNA anddoxorubicin (DOX)-loaded Se NP in GBM therapy [165]. The RGD functionalization of PAMAM enhances the uptake of siRNA dendrimers by cancer cells [165]. The nanocarriers were able to penetrate a BBB model in vitro, developed to deliver the drug and enhance the antitumor activity [165]. Moreover, chitosan lipidic nanocapsules were used for galectin-1 and EGFR-siRNAs' delivery in nude mice-bearing orthotopic U87 MG GBM cells [166]. The mean survival time increased in the mice treated 14 days after tumor implantation with both anti-EGFR and anti-Galectin-1 siRNAs plus TMZ (39 days), in comparison to untreated mice (32 days), or EGFR siRNA plus TMZ or anti-Galectin-1 siRNA plus TMZ (34 days), representing a promising strategy to induce anti-tumor effects in GBM [166]. Furthermore, CXCR4-targeted peptide carriers for VEGF-siRNA delivery were tested in GBM therapy [167]. The peptide carriers were able to condense and protect siRNA from RNAse degradation and induced a 2–6-fold decrease in VEGF expression in the cells, indicating that the surface modification of the nanocarriers can improve their specificity towards GBM cells [167]. However, more studies to develop safe and well-tolerated nanocarriers for siRNA delivery are needed. Another therapy that appeared to be very powerful and hopeful is immunotherapy, in which drug delivery systems are extensively used.

6.1.2. Immunotherapies

After the success achieved for treating various other cancers, immunotherapies have been considerably investigated to translate the same achievements in GBM treatment. Immunotherapy consists of harnessing the immune system to eradicate the tumor cells and is quite efficient in the treatment of high mutational burden tumors. Since GBM has a low tumor mutational burden and an immunosuppressive environment, various strategies have been explored to boost host immunity against GBM [168].

Among them, immune checkpoint inhibitors release the inhibitory brakes of T cells, activating the immune system to induce anti-tumor responses [169]. When the binding to their ligand is inhibited, the checkpoint receptors can promote an effective cell response against GBM [170]. Targeted checkpoint molecules such as Nivolumab (Opdivo®), pembrolizumab (Keytruda®), durvalumab (Imfinzi®), and atezolizumab (Tecentriq®) (an anti-programmed death-ligand 1) have been approved to treat several types of cancer and are currently trialed in GBM treatment [171,172]. For example, Gardell et al. used human monocyte-derived macrophages genetically modified for bispecific T cell engager (BiTE) and proinflammatory cytokine IL-12 secretion [173]. BiTE is specific for the mutation of epidermal growth factor receptor variant 3 (EGFRV3), expressed by the GBM cell. The secreted BiTE, by binding to the tumor antigen, was able to activate T cells as well as their proliferation and degranulation, leading to the elimination of the antigen-specific tumor cells in in vitro and in vivo models. BiTE secretion promotes a reduction in the tumor burden [173]. However, the kinetics release of BiTE protein from the cells still needs to be improved which reveal the importance of the platform optimization in the development of therapeutic approaches. Further, chimeric antigen receptors (CAR), that consist of the use of genetically modified T cells to express CAR genes, have been approved by the FDA for the treatment of hematologic malignancies [174]. O'Rourke et al. were the first to use autologous T cells redirected to the EGFRV3 mutation by CARs on human GBM patients [175]. They demonstrated that the use of CART-EGFRV3 (10 patients) is feasible and safe, since no toxicity was observed [175]. Seven patients had surgery after CART-EGFRV3 treatment, which allowed us to gather more information: (a) The trafficking of CART-EGFRV3 cells was observed in the direction of the tumor within the first 2 weeks of treatment. (b) The in-situ studies of the tumor environment also showed an up-regulation of immunosuppressive molecules, such as indoleamine 2,3-dioxygenase 1 (IDO1), programmed cell death ligand 1 (PD-L1) and IL-10, as well as the recruitment of immunosuppressive regulatory T cells expressing FoxP3. Thus, CART therapy for GBM still needs more investigation because of the immunosuppressive tumor microenvironment, cell trafficking, and risks of CNS toxicity [175].

Some approaches based on vaccines are also investigated as a potential adaptive immunotherapy for GBM. An autologous tumor lysate-pulsed dendritic cell vaccine called DCVax®-L, produced by Northwest Biotherapeutics, Inc., Bethesda, MD, USA [176], has been used against glioblastoma and appears to be safe. DCVax-L has been approved for GBM treatment in Switzerland, but is still under clinical trials in the United States [177]. Additionally, a phase 3 trial is ongoing to evaluate the long-term effects of the DCVax®-L vaccine in patients after surgery and chemoradiotherapy [178].

On another scale of immunotherapies targeting GBM, viral-based therapy involves genes delivery via viral vectors. For example, Desjardins et al. focused on the use of the convection-enhanced intratumoral delivery of the recombinant nonpathogenic polio-rhinovirus chimera (PVSRIPO) which recognizes the neurotropic poliovirus receptor CD155 widely expressed by GBM cells and improves the survival rate of the patients [179]. In summary, immunotherapies demonstrated promising results in terms of feasibility, safety, and even signs of efficacy. The challenges ahead are still numerous, including the optimization of the dosing, the modulation of immunosuppressive tumor microenvironment, the molecular marked heterogeneity of GBM and the understanding of the chemokines network. Thus, drug delivery systems have emerged to overcome some of those limitations.

6.2. Drugs Delivery Systems for Glioblastoma Treatments

6.2.1. Systemic Delivery

The BBB is considered as the major hurdle in drug delivery-based therapies because of its low permeability that hampers the passage of anti-cancer agents (ACA). The transport of ACA is achieved via two mechanisms: (a) passive transport (diffusion of water-soluble compounds and lipophilic molecules with a molecular weight less than 500 Da), and (b) active transport (mediated by membrane protein carriers of small molecules) [180]. Therefore, in order to promote the passage of ACA, different strategies have been explored, including small molecules capable of crossing the BBB, chemical modification of ACA, drug-loaded nanocarriers, and cell delivery systems [181].

Cell-Mediated Delivery:

Cell-mediated delivery utilizes cells such as leukocytes and stem cells to carry drug carriers themselves [182]. The strategy had several advantages such as long circulation times, flexible morphology, and cellular signaling [183]. The drugs can be loaded into the cells through biological pathways (endocytosis, ligand-receptor interactions), physical approaches (hypotonic hemolysis, electroporation), or chemical modifications (covalent conjugation onto surface markers, biotinylation, click chemistry) [184].

Macrophages are commonly used because of their particularity to migrate to the tumor side in response to the secretion of cytokines and chemokines [184]. Cell-mediated delivery has been widely explored in GBM. For example, neural stem cells (NSC) have been used to secrete and deliver the proapoptotic protein TRAIL to human intracranial glioma xenografts [185]. The use of high doses of TRAIL in patients can induce issues of toxicity and a danger of excessive antiviral host immune responses; for this reason, the molecule was delivered by NSCs. NSCs were able to migrate to the tumor site and secrete TRAIL, resulting in the apoptosis of the cancer cells without toxicity for the normal brain parenchyma. They also induced a significant reduction in the tumor size [185]. Wang et al. found that monocyte-mediated DOX (also known as Adriamycin®) delivery through NPs, with the surface coated with polyglycerol and RGD peptides for GBM treatment, caused tumor cell damage both in vitro and in vivo in mice orthotopic GBM xenografts. [182]. In the same context, Pang et al. loaded NPs into macrophages such as "Trojan horses" to deliver DOX for GBM treatment [186]. The viability of the cells encapsulating the NPs was not affected and an improvement of the macrophages' penetration into the core of the spheroids model was observed, which mimics the behavior of the cells in an in vivo model [186]. To conclude, the tumor targeting was enhanced after loading the NPs into the cells, which indicates that macrophages can improve glioma therapy and underline the importance of using NPs [186].

Nanocarriers:

Nanotechnology and nanocarrier-based drug delivery have recently gained remarkable attention due to their characteristics of biosafety, sustained drug release, and enhanced drug bioactivity and BBB penetrability [187]. Based on preparation methods, nanocarriers can be classified into nanocapsules, nanospheres, and NPs that are the mostly used in GBM treatment.

Nanocapsules are small vesicles of 100–200 nm in which hydrophobic drugs are encapsulated in the empty space by a polymer membrane. Polymers such as poly(lactic acid) (PLA) and Poly Lactic-co-Glycolic Acid (PLGA) can be used to prepare these nanomaterials [188]. NPs can be loaded by different therapeutic agents and are characterized by particular properties that allow them to pass the BBB [189] and achieve the tumor site. The particle size, surface charge, hydrophobicity, and coating material are the NPs' physiochemical properties that play an important role in the targeting process [190]. The size of the NPs is a critical factor for the NPs' delivery; small size NPs < 200 nm are preferred and suitable for systemic administration and can smoothly reach the leaky blood vessels of the tumor microenvironment [191–193]. The shape, stability, and charge of the NPs are also important due to their implication in fluid dynamics and their interaction with cell charge membranes and proteins [194,195]. Based on their composition and characteristics, NPs can be classified into lipidic NPs, organic NPs, and inorganic NPs [196–198].

Lipid-based nanocarriers regroup liposomes, nanostructured lipid carriers, solid lipid NPs, and lipid micelles (Figure 5). Liposomes are small vesicles composed of a phospholipidic bilayer that surrounds a water-soluble core similar to the cell membrane [199]. Liposomes are characterized by an easy encapsulation of ACA, an easy preparation, biodegradability, and a favorable biocompatibility [200]. Nanostructured lipid carriers (NLCs) are composed of a matrix with solid and liquid lipids forming an unordered matrix, providing a large space for drug incorporation [201]. Solid lipids NPs (SLNs) are formed from a solid hydrophobic lipid core and have demonstrated a higher stability compared with liposomes [202]. Further, SLNs have the ability to cross the BBB and deliver a wide spectrum of GBM-targeted ACAs, such as large molecules, genes, oligonucleotides, and enzymes [203]. Finally, lipidic micelles are spherical amphiphilic aggregates with a hydrophobic core and a hydrophilic shell in which drugs are loaded in the central core or can be linked to the lipids [201].

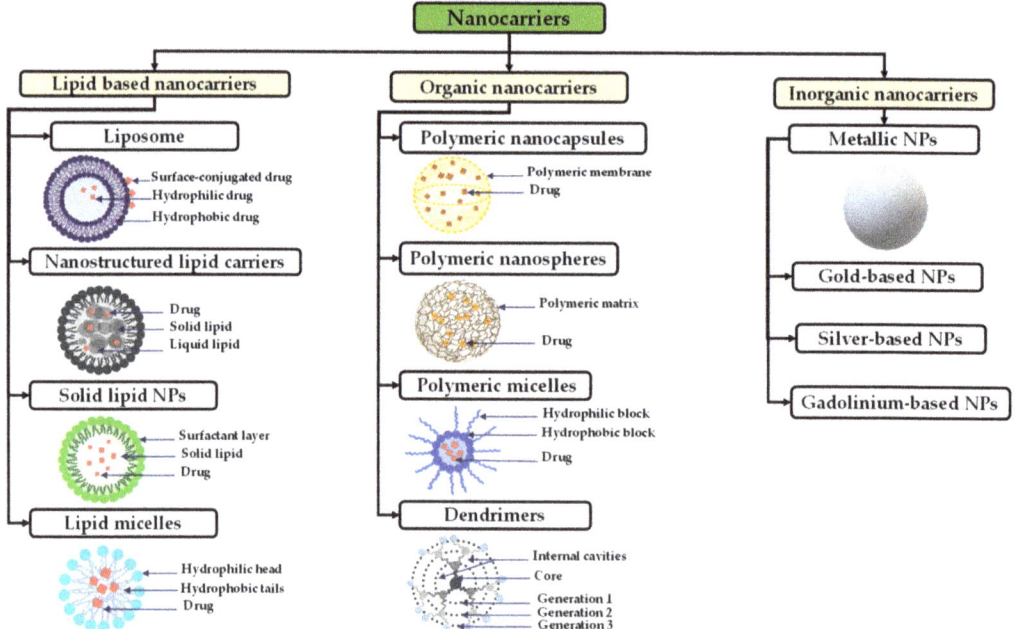

Figure 5. Schematic representation of different types of nanocarriers and their structures used in GBM treatment.

Inorganic NPs are generally composed of mineral compounds, such as metals. Among various inorganic NPs: iron oxide NPs are commonly used as contrast agents for MRI, and gold NPs are used to improve photothermal therapy [204–206].

For example, Liu et al. prepared magnetic iron-based NPs (MNP) modified by PEG-transferrin (Tf-PEG) and polylysine (PLL) to condense small interference RNA against polo-like kinase I (PLK1) (Tf-PEG-PLL/MNP@siPLK1). The Tf was used to target GBM cells since they express a high amount of transferrin receptors. PLK1 is involved in G2/M transition in the cell cycle and is related to tumor progression and recurrence [207]. They found that Tf-PEG-PLL/MNP@siPLK1 at the dose of 1.6 mg/kg prolonged the survival time of GBM mice, 80% of them being alive at three months. In contrast, a median survival time of about one month was observed in Tf-PEG-PLL/MNP@Scrambled PLK1-treated GBM-mice [207]. On the other hand, Zhu et al. developed ruthenium Tf and aptamer AS1411 co-grafted NPs loaded with [Ru(bpy)2(tip)]2+ (RBT), an antitumor drug for cell apoptosis. Using photodynamic therapy for GBM, they proved that RBT@MRN-SS-Tf/Apt killed glioma cells in vivo and in vitro under laser irradiation, prolonging the median survival rate [208].

Polymeric nanoparticles can be prepared using a different range of materials and are used as carriers for different drugs, such as chemotherapeutic drugs [188,209]. Polymeric nanoparticles are more advantageous over other types of NPs because of their biocompatibility, biodegradability, and the improvement they achieved in the kinetics release as reported in many reviews on the subject [210,211]. Polymeric NPs preparation can be very flexible in terms of composition, structure, and properties [212]. Polymeric NPs can be prepared using: (a) Synthetic polymer NPs such as PLA, poly(ε-caprolactone) (PCL), poly(glycolic acid) (PGA), PLGA, and poly (amino acids) [209,213,214], these polymers are biocompatible and degrade hydrolytically [215]. (b) Natural polymers which are composed of polymers such alginate [216,217], chitosan [216,217], dextran [218], and HA [219].

Polymeric micelles are highly biocompatible amphiphilic nanoparticles capable of delivering different therapeutic agents and characterized by their flexibility in terms of design modification [220]. Polymeric micelles have core–shell-type NPs formed through the self-assembly of block copolymers, and which have a controllable size range of 10–100 nm [221]. Biodegradable polyesters such as PCL, poly (D,L-lactide) (PDLA), and poly (D,L-lactide-co-glycolide) (P(DLA-co-G) are commonly used to form the core which helps to prolong the half-life of the loaded drugs for more than 10 h [196,222]. Dendrimers are small particles with sizes less than 12 nm, composed of repeating monomeric or oligomeric units with an internal cavity surrounded by reactive terminal groups [223]. Dendrimers are used to encapsulate different drug agents, such as siRNA, and are highly efficient for BBB crossing, but are toxic to normal tissue because of their interactions with the cell membrane and their less controllable release behavior [224].

The use of nanocarriers has been well established over the past decade both in pharmaceutical research and clinical settings to enhance the in vivo treatment efficiency [225]. For GBM, such treatments are in development as well.

- Lipid-Based Nanocarriers for Glioblastoma Treatment

Lipid based NPs have been extensively used to target GBM. They can efficiently encapsulate multiple drugs that act synergistically to kill GBM cells or drugs with poor physicochemical properties (e.g., poor water-soluble drugs). For example, in a study conducted by Zhang et al., glucose-functionalized liposomes (gLTP) that co-load TMZ and pro-apoptotic peptide (PAP) can cross the BBB through the glucose–GLUT1 pathway to deliver these drugs to the tumor site. PAP affects the mitochondria reducing ATP generation, while enhancing the sensitivity of GBM cells to TMZ [226]. In the same way, Papachristdoulou et al. delivered, via liposomes, O6-(4-bromothenyl) guanine derivatives (O6BTG) targeting MGMT to enhance TMZ efficacy in vitro [227]. The magnetic resonance image-guided microbubble was also used to enhance the low-intensity pulsed focused ultrasound that permits the opening of the BBB and better deliver the liposomes [227].

The O6BTG-liposomes combined with TMZ reduced the tumor growth and increased mice survival [227].

In another study, Jhaveri et al. encapsulated RES, a natural polyphenol with poor physicochemical properties, at a drug loading efficiency of around 70% in PEGylated liposomes. These liposomes were modified with Tf moieties to increase their interaction with GBM cells (Tf-RES-L) [228]. They found that liposomes prolong the drug-release in vitro, and delivered RES induces GBM cell cycle arrest at the S-phase and activates their apoptosis through caspases 3/7 [228]. Tf-RES-L also permits an inhibition of GBM tumor growth in vivo, improving survival in mice [228].

Among many types of lipid-based nanoparticles, NLCs and SLNs gained an extreme focus for developing GBM treatments, especially in the delivery of GBM-targeted ACA [196,229,230]. Song et al. prepared dual-ligand-commodified NLCs using both lactoferrin, a member of the Tf family, and RGD peptides recognized by integrins overexpressed in GBM cells. They demonstrated that the use of these dual-ligand-comodified NLCs (139 nm) for TMZ and vincristine delivery induce a higher cytotoxic effect in vitro on human GBM cells (U87MG cells) compared to single-drug-loaded NLCs or free drugs. The same results were gained in vivo on the inhibition of tumor growth in U87 MG cell-bearing nude mice [231]. Furthermore, the size of the tumor treated by dual lactoferrin/RGD-NLCs was reduced compared to the tumor treated by single-ligand NLCs [231]. The use of dual ligands improves the GBM cell targeting in the brain. However, the lipid composition of NLCs can also greatly influence the ability of the liposome to cross the BBB and target GBM cells. Zwain et al. prepared NLCs using four liquid lipids alone or in combination (propylene glycol monolaurate, propylene glycol monocaprylate, caprylocaproylmacrogol-8-glycerides, and/or polyox-yl-15-hydroxystearate) to encapsulate the poorly water-soluble docetaxel (DTX), also known as Taxotere®. They observed that NLCs composed of the four lipids had not only the highest drug loading (almost 89%), but they also crossed the BBB in the in vitro model without the loss of the barrier integrity [232]. These NLCs, with an average particle size of 123.3 nm, were internalized more efficiently by U87MG cells compared with non-cancerous cells. They were also more efficient to reduce the size of U87MG spheroids than the free drug, by inhibiting both the cell cycle via the G2/M phase and mitochondria activity [232]. Another strategy to target GBM cells is the use of antibodies against specific growth factor receptors such as the epidermal growth factor receptor (EGFR). For example, carmustine-loaded cationic SLNs grafted with an anti-EGFR permit and affective delivery of the drug resulting in an antiproliferative efficacy against the tumor growth [233].

SLNs and NLCs are effective as drug carriers for GBM. However, despite all the promising results in the literature, none of these carriers have been successfully developed by a pharmaceutical company. Therefore, more efforts should be focused on the development of reproducible nanocarriers.

- Polymeric-Based Nanocarriers for Glioblastoma Treatment

Due to their biocompatibility, low toxicity, and biodegradability, polymers offer many advantages [234]. Han et al., in a recent study, used paclitaxel (Taxol®)-loaded into dextran NPs coated with RVG29 peptide for targeted chemotherapy in glioma [235]. RVG29 is a peptide with a high affinity to the nicotinic acetylcholine receptor (nAchR) on neuronal cells and is highly implicated in drug resistance [235]. The use of NPs either in vitro or in vivo exhibited a higher cell growth inhibition rate against C6 cells compared with the non-grafted NPs [235]. To our knowledge, these polymers are not used much in the context of GBM treatment compared to other cancers such as breast cancer [236], cervical cancer [237], and lung cancer [238].

On the other side, PLGA, PLA, and PGA-based nanocarriers are the most extremely used polymers in brain delivery (Table 3) [239]. In the context of GBM, these nanocarriers are mainly used for the encapsulation of chemotherapeutic molecules to control their release. For example, DOX-loaded PLGA-PEG NPs with a size around 200 nm were prepared for the in vitro study of the drug kinetic release, no burst release was observed, and a sustained release was maintained for up to 96 h [240]. Ramalho et al. used PLGA-NPs functionalized with OX26, a monoclonal antibody for a transferrin receptor, and loaded with TMZ for targeting U215 and U87 cell lines. The NPs showed an encapsulation efficiency of 48% and a size of 194 nm, both free and encapsulated TMZ induced a decrease of cell growth in the studied lines, but the use of NPs exhibits a longer and stronger action on the cells [241]. Caban-Toktas et al. studied paclitaxel co-loaded in PLGA NPs with R-Flurbiprofen, a nonsteroidal anti-inflammatory drug known for its strong anticancer activity [242]. In the same study, chitosan-modified PLGA NPs were also co-loaded with paclitaxel and R-Flurbiprofen for an efficient delivery to the tumor site [242]. Sixty percent of the paclitaxel was released from the NPs for five days until reaching the pseudo-plateau. On the other hand, R-flurbiprofen was released quickly in the firsts 6 h. Additionally, the NPs showed efficient cytotoxic activity and were well integrated by the tumor cells, resulting in anti-tumoral activity against glioma [242]. The in vivo studies confirmed that the use of paclitaxel-loaded NPs with R-flurbiprofen-loaded NPs induces a significantly higher reduction of the tumor compared to when the drug-NPs are used individually [242].

Due to the protection they provide, NPs can also be used to encapsulate and deliver peptides and small proteins, such as CXCL12, in the aim of controlling GBM cell migration as a therapeutic approach. Our team strongly believe that the control of GBM cells migration via the CXCL12–CXCR4 axis can be a promising approach to rule the spread of those cells and facilitate their elimination. For this aim, we have developed composite alginate–chitosan NPs with an average size of 250 nm for CXCL12 encapsulation which, upon its release, increases GBM cell migration [243]. Three initial mass loadings were tested (0.372 µg/mg NPs, 0.744 µg/mg NPs, and 1.490 µg/mg NPs). Our results showed that the alginate–chitosan NPs entrapped CXCL12 with a percentage of ~98% without loss of the molecule [243]. For all the conditions tested, a burst released in the first 2 h was observed, followed by a sustained release that reach a pseudo-plateau after 72 h without a complete release of the chemokine [243]. The releasing profile observed was coherent with a diffusion-based system which led us to evaluate the driving mass transport phenomenon [243]. Using the experimental data, we performed mathematical modeling using Fick's second law of diffusion for a spherical geometry, which considered the size distribution of NPs (class method) and boundary conditions that allowed us to model the interactions between the CXCL12 molecules and the NPs. The cumulative mass release vs. time and position equation was solved using a finite difference approach and mechanistic parameters (effective diffusion coefficient, D_{eff}; overall mass transfer coefficient at the surface, k) which were estimated using an evolutionary algorithm, leading to coefficients of a determination > 0.97 [243]. Small values of D_{eff} (~2×10^{-19} m^2/s) were obtained, which can be associated with the presence of electrostatic interactions between the positive charge of CXCL12 and the negative one of the alginates composing the NPs [243]. However, since our experiments were conducted in static conditions, it is impossible to deny that in vivo, other types of mass transport phenomena may occur, such as convective interstitial brain fluid flow, that may be a reason for an increased releasing rate. Furthermore, our migration assays proved that CXCL12 significantly controlled the invasion of the F98 cell line, which highlights the importance of using CXCL12 in delivery systems for GBM targeting [243].

In the same way, Mansor et al. used PLGA and the PLGA-PEG co-polymer for CXCL12 encapsulation [213]. They used a different proportion of PLGA, an encapsulation efficiency of 67% was observed for 0% PLGA-COOH, and for the two other proportions (17% and 67% PLGA-COOH), the encapsulation was surprisingly above 100% [213]. The highest percentage of CXCL12 released was 43%, achieved with a 33% proportion of PLGA-COOH in a physiologically relevant solution (pH 7.4). This percentage increased when the medium was changed to an acidic medium buffer (pH 4). As another example, Alghamri et al. developed synthetic protein NPs coated with iRGD to target the CXCL12–CXCR4 axis in GBM. The NPs blocked CXCR4 via its inhibitor in both in vitro and in vivo models. The treatment inhibits GBM proliferation and the induction of immunogenic tumor cell death.

Further, the use of radiotherapy with the treatment inhibited GBM progression, leading to a 60% increased survival rate compared to the controls [244].

Table 3. Some examples of polymeric-based NPs.

Polymer Type	Drug/Molecule Loaded	Particle Size (nm)	Ref
PLGA	DOX	~120	[245]
PLGA	TMZ	~194	[241]
PLGA-PEG	DOX	~50	[240]
PLGA-PEG-chitosan	Paclitaxel and R-flurbiprofen	150–190	[242]
PLGA	DTX and indocyanine green	~220	[246]
PLGA/PEG-PLGA	CXCL12	200–250	[213]
Chitosan-Alginate	CXCL12	~250	[243]
Chitosan-modified PLGA NPs	R-Flurbiprofen and Paclitaxel	150–190	[100]
Dextran	Paclitaxel	~60	[235]
Silk fibroin	Indocyanine green	~209	[247]
Synthetic protein	AMD3100	37–98	[244]

NPs provide a series of advantages for delivery applications to enhance the therapeutic efficiency of the drugs, but the major challenge remaining is the transport to the tumor site without degradation [248]. Despite all the advantages of systemic drug delivery across the BBB, systemic delivery needs to address different challenges for further improvement. The long distance between the delivery route and the target site and the drug digestion remain the biggest limitations of systemic delivery.

6.2.2. Local Delivery

Local delivery consists of delivering chemotherapeutic agents in the surgical cavity after the tumor resection for GBM therapy improvement [41]. A series of factors make local delivery advantageous in GBM treatment [249]. Metastasis occurs within approximately ~2 cm of the tumor's original site, which means it is close to where the drugs were loaded locally; the administration of the drugs will no longer face the BBB limitations [249]. Different strategies for local delivery to improve the GBM survival rate have been developed, including intranasal drugs delivery, convection enhanced delivery, and direct injection of the drugs including rigid implants and hydrogels [250].

Intranasal Drugs Delivery:

The intranasal route can bypass the BBB and achieve reaching the brain for the delivery of drugs. It is important to understand the anatomy of the nasal cavity and the mechanisms of compound transport through the intranasal route. Bruinsmann et al., described this aspect in detail [251]. In this paragraph, we focus on discussing the different GBM treatments via the intranasal approach to deliver drugs to the tumor.

Blacher et al. used "anthranoid 4,5-dihydroxyanthraquinone-2-carboxylic acid", also known as rhein, to inhibit CD38 by intranasal injection in mice. CD38 deficiency is known to regulate microglial activation and attenuates glioma progression [252–254]. The tumor in the mice treated decreased, concluding that the intranasal drugs' administration is effective and rhein can be a therapeutic target in GBM [252]. Li et al. used intranasal drug delivery to administer TMZ in a rat model bearing orthotopic C6 glioma xenografts showing a significantly reduction in the tumor growth compared with intravenous injection or gavage [255]. The results suggest that the intranasal route should be further considered as an option for TMZ delivery into the brain [255]. However, different therapeutic agents are under investigation for GBM treatment, but the use of a delivery system has been proved to be more beneficial in term of maintaining the drug release.

NPs are also good vehicles to control the drug release and overcome some limitations of the intranasal drug delivery, such as the poor capacity of crossing the nasal mucosa and enzymatic degradation [251]. Polymeric NPs (PLGA-based [251,256], PCL-based [257,258]) and lipid-based NPs are the most commonly used for nose-to-brain delivery [196,259]. For instance, PLGA and oligomeric chitosan composite NPs were designed to co-deliver alpha-cyano-4-hydroxycinnamic acid (CHC) and the monoclonal antibody cetuximab (CTX) into the brain by nasal administration to ensure the therapeutic efficacy for GBM treatment [256]. CHC and CTX are known to have a therapeutic effect against angiogenesis, cancer cell invasion, and metastasis [256]. In vitro assays using a chicken chorioallantoic membrane assay showed no reduction of cell viability for U251 and SW1088 glioma cell lines, but the designed NPs showed a stability that reached three months and a high encapsulation of the drugs was reached [256]. More recently, they designed a new platform using PLGA and chitosan composite NPs to carry CHC. CHC-NPs were covalently coated with CTX. An ex vivo study using a porcine mucosa demonstrated the capacity of the NPs to promote CHC and CTX permeation, whereas the chicken chorioallantoic membrane assay demonstrated its capacity to reduce the tumor size [260]. Sousa et al. also used PLGA-based NPs to administer the monoclonal antibody bevacizumab, an anti-VEGF used as an anti-cancer drug, intranasally in mice [261]. The use of bevacizumab-loaded NPs when administered intranasally into CD-1 mice showed higher brain bioavailability compared to the free drug. Furthermore, used in a GBM nude mouse model, the NPs-based delivery system also induced a reduction in the tumor growth after 14 days, with a high anti-angiogenic effect of bevacizumab compared to free drug administration [261]. PCL-based NPs have also been used to route drugs addressing the brain tissue intranasally. De Oliveira et al. used PCL based NPs loaded with melatonin to target the U87 MG GBM cell line [258]. The NPs revealed to be non-cytotoxic on healthy cells (MRC-5) and increased the water solubility of the drug in addition to promoting strong activity against U87 MG cells. In vivo assays in rats through intranasal injection increased the drug uptake in the brain compared to when administered directly without nanocarriers [258]. Conversely, Alex et al. develop PCL-based NPs to encapsulate the anticancer drug carboplatin to target GBM via the nasal route [257]. The optimized formulation was a 311.6 nm particle size, and they observed a burst release of the drug followed by a slow continued release. However, ex vivo permeation studies through sheep nasal mucosa showed a lower drug permeation, which was attributed to the nasal mucosa complexity. While improving the delivery and accumulation of drugs to the brain, those results highlight the complexity of the nose-to-brain route. Despite all the advantages given by intranasal delivery, the low volumes of the drugs delivered remain the main problem that limits its use.

Convection Enhanced Delivery:

Convection enhanced delivery (CED) is a local therapeutic method that aims to enhance intracerebral drugs diffusion to the CNS by bypassing the BBB, allowing the introduction of high doses of therapeutic agents with different ranges of molecular weight through the interstitial spaces [262]. CED is based on the principles of "bulk flow" which refer to the extracellular flow of fluid delivered via a pressure gradient rather than the normal passive diffusion transport [262]. CED fundamental procedures consist of the stereotactic placement of a microcatheter directly into the tumor and generating an external pressure using a motor-driven pump to induce fluid convection in the brain [263]. CED permits a deeper penetration and distribution of the drugs, eliminating the problem of depletion frequently seen using the direct injection [264]. In addition, CED is used even with agents with a high molecular weight, including proteins, nucleic acids, and antibodies [265,266].

Several studies have proved the safety and feasibility of CED [106,263,267]. Additionally, drug encapsulation into nano-sized carriers proved to be more beneficial to increase the efficiency of delivery. For instance, Séhédic et al. developed lipid nanocapsules (LNCs) to incorporate radionuclides and implant them in the brain using stereotactic injections for locoregional therapy [268]. Using the CED, they demonstrated that lipophilic thiobenzoate complexes of rhenium-188 loaded in LNCs (LNC188Re) with a function-blocking antibody (12G5) directed at the CXCR4 on its surface enhance the median survival and show major clinical improvement in Scid mice [268]. The retention of rhenium in the brain and the outcomes achieved (distribution, efficacy, gradient) were principally ensured by LNCs, which accentuate the interest of using nanocarriers. Zhang et al. used cisplatin-loaded NPs of 70 nm in diameter functionalized with PEG for administration by CED to control the release of cisplatin and kill the tumor cells that they reach without causing toxicity [269]. Their small size and dense PEG corona prevented them from being trapped as they moved within the brain tissue while controlling the delivery of the drug, making them efficient brain-penetrating drug delivery vehicles. Their results also showed a significant increase in the survival rate of a GBM rat brain tumor model, thus highlighting the advantages of using NPs. CED, combined with the delivery of the favorable physicochemical properties ensured by NPs, has demonstrated a great potential to improve clinical outcomes. For instance, Stephen et al. used magnetic NPs coated with a chitosan-PEG copolymer to deliver MGMT inhibitor O6-benzylguanine via CED for GBM targeting as a treatment for GBM patients showing resistance to TMZ [270]. They showed that the distribution of the NPs in the mice's brains was excellent, whereas the activity of MGMT decreased significantly, which, in the presence of TMZ, increased the median survival rate [270]. In another study, Chen et al. proved that the nanoliposomal formulation of irinotecan with CED technology enhanced the survival time of the treated mice when combined with radiation, as compared with the systemic injection of irinotecan plus radiotherapy [271]. CED for GBM treatment has been also reported in clinical trials. Cruickshank et al. injected irinotecan drug-loaded beads suspended in an alginate solution into patients after surgical resection. Studies are still under investigation, however, only one patient has died, due to causes which were not associated with the treatment, thus suggesting that the use of irinotecan drug-loaded beads may be a promising, stable, and safe platform to assess the local delivery of new agents [272]. All these studies focus on combining CED with nanocarriers for a better control of the drug release in the aim of increasing survival. Despite the promising results achieved, different physical and technical limitations and challenges are still to be overcome. The main obstacle occurring is the backflow, sometimes referred as reflux, that takes place when the perfusate is not well penetrated in the tissues [262]. Hopefully, backflow resistant catheters have been developed, which may solve this issue.

Direct Drug Injection:

The direct drug injection for the delivery of ACA within the tumor resection cavity emerged to resolve the bypassing BBB limitations and increase the drugs' concertation in the tumor site. This method has lot of advantages, including side effects reduction, safe administration of different molecules, and the depletion of toxicity actions [273].

- Rigid Implants:

The direct drug injection opens the doors for local implant-based GBM treatments. The only local delivery system approved by the FDA and currently used for GBM treatment is the polifeprosan 20 with the carmustine-loaded wafer Gliadel® [274]. Gliadel® wafers are 14.5 mm in diameter and 1 mm in thickness, the wafer is made from a biodegradable hydrophobic co-polymer 1,3-bis-(p-carboxyphenoxy)propane (pCPP) and sebacic acid [274]. When in contact with aqueous fluids, the wafers start releasing the carmustine into the surrounding tissue [275]. After approving Gliadel® wafers, several chemotherapeutic agents have been tested in preclinical models such as paclitaxel [276], acriflavine [277], and DOX [278]. Due to the rigidity of the device compared with the soft nature of the brain tissue, different adverse reactions occur such as necrosis, infection, and convulsions [277]. The main problem remaining using these wafers is the drug release profile. For this, many studies have explored the possibility of reducing the burst release profile and sustaining the release for a long period [250,279,280]. For example, Shapira-Furman et al. used Gliadel wafers co-loaded with 50% w/w of TMZ and BCNU in PLGA for sustaining the release of the drugs for four weeks [281]. The drugs were first coated with the polymer to form core–shell particles, in which the coating shell served as a membrane for the drug particles [281]. The median survival was 15 days in the group treated with BCNU wafers alone, whereas the group with TMZ wafers alone had a median survival of 19 days [281]. The group treated with combined BCNU and TMZ wafers had a median survival of 28 days, suggesting that the combination of drugs can achieve a big improvement for local drug delivery [281]. However, rapid drug release, cell migration, drug resistance, and side effects are different problems that prevent Gliadel wafers from being an effective option to treat GBM.

- New Innovative Drug-Delivery Approaches in Glioblastoma Treatments:

Hydrogels:

Hydrogels can be defined as 3D polymeric hydrophilic networks within an aqueous medium [282]. Due to their ability to encapsulate different agents and control their release, hydrogels are used for different biomedical applications and medicine such as artificial skin, membranes for biosensors, 3D platforms, and drug delivery devices [283–285]. Further, the use of hydrogels can be more beneficial than the Gliadel wafers because of their ability to mimic the mechanical properties and the softness of the brain tissue. For instance, Wang et al. have shown, using PEG-based hydrogels bearing GRGDS adhesion peptides and U87 human GBM cells, that matrix stiffness induces differential GBM cell proliferation, morphology, and migration [286]. Increasing the matrix stiffness (associated with tumor-like mechanical properties) led to delayed U87 cell proliferation, but the authors observed that cells formed denser spheroids with extended cell protrusions.

Various studies explored the use of hydrogels for GBM treatments in this context [286–289]. Bastiancich et al. reviewed the different types of hydrogels as drug delivery systems for GBM local treatment recently used in preclinical and clinical studies, suggesting that loaded hydrogels with one or many chemotherapeutic agents are advantageous for GBM treatment [290]. Hydrogels fill the gap between the tumor resection and the administration of chemotherapy and radiotherapy, allowing a sustained release of the drugs, which may lead to better results than a conventional CED approach [290]. Akbar et al. developed a biodegradable hydrogel from PLGA:plasticizers with a ratio of 40:60 for TMZ delivery in C6 glioma rats [291]. A significant reduction of the tumor was observed, and no mortality was associated with the gel matrix treatment, concluding that the gels can be safe and effective when used in vivo [291]. In another recent study, hydrogel loaded with the quisinostat drug and radiopaque gold NPs (AuNP) has been explored in GBM. Radiopaque NPs were used as the contrast agent that would release the drugs when irradiated. The release of quisinostat in vitro was high, which inhibited the tumor growth in the in vivo mice model bearing xenografted human GBM tumors [292]. The platform developed can also be used simultaneously for radiation therapy. OncoGel™ is a PLGA-PEG-based thermo-sensitive hydrogel used for paclitaxel delivery in GBM treatment, which has been shown to prolong the survival in a rodent glioma model [293]. OncoGel™ provides a sustained release of paclitaxel for 50 days, maintaining a high local concentration and biodegrades after four to six weeks [294]. In 2007, the first clinical trial (NCT00479765) using OncoGel™ for recurrent glioma in order to evaluate the safety and tolerability of the system in the patients started, but could not be ended for sponsor businesses [290]. Déry et al. used a biodegradable hydrogel (GlioGel) loaded with three chemoattractants (CXCL10, CCL2, and CCL11) to attract murine F98 and U87 GBM cells toward a therapeutic trap using an agarose drop assay [295]. The zones with high concentrations of CXCL10 display the highest number of the cells attracted compared to the control due to the chemoattractant gradient. CCL2 showed a very similar response to CXCL10 for the F98 cells, but the U87MG cells were less responsive, and both cells did not show any significant effect on chemotaxis to CCL11 [295]. The team performed in vivo assays using an orthotopic syngeneic F98-Fischer rat model. Three days after the implantation of the F98 tumor cells, the GlioGels containing the chemoattractant were inoculated. Many peritumoral clusters were observed when CXCL10, CCL2, and CCL11 were implanted in the controlateral hemisphere compared to those implanted in ipsilateral hemisphere [295]. These results support the hypothesis that the use of the GlioGel with chemokines can modify the migration behavior of the GBM cells.

Nonetheless, for a sustained controlled release of chemotherapeutic drugs, nanocarriers can be confined in a hydrogel. Several reviews have highlighted that a better controlled release can be obtained when NPs are loaded in hydrogels [296,297]. For instance, Brachi et al. have shown that a multi-component system composed of polymeric NPs BODIPY-loaded and embedded within a thermosensitive hydrogel, revealed to be more efficient in terms of drug retention within the tumor in an orthotopic GBM mice model compared to NPs alone [298]. Zhao et al. used PLGA NPs for paclitaxel encapsulation, then loaded them into photopolymerizable hydrogels that had been implanted in the resection cavity [299]. They found that the system enhanced long-term survival (<150 days) in the U87 cells in vivo mice model compared with the mice where the hydrogels were implanted empty (they tolerated the hydrogels and had a long healthy life for up to four months) [299]. Furthermore, for biocompatibility, biodegradability, a better control of the gelation time, and a sustained release of hydrophobic and hydrophilic drugs, some prepolymer hydrogels have shown remarkable results, but still need to be investigated in GBM [300–302]. However, because of the many advantages of combining NPs to hydrogels, this approach can also be transposed to the development of a chemoattractant releasing device as part of cancer cell traps.

Cancer Cells Trap:

Najberg et al. proposed, in 2019, trapping cancer cells within one confined area to facilitate their removal [297]. In the paper, different strategies for cell trapping, such as the use of chemotaxis to attract cancer cells expressing CXCR4, were proposed [297]. Giarra et al. used this technique for preparing a fake metastatic niche made of CXCL12-loaded thermoresponsive hydrogels based on methylcellulose or polaxamers with or without HA [303]. Only gels based on methylcellulose embedded with CXCL12 allowed GBM CXCR4-expressing cells to migrate in the direction of the hydrogel and finally be captured within [303]. They also demonstrated that the cancerous cell migration depended on the mechanical properties of the hydrogel; softer hydrogel made of methylcellulose promotes better cell migration as opposed to stiffer poloxamers hydrogels [303]. Similarly, Molina-Peña et al. loaded CXCL12 in PLGA and PEG-PLGA NPs to integrate the system into a chitosan solution with fiber-forming additive polyethylene oxide for producing a nanofibrous scaffold by electrospinning [304]. The use of the nanofibrous scaffolds with the NPs allowed a sustained release for up to 35 days instead of 5 days for the NPs alone, and an attenuation of the burst release [304]. They have also assessed this system in vivo with blank-NP-loaded nanofibrous scaffold and found no difference between the rats with the scaffolds implanted and the controls, suggesting an excellent biocompatibility of the scaffold during the first week of the treatment [304]. In the same context, our research group has recently developed an alginate-based macroporous hydrogel as a potential device for GBM cell trapping [29]. Since the main cause of GBM recurrence is the infiltrated GBM cells that migrate from the tumor, as discussed earlier, we propose to inverse the direction of GBM cell migration towards a well confined area in which they will be trapped and can be eliminated with localized radiotherapy using a chemoattractant gradient of CXCL12 (Figure 6).

The device proposed takes the name of gliotrap (GBM-trapping), and it combines an alginate macroporous hydrogel functionalized with RGD peptides (for cells catching) and alginate–chitosan composite NPs encapsulating CXCL12 (for cells attraction). The functionalization of the hydrogel with RGD peptides aims to promote the GBM cell adhesion inside the matrices via the interactions between the peptides and the $\alpha v \beta 3$ and $\alpha v \beta 5$ integrins widely expressed by those cells, as discussed above [29]. Hydrogels will be loaded with the NPs' delivery system and implanted into the surgical cavity of the tumor after its resection to ensure a CXCL12 gradient maintained for a very long period. The NPs are designed to promote a controlled release of CXCL12 and so create a cancer cell attracting gradient. This will help to maintain the CXCL12 gradient under a fast release that could happen because of the fluid flow in the brain.

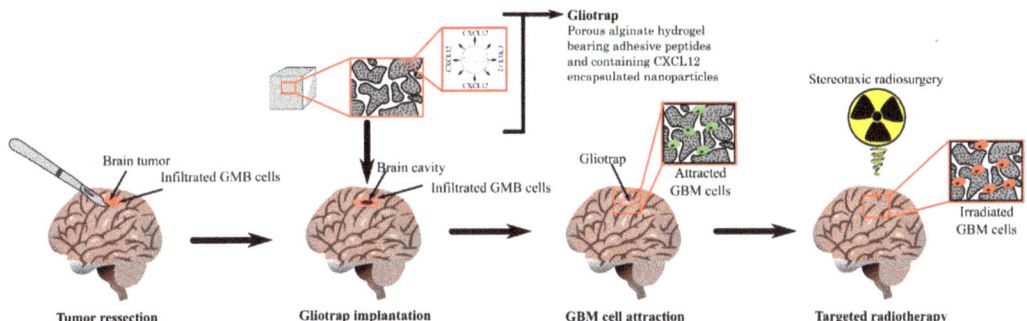

Figure 6. The strategy proposed by our team for GBM treatment.

So far, we have demonstrated using Transwell™ chemotaxis assays, that the NPs loaded with CXCL12 alone are capable of increasing the invasion of F98 cells [243]. Further, we previously developed an RGD-functionalized macroporous matrix in which the GB cells can accumulate and be retained [29]. Using an F98 GB cell line, it was demonstrated that the macroporous matrix can possibly accumulate and retain the F98 cells. These cells could then be effectively eliminated using local stereotaxic radiotherapy [29]. The main challenge remaining is to combine the two systems by loading the NPs-CXCL12 into the macroporous hydrogel. The release kinetics of CXCL12-AF647 encapsulated in alginate–chitosan NPs from the macroporous matrix will be investigated in the next step. Additionally, we will investigate the effect of a simulated brain fluid flow on CXCL12 release from the porous matrices using a custom-made 3D in vitro model that considers the fluid flow impact. The conception of a 3D in vitro model that mimics the brain fluid dynamics will provide a better understanding of the impact of the interstitial fluid flow on the release profile of CXCL12 for further optimization.

7. Conclusions

The present review discussed different novel strategies for GBM treatment that have emerged during the last decades. The standard treatments for the disease lack specificity and are very limited, mostly due to their incapacity to target cancerous cells that migrate out of the tumor to the surrounding parenchyma. We have also highlighted, as interesting therapeutic targets, several phenomena that are known to have a strong impact on GBM cell migration, such as the CXCL12–CXCR4 axis, the ECM composition, as well as the interstitial fluid flow. Additionally, we have discussed different drug delivery systems currently used in the development of GB treatments. Systemic administration has shown to be very beneficial. The use of NPs particularly opened a new horizon as they can promote drug accumulation at the site of the tumor and have shown better results when combined with other treatments such as immunotherapies, or with another drug delivery system, such as cells. Although there is still a lot of research to do in this field, the type of drug used, its administration, and the complexity of the body's reaction to the treatment require the development of new pre-clinical models that mimic the complexity of the human brain. Local administration of drug delivery systems, such as intranasal drug delivery, CED, and the implantation of polymer-based biomaterials (rigid implants and hydrogels), have proved to be even more effective. More precisely, hydrogels also proved to be advantageous compared to the rigid implants because of their unique characteristics, including biocompatibility, biodegradability, and their response to stimuli. Hydrogels can be implanted into the surgical cavity after the tumor resection to ensure a high local concentration of the therapeutic drug and a sustained release in the tumor site, especially when combined with NPs. New strategies in drug delivery devices addressing GBM are also focusing on the development of GBM cancer cell traps, which comprises of a hydrogel with embedded NPs used to trigger cell chemotaxis, while the hydrogel itself acts as a cell capturing device. Finally, we highlighted with our ongoing research that, as promising as these new technologies are, there are still many challenges remaining.

Author Contributions: M.-A.L., B.P., B.M., N.F. and N.V. secured the funding. M.-A.L. and N.F. supervised and conceptualized the study. W.E.K. wrote the original draft. M.-A.L. and N.F. reviewed and edited the manuscript. All authors have read and agreed to the published version of the manuscript.

Funding: This work was supported by the New Frontiers in the Research Fund grant # NFRFE-2018-00764 and Fonds de Recherche du Québec—Nature et Technologie grant #299713.

Institutional Review Board Statement: Not applicable.

Informed Consent Statement: Not applicable.

Data Availability Statement: Not applicable.

Conflicts of Interest: The authors declare no conflict of interest.

References

1. Bray, F.; Ferlay, J.; Soerjomataram, I.; Siegel, R.L.; Torre, L.A.; Jemal, A. Global cancer statistics 2018: GLOBOCAN estimates of incidence and mortality worldwide for 36 cancers in 185 countries. *CA Cancer J. Clin.* **2018**, *68*, 394–424. [CrossRef] [PubMed]
2. Sung, H.; Ferlay, J.; Siegel, R.L.; Laversanne, M.; Soerjomataram, I.; Jemal, A.; Bray, F. Global Cancer Statistics 2020: GLOBOCAN Estimates of Incidence and Mortality Worldwide for 36 Cancers in 185 Countries. *CA Cancer J. Clin.* **2021**, *71*, 209–249. [CrossRef] [PubMed]
3. Schwartzbaum, J.A.; Fisher, J.L.; Aldape, K.D.; Wrensch, M. Epidemiology and molecular pathology of glioma. *Nat. Clin. Pract. Neurol.* **2006**, *2*, 494–503. [CrossRef] [PubMed]
4. Louis, D.N.; Perry, A.; Wesseling, P.; Brat, D.J.; Cree, I.A.; Figarella-Branger, D.; Hawkins, C.; Ng, H.K.; Pfister, S.M.; Reifenberger, G.; et al. The 2021 WHO Classification of Tumors of the Central Nervous System: A summary. *Neuro-Oncology* **2021**, *23*, 1231–1251. [CrossRef]
5. Patel, A.P.; Fisher, J.L.; Nichols, E.; Abd-Allah, F.; Abdela, J.; Abdelalim, A.; Abraha, H.N.; Agius, D.; Alahdab, F.; Alam, T.; et al. Global, regional, and national burden of brain and other CNS cancer, 1990–2016: A systematic analysis for the Global Burden of Disease Study 2016. *Lancet Neurol.* **2019**, *18*, 376–393. [CrossRef]
6. Dolecek, T.A.; Propp, J.M.; Stroup, N.E.; Kruchko, C. CBTRUS Statistical Report: Primary Brain and Central Nervous System Tumors Diagnosed in the United States in 2005–2009. *Neuro-Oncology* **2012**, *14*, v1–v49. [CrossRef]
7. Ostrom, Q.T.; Gittleman, H.; Truitt, G.; Boscia, A.; Kruchko, C.; Barnholtz-Sloan, J.S. CBTRUS statistical report: Primary brain and other central nervous system tumors diagnosed in the United States in 2011–2015. *Neuro-Oncology* **2018**, *20*, iv1–iv86. [CrossRef]
8. Chakrabarti, I.; Cockburn, M.; Cozen, W.; Wang, Y.-P.; Preston-Martin, S. A population-based description of glioblastoma multiforme in Los Angeles County, 1974–1999. *Cancer* **2005**, *104*, 2798–2806. [CrossRef]
9. Tamimi, A.F.; Juweid, M. Epidemiology and outcome of glioblastoma. *Exon Publ.* **2017**, 143–153. [CrossRef]
10. Lah, T.T.; Novak, M.; Breznik, B. Brain malignancies: Glioblastoma and brain metastases. *Semin. Cancer Biol.* **2020**, *60*, 262–273. [CrossRef]
11. Al-Rikabi, A.C.; Al-Sohaibani, M.O.; Jamjoom, A.; Al-Rayess, M.M. Metastatic deposits of a high-grade malignant glioma in cervical lymph nodes diagnosed by fine needle aspiration (FNA) cytology-Case report and literature review. *Cytopathology* **1997**, *8*, 421–427. [CrossRef] [PubMed]
12. Widjaja, A.; Mix, H.; Gölkel, C.; Flemming, P.; Egensperger, R.; Holstein, A.; Rademaker, J.; Becker, H.; Hundt, M.; Wagner, S.; et al. Uncommon metastasis of a glioblastoma multiforme in liver and spleen. *Digestion* **2000**, *61*, 219–222. [CrossRef]
13. Lin, C.; Liu, L.; Zeng, C.; Cui, Z.-K.; Chen, Y.; Lai, P.; Wang, H.; Shao, Y.; Zhang, H.; Zhang, R.; et al. Activation of mTORC1 in subchondral bone preosteoblasts promotes osteoarthritis by stimulating bone sclerosis and secretion of CXCL12. *Bone Res.* **2019**, *7*, 5. [CrossRef] [PubMed]
14. Arora, S.; Bhardwaj, A.; Singh, S.; Srivastava, S.K.; McClellan, S.; Nirodi, C.S.; Piazza, G.A.; Grizzle, W.E.; Owen, L.B.; Singh, A.P. An undesired effect of chemotherapy: Gemcitabine promotes pancreatic cancer cell invasiveness through reactive oxygen species-dependent, nuclear factorκb- and hypoxia-inducible factor 1α-mediated up-regulation of CXCR4. *J. Biol. Chem.* **2013**, *288*, 21197–21207. [CrossRef] [PubMed]
15. Behnan, J.; Finocchiaro, G.; Hanna, G. The landscape of the mesenchymal signature in brain tumours. *Brain* **2019**, *142*, 847–866. [CrossRef] [PubMed]
16. Ghosh, D.; Nandi, S.; Bhattacharjee, S. Combination therapy to checkmate Glioblastoma: Clinical challenges and advances. *Clin. Transl. Med.* **2018**, *7*, 33. [CrossRef] [PubMed]
17. Scherer, H.J. Structural Development in Gliomas. *Am. J. Cancer* **1938**, *34*, 333–351.
18. Singh, S.K.; Hawkins, C.; Clarke, I.D.; Squire, J.A.; Bayani, J.; Hide, T.; Henkelman, R.M.; Cusimano, M.D.; Dirks, P.B. Identification of human brain tumour initiating cells. *Nature* **2004**, *432*, 396–401. [CrossRef]

19. Barone, D.G.; Lawrie, T.A.; Hart, M.G. Image guided surgery for the resection of brain tumours. *Cochrane Database Syst. Rev.* **2014**, *2014*, CD009685. [CrossRef]
20. Mrugala, M.M. Advances and challenges in the treatment of glioblastoma: A clinician's perspective. *Discov. Med.* **2013**, *15*, 221–230.
21. Azagury, D.E.; Dua, M.M.; Barrese, J.C.; Henderson, J.M.; Buchs, N.C.; Ris, F.; Cloyd, J.M.; Martinie, B.J.; Razzaque, S.; Nicolau, S.; et al. Image-guided surgery. *Curr. Probl. Surg.* **2015**, *52*, 476–520. [CrossRef]
22. Klimberg, V.S.; Rivere, A. Ultrasound image-guided core biopsy of the breast. *Chin. Clin. Oncol.* **2016**, *5*, 33. [CrossRef]
23. Davis, M.E. Glioblastoma: Overview of Disease and Treatment. *Clin. J. Oncol. Nurs.* **2016**, *20*, S2–S8. [CrossRef]
24. Desmarais, G.; Fortin, D.; Bujold, R.; Wagner, R.; Mathieu, D.; Paquette, B. Infiltration of glioma cells in brain parenchyma stimulated by radiation in the F98/Fischer rat model. *Int. J. Radiat. Biol.* **2012**, *88*, 565–574. [CrossRef]
25. Mann, J.; Ramakrishna, R.; Magge, R.; Wernicke, A.G. Advances in radiotherapy for glioblastoma. *Front. Neurol.* **2018**, *8*, 748. [CrossRef]
26. Fuller, C.D.D.; Choi, M.; Forthuber, B.; Wang, S.J.J.; Rajagiriyil, N.; Salter, B.J.J.; Fuss, M. Standard fractionation intensity modulated radiation therapy (IMRT) of primary and recurrent glioblastoma multiforme. *Radiat. Oncol.* **2007**, *2*, 26. [CrossRef] [PubMed]
27. Weller, M.; Fisher, B.; Taphoorn, M.J.B.; Belanger, K.; Brandes, A.A.; Marosi, C.; Bogdahn, U.; Curschmann, J.; Janzer, R.C. Radiotherapy plus Concomitant and Adjuvant Temozolomide for Glioblastoma. *N. Engl. J. Med.* **2005**, *352*, 987–996.
28. Hatoum, A.; Mohammed, R.; Zakieh, O. The unique invasiveness of glioblastoma and possible drug targets on extracellular matrix. *Cancer Manag. Res.* **2019**, *11*, 1843–1855. [CrossRef]
29. Solano, A.G.; Dupuy, J.; Therriault, H.; Liberelle, B.; Faucheux, N.; Lauzon, M.-A.; Virgilio, N.; Paquette, B. An alginate-based macroporous hydrogel matrix to trap cancer cells. *Carbohydr. Polym.* **2021**, *266*, 118115. [CrossRef]
30. Desmarais, G.; Charest, G.; Therriault, H.; Shi, M.; Fortin, D.; Bujold, R.; Mathieu, D.; Paquette, B. Infiltration of F98 glioma cells in Fischer rat brain is temporary stimulated by radiation. *Int. J. Radiat. Biol.* **2016**, *92*, 444–450. [CrossRef]
31. Combs, S.E.; Widmer, V.; Thilmann, C.; Hof, H.; Debus, J.; Schulz-Ertner, D. Stereotactic radiosurgery (SRS): Treatment option for recurrent glioblastoma multiforme (GBM). *Cancer* **2005**, *104*, 2168–2173. [CrossRef] [PubMed]
32. Yamamoto, T.; Nakai, K.; Matsumura, A. Boron neutron capture therapy for glioblastoma. *Cancer Lett.* **2008**, *262*, 143–152. [CrossRef] [PubMed]
33. Norden, A.D.; Wen, P.Y. Glioma therapy in adults. *Neurologist* **2006**, *12*, 279–292. [CrossRef]
34. Williams, B.J.; Suki, D.; Fox, B.D.; Pelloski, C.E.; Maldaun, M.V.C.; Sawaya, R.E.; Lang, F.F.; Rao, G. Stereotactic radiosurgery for metastatic brain tumors: A comprehensive review of complications: Clinical article. *J. Neurosurg. JNS* **2009**, *111*, 439–448. [CrossRef]
35. Alphandéry, E. Glioblastoma treatments: An account of recent industrial developments. *Front. Pharmacol.* **2018**, *9*, 879. [CrossRef]
36. Neuwelt, E.A.; Rapoport, S.I. Modification of the blood-brain barrier in the chemotherapy of malignant brain tumors. *Fed. Proc.* **1984**, *43*, 214–219.
37. Sayegh, E.T.; Kaur, G.; Bloch, O.; Parsa, A.T. Systematic review of protein biomarkers of invasive behavior in glioblastoma. *Mol. Neurobiol.* **2014**, *49*, 1212–1244. [CrossRef]
38. Wu, W.; Klockow, J.L.; Zhang, M.; Lafortune, F.; Chang, E.; Jin, L.; Wu, Y.; Daldrup-Link, H.E. Glioblastoma multiforme (GBM): An overview of current therapies and mechanisms of resistance. *Pharmacol. Res.* **2021**, *171*, 105780. [CrossRef]
39. O'Reilly, S.M.; Newlands, E.S.; Brampton, M.; Glaser, M.G.; Rice-Edwards, J.M.; Illingworth, R.D.; Richards, P.G.; Kennard, C.; Colquhoun, I.R.; Lewis, P.; et al. Temozolomide: A new oral cytotoxic chemotherapeutic agent with promising activity against primary brain tumours. *Eur. J. Cancer* **1993**, *29*, 940–942. [CrossRef]
40. Witthayanuwat, S.; Pesee, M.; Supaadirek, C.; Supakalin, N.; Thamronganantasakul, K.; Krusun, S. Survival analysis of Glioblastoma Multiforme. *Asian Pac. J. Cancer Prev.* **2018**, *19*, 2613–2617.
41. Stupp, R.; Hegi, M.E.; Mason, W.P.; van den Bent, M.J.; Taphoorn, M.J.; Janzer, R.C.; Ludwin, S.K.; Allgeier, A.; Fisher, B.; Belanger, K.; et al. Effects of radiotherapy with concomitant and adjuvant temozolomide versus radiotherapy alone on survival in glioblastoma in a randomised phase III study: 5-year analysis of the EORTC-NCIC trial. *Lancet Oncol.* **2009**, *10*, 459–466. [CrossRef]
42. Gerber, D.E.; Grossman, S.A.; Zeltzman, M.; Parisi, M.A.; Kleinberg, L. The impact of thrombocytopenia from temozolomide and radiation in newly diagnosed adults with high-grade gliomas1. *Neuro-Oncology* **2007**, *9*, 47–52. [CrossRef] [PubMed]
43. Anand, U.; Dey, A.; Chandel, A.K.S.; Sanyal, R.; Mishra, A.; Pandey, D.K.; De Falco, V.; Upadhyay, A.; Kandimalla, R.; Chaudhary, A.; et al. Cancer chemotherapy and beyond: Current status, drug candidates, associated risks and progress in targeted therapeutics. *Genes Dis.* **2022**, in press. [CrossRef]
44. Grossman, S.A.; Reinhard, C.; Colvin, O.M.; Chasin, M.; Brundrett, R.; Tamargo, R.J.; Brem, H. The intracerebral distribution of BCNU delivered by surgically implanted biodegradable polymers. *J. Neurosurg.* **1992**, *76*, 640–647. [CrossRef]
45. Bartzatt, R. Lomustine Analogous Drug Structures for Intervention of Brain and Spinal Cord Tumors: The Benefit of In Silico Substructure Search and Analysis. *Chemother. Res. Pract.* **2013**, *2013*, 360624. [CrossRef]
46. Binabaj, M.M.; Bahrami, A.; ShahidSales, S.; Joodi, M.; Joudi Mashhad, M.; Hassanian, S.M.; Anvari, K.; Avan, A. The prognostic value of MGMT promoter methylation in glioblastoma: A meta-analysis of clinical trials. *J. Cell. Physiol.* **2018**, *233*, 378–386. [CrossRef]

47. Illic, R.; Somma, T.; Savic, D.; Frio, F.; Milicevic, M.; Solari, D.; Nikitovic, M.; Lavrnic, S.; Raicevic, S.; Milosevic, S.; et al. A Survival Analysis with Identification of Prognostic Factors in a Series of 110 Patients with Newly Diagnosed Glioblastoma Before and After Introduction of the Stupp Regimen: A Single-Center Observational Study. *World Neurosurg.* **2017**, *104*, 581–588. [CrossRef]
48. Taphoorn, M.J.B.; Stupp, R.; Coens, C.; Osoba, D.; Kortmann, R.; van den Bent, M.J.; Mason, W.; Mirimanoff, R.O.; Baumert, B.G.; Eisenhauer, E. Health-related quality of life in patients with glioblastoma: A randomised controlled trial. *Lancet Oncol.* **2005**, *6*, 937–944. [CrossRef]
49. Huijbers, I.J.; Iravani, M.; Popov, S.; Robertson, D.; Al-Sarraj, S.; Jones, C.; Isacke, C.M. A role for fibrillar collagen deposition and the collagen internalization receptor endo180 in glioma invasion. *PLoS ONE* **2010**, *5*, e9808. [CrossRef]
50. Joo, K.M.; Jin, J.; Kim, E.; Kim, K.H.; Kim, Y.; Kang, B.G.; Kang, Y.J.; Lathia, J.D.; Cheong, K.H.; Song, P.H.; et al. MET signaling regulates glioblastoma stem cells. *Cancer Res.* **2012**, *72*, 3828–3838. [CrossRef]
51. Veeravalli, K.K.; Rao, J.S. MMP-9 and uPAR regulated glioma cell migration. *Cell Adhes. Migr.* **2012**, *6*, 509–512. [CrossRef]
52. Pencheva, N.; de Gooijer, M.C.; Vis, D.J.; Wessels, L.F.A.A.; Würdinger, T.; van Tellingen, O.; Bernards, R. Identification of a Druggable Pathway Controlling Glioblastoma Invasiveness. *Cell Rep.* **2017**, *20*, 48–60. [CrossRef] [PubMed]
53. Theocharis, A.D.; Skandalis, S.S.; Gialeli, C.; Karamanos, N.K. Extracellular matrix structure. *Adv. Drug Deliv. Rev.* **2016**, *97*, 4–27. [CrossRef]
54. Mohiuddin, E.; Wakimoto, H. Extracellular matrix in glioblastoma: Opportunities for emerging therapeutic approaches. *Am. J. Cancer Res.* **2021**, *11*, 3742–3754.
55. Li, G.; Qin, Z.; Chen, Z.; Xie, L.; Wang, R.; Zhao, H. Tumor microenvironment in treatment of glioma. *Open Med.* **2017**, *12*, 247–251. [CrossRef]
56. de Gooijer, M.C.; Guillén Navarro, M.; Bernards, R.; Wurdinger, T.; van Tellingen, O. An Experimenter's Guide to Glioblastoma Invasion Pathways. *Trends Mol. Med.* **2018**, *24*, 763–780. [CrossRef]
57. Tamkun, J.W.; DeSimone, D.W.; Fonda, D.; Patel, R.S.; Buck, C.; Horwitz, A.F.; Hynes, R.O. Structure of integrin, a glycoprotein involved in the transmembrane linkage between fibronectin and actin. *Cell* **1986**, *46*, 271–282. [CrossRef]
58. Humphries, J.D.; Askari, J.A.; Zhang, X.-P.; Takada, Y.; Humphries, M.J.; Mould, A.P. Molecular Basis of Ligand Recognition by Integrin 5. *J. Biol. Chem.* **2000**, *275*, 20337–20345. [CrossRef]
59. Bouvard, D.; Pouwels, J.; De Franceschi, N.; Ivaska, J. Integrin inactivators: Balancing cellular functions in vitro and in vivo. *Nat. Rev. Mol. Cell Biol.* **2013**, *14*, 430–442. [CrossRef]
60. Takada, Y.; Ye, X.; Simon, S. The integrins. *Genome Biol.* **2007**, *8*, 215. [CrossRef]
61. Banères, J.L.; Roquet, F.; Green, M.; LeCalvez, H.; Parello, J. The cation-binding domain from the α subunit of integrin $\alpha 5\beta 1$ is a minimal domain for fibronectin recognition. *J. Biol. Chem.* **1998**, *273*, 24744–24753. [CrossRef]
62. Hynes, R.O. Integrins: Bidirectional, Allosteric Signaling Machines. *Cell* **2002**, *110*, 673–687. [CrossRef]
63. Varner, J.A.; Cheresh, D.A. Integrins and cancer. *Curr. Opin. Cell Biol.* **1996**, *8*, 724–730. [CrossRef]
64. Paolillo, M.; Serra, M.; Schinelli, S. Integrins in glioblastoma: Still an attractive target? *Pharmacol. Res.* **2016**, *113*, 55–61. [CrossRef]
65. Muradashvili, N.; Lominadze, D. Role of fibrinogen in cerebrovascular dysfunction after traumatic brain injury. *Brain Inj.* **2013**, *27*, 1508–1515. [CrossRef] [PubMed]
66. Gritsenko, P.G.; Ilina, O.; Friedl, P. Interstitial guidance of cancer invasion. *J. Pathol.* **2012**, *226*, 185–199. [CrossRef]
67. Zimmermann, D.R.; Dours-Zimmermann, M.T. Extracellular matrix of the central nervous system: From neglect to challenge. *Histochem. Cell Biol.* **2008**, *130*, 635–653. [CrossRef]
68. Maglott, A.; Bartik, P.; Cosgun, S.; Klotz, P.; Rondé, P.; Fuhrmann, G.; Takeda, K.; Martin, S.; Dontenwill, M. The Small $\alpha_5 \beta_1$ Integrin Antagonist, SJ749, Reduces Proliferation and Clonogenicity of Human Astrocytoma Cells. *Cancer Res.* **2006**, *66*, 6002–6007. [CrossRef]
69. Mallawaaratchy, D.M.; Buckland, M.E.; McDonald, K.L.; Li, C.C.Y.; Ly, L.; Sykes, E.K.; Christopherson, R.I.; Kaufman, K.L. Membrane Proteome Analysis of Glioblastoma Cell Invasion. *J. Neuropathol. Exp. Neurol.* **2015**, *74*, 425–441. [CrossRef]
70. Nakada, M.; Nambu, E.; Furuyama, N.; Yoshida, Y.; Takino, T.; Hayashi, Y.; Sato, H.; Sai, Y.; Tsuji, T.; Miyamoto, K.; et al. Integrin $\alpha 3$ is overexpressed in glioma stem-like cells and promotes invasion. *Br. J. Cancer* **2013**, *108*, 2516–2524. [CrossRef]
71. Schnell, O.; Krebs, B.; Wagner, E.; Romagna, A.; Beer, A.J.; Grau, S.J.; Thon, N.; Goetz, C.; Kretzschmar, H.A.; Tonn, J.-C.; et al. Expression of Integrin $\alpha v \beta 3$ in Gliomas Correlates with Tumor Grade and Is not Restricted to Tumor Vasculature. *Brain Pathol.* **2008**, *18*, 378–386. [CrossRef] [PubMed]
72. Blandin, A.-F.; Noulet, F.; Renner, G.; Mercier, M.-C.; Choulier, L.; Vauchelles, R.; Ronde, P.; Carreiras, F.; Etienne-Selloum, N.; Vereb, G.; et al. Glioma cell dispersion is driven by $\alpha 5$ integrin-mediated cell–matrix and cell–cell interactions. *Cancer Lett.* **2016**, *376*, 328–338. [CrossRef] [PubMed]
73. Amano, S.; Akutsu, N.; Matsunaga, Y.; Kadoya, K.; Nishiyama, T.; Champliaud, M.-F.; Burgeson, R.E.; Adachi, E. Importance of Balance between Extracellular Matrix Synthesis and Degradation in Basement Membrane Formation. *Exp. Cell Res.* **2001**, *271*, 249–262. [CrossRef] [PubMed]
74. Kubiatowski, T.; Jang, T.; Lachyankar, M.B.; Salmonsen, R.; Nabi, R.R.; Quesenberry, P.J.; Litofsky, N.S.; Ross, A.H.; Recht, L.D. Association of increased phosphatidylinositol 3-kinase signaling with increased invasiveness and gelatinase activity in malignant gliomas. *J. Neurosurg.* **2001**, *95*, 480–488. [CrossRef]

75. Qiu, X.Y.; Hu, D.X.; Chen, W.-Q.; Chen, R.Q.; Qian, S.R.; Li, C.Y.; Li, Y.J.; Xiong, X.X.; Liu, D.; Pan, F.; et al. PD-L1 confers glioblastoma multiforme malignancy via Ras binding and Ras/Erk/EMT activation. *Biochim. Biophys. Acta-Mol. Basis Dis.* **2018**, *1864*, 1754–1769. [CrossRef]
76. Desgrosellier, J.S.; Cheresh, D.A. Integrins in cancer: Biological implications and therapeutic opportunities. *Nat. Rev. Cancer* **2010**, *10*, 9–22. [CrossRef]
77. Mikheev, A.M.; Mikheeva, S.A.; Trister, A.D.; Tokita, M.J.; Emerson, S.N.; Parada, C.A.; Born, D.E.; Carnemolla, B.; Frankel, S.; Kim, D.-H.; et al. Periostin is a novel therapeutic target that predicts and regulates glioma malignancy. *Neuro-Oncology* **2015**, *17*, 372–382. [CrossRef]
78. Serres, E.; Debarbieux, F.; Stanchi, F.; Maggiorella, L.; Grall, D.; Turchi, L.; Burel-Vandenbos, F.; Figarella-Branger, D.; Virolle, T.; Rougon, G.; et al. Fibronectin expression in glioblastomas promotes cell cohesion, collective invasion of basement membrane in vitro and orthotopic tumor growth in mice. *Oncogene* **2014**, *33*, 3451–3462. [CrossRef]
79. Xiong, J.; Balcioglu, H.E.; Danen, E.H.J. Integrin signaling in control of tumor growth and progression. *Int. J. Biochem. Cell Biol.* **2013**, *45*, 1012–1015. [CrossRef]
80. Balkwill, F. Cancer and the chemokine network. *Nat. Rev. Cancer* **2004**, *4*, 540–550. [CrossRef]
81. Hughes, C.E.; Nibbs, R.J.B. A guide to chemokines and their receptors. *FEBS J.* **2018**, *285*, 2944–2971. [CrossRef]
82. Kulbe, H.; Levinson, N.R.; Balkwill, F.; Wilson, J.L. The chemokine network in cancer-Much more than directing cell movement. *Int. J. Dev. Biol.* **2004**, *48*, 489–496. [CrossRef]
83. Balestrieri, M.L.; Balestrieri, A.; Mancini, F.P.; Napoli, C. Understanding the immunoangiostatic CXC chemokine network. *Cardiovasc. Res.* **2008**, *78*, 250–256. [CrossRef]
84. Bockaert, J.; Pin, J.P. Molecular tinkering of G protein-coupled receptors: An evolutionary success. *EMBO J.* **1999**, *18*, 1723–1729. [CrossRef]
85. Bonavia, R.; Bajetto, A.; Barbero, S.; Pirani, P.; Florio, T.; Schettini, G. Chemokines and their receptors in the CNS: Expression of CXCL12/SDF-1 and CXCR4 and their role in astrocyte proliferation. *Toxicol. Lett.* **2003**, *139*, 181–189. [CrossRef]
86. Johnson, G.L.; Dhanasekaran, N. The G-protein family and their interaction with receptors. *Endocr. Rev.* **1989**, *10*, 317–331. [CrossRef]
87. L'Allemain, G.; Pouyssegur, J.; Weber, M.J. p42/mitogen-activated protein kinase as a converging target for different growth factor signaling pathways: Use of pertussis toxin as a discrimination factor. *Cell Regul.* **1991**, *2*, 675–684. [CrossRef]
88. Huang, Z.; Cheng, L.; Guryanova, O.A.; Wu, Q.; Bao, S. Cancer stem cells in glioblastoma—molecular signaling and therapeutic targeting. *Protein Cell* **2010**, *1*, 638–655. [CrossRef]
89. Liu, R.; Tian, B.; Gearing, M.; Hunter, S.; Ye, K.; Mao, Z. Cdk5-mediated regulation of the PIKE-A-Akt pathway and glioblastoma cell invasion. *Proc. Natl. Acad. Sci. USA* **2008**, *105*, 7570–7575. [CrossRef]
90. Roland, J.; Murphy, B.J.; Ahr, B.; Robert-Hebmann, V.; Delauzun, V.; Nye, K.E.; Devaux, C.; Biard-Piechaczyk, M. Role of the intracellular domains of CXCR4 in SDF-1–mediated signaling. *Blood* **2003**, *101*, 399–406. [CrossRef]
91. Würth, R.; Bajetto, A.; Harrison, J.K.; Barbieri, F.; Florio, T. CXCL12 modulation of CXCR4 and CXCR7 activity in human glioblastoma stem-like cells and regulation of the tumor microenvironment. *Front. Cell. Neurosci.* **2014**, *8*, 144. [CrossRef] [PubMed]
92. Décaillot, F.M.; Kazmi, M.A.; Lin, Y.; Ray-Saha, S.; Sakmar, T.P.; Sachdev, P. CXCR7/CXCR4 heterodimer constitutively recruits β-arrestin to enhance cell migration. *J. Biol. Chem.* **2011**, *286*, 32188–32197. [CrossRef] [PubMed]
93. Liu, Y.; Carson-Walter, E.; Walter, K.A. Targeting chemokine receptor CXCR7 inhibits glioma cell proliferation and mobility. *Anticancer Res.* **2015**, *35*, 53–64.
94. Groblewska, M.; Litman-Zawadzka, A.; Mroczko, B. The role of selected chemokines and their receptors in the development of gliomas. *Int. J. Mol. Sci.* **2020**, *21*, 3704. [CrossRef] [PubMed]
95. Lepore, F.; D'Alessandro, G.; Antonangeli, F.; Santoro, A.; Esposito, V.; Limatola, C.; Trettel, F. CXCL16/CXCR6 axis drives microglia/macrophages phenotype in physiological conditions and plays a crucial role in glioma. *Front. Immunol.* **2018**, *9*, 2750. [CrossRef]
96. Novak, M.; Koprivnikar Krajnc, M.; Hrastar, B.; Breznik, B.; Majc, B.; Mlinar, M.; Rotter, A.; Porčnik, A.; Mlakar, J.; Stare, K.; et al. CCR5-Mediated Signaling is Involved in Invasion of Glioblastoma Cells in Its Microenvironment. *Int. J. Mol. Sci.* **2020**, *21*, 4199. [CrossRef] [PubMed]
97. Lee, S.; Latha, K.; Manyam, G.; Yang, Y.; Rao, A.; Rao, G. Role of CX3CR1 signaling in malignant transformation of gliomas. *Neuro-Oncology* **2020**, *22*, 1463–1473. [CrossRef]
98. Rodero, M.; Marie, Y.; Coudert, M.; Blondet, E.; Mokhtari, K.; Rousseau, A.; Raoul, W.; Carpentier, C.; Sennlaub, F.; Deterre, P. Polymorphism in the microglial cell-mobilizing CX3CR1 gene is associated with survival in patients with glioblastoma. *J. Clin. Oncol.* **2008**, *26*, 5957–5964. [CrossRef]
99. Munson, J.M.; Bellamkonda, R.V.; Swartz, M.A. Interstitial flow in a 3d microenvironment increases glioma invasion by a cxcr4-dependent mechanism. *Cancer Res.* **2013**, *73*, 1536–1546. [CrossRef]
100. Calatozzolo, C.; Canazza, A.; Pollo, B.; Di Pierro, E.; Ciusani, E.; Maderna, E.; Salce, E.; Sponza, V.; Frigerio, S.; Di Meco, F.; et al. Expression of the new CXCL12 receptor, CXCR7, in gliomas. *Cancer Biol. Ther.* **2011**, *11*, 242–253. [CrossRef]

101. Balabanian, K.; Lagane, B.; Infantino, S.; Chow, K.Y.C.; Harriague, J.; Moepps, B.; Arenzana-Seisdedos, F.; Thelen, M.; Bachelerie, F. The Chemokine SDF-1/CXCL12 Binds to and Signals through the Orphan Receptor RDC1 in T Lymphocytes. *J. Biol. Chem.* **2005**, *280*, 35760–35766. [CrossRef]
102. Li, M.; Lu, Y.; Xu, Y.; Wang, J.; Zhang, C.; Du, Y.; Wang, L.; Li, L.; Wang, B.; Shen, J.; et al. Horizontal transfer of exosomal CXCR4 promotes murine hepatocarcinoma cell migration, invasion and lymphangiogenesis. *Gene* **2018**, *676*, 101–109. [CrossRef]
103. Bai, R.; Jie, X.; Sun, J.; Liang, Z.; Yoon, Y.; Feng, A.; Oum, Y.; Yu, W.; Wu, R.; Sun, B.; et al. Development of CXCR4 modulators based on the lead compound RB-108. *Eur. J. Med. Chem.* **2019**, *173*, 32–43. [CrossRef]
104. Brickute, D.; Braga, M.; Kaliszczak, M.A.; Barnes, C.; Lau, D.; Carroll, L.; Stevens, E.; Trousil, S.; Alam, I.S.; Nguyen, Q.-D.; et al. Development and Evaluation of an 18F-Radiolabeled Monocyclam Derivative for Imaging CXCR4 Expression. *Mol. Pharm.* **2019**, *16*, 2106–2117. [CrossRef]
105. Truogo, D.; Fiorelli, R.; Barrientos, E.S.; Melendez, E.L.; Sanai, N.; Mehta, S.; Nikkhah, M. A three-dimensional (3D) organotypic microfluidic model for glioma stem cells–Vascular interactions. *Biomaterials* **2019**, *198*, 63–77. [CrossRef]
106. Cornelison, R.C.; Brennan, C.E.; Kingsmore, K.M.; Munson, J.M. Convective forces increase CXCR4-dependent glioblastoma cell invasion in GL261 murine model. *Sci. Rep.* **2018**, *8*, 17054. [CrossRef]
107. Mortezaee, K. CXCL12/CXCR4 axis in the microenvironment of solid tumors: A critical mediator of metastasis. *Life Sci.* **2020**, *249*, 117534. [CrossRef]
108. Domanska, U.M.; Kruizinga, R.C.; Nagengast, W.B.; Timmer-Bosscha, H.; Huls, G.; De Vries, E.G.E.; Walenkamp, A.M.E. A review on CXCR4/CXCL12 axis in oncology: No place to hide. *Eur. J. Cancer* **2013**, *49*, 219–230. [CrossRef]
109. Duan, Y.; Zhang, S.; Wang, L.; Zhou, X.; He, Q.; Liu, S.; Yue, K.; Wang, X. Targeted silencing of CXCR4 inhibits epithelial-mesenchymal transition in oral squamous cell carcinoma. *Oncol. Lett.* **2016**, *12*, 2055–2061. [CrossRef]
110. Fu, Z.; Zhang, P.; Luo, H.; Huang, H.; Wang, F. CXCL12 modulates the radiosensitivity of cervical cancer by regulating CD44. *Mol. Med. Rep.* **2018**, *18*, 5101–5108. [CrossRef]
111. Duda, D.G.; Kozin, S.V.; Kirkpatrick, N.D.; Xu, L.; Fukumura, D.; Jain, R.K. CXCL12 (SDF1α)-CXCR4/CXCR7 Pathway Inhibition: An Emerging Sensitizer for Anticancer Therapies? *Clin. Cancer Res.* **2011**, *17*, 2074–2080. [CrossRef] [PubMed]
112. Ping, Y.; Yao, X.; Jiang, J.; Zhao, L.; Yu, S.; Jiang, T.; Lin, M.C.M.; Chen, J.; Wang, B.; Zhang, R. The chemokine CXCL12 and its receptor CXCR4 promote glioma stem cell-mediated VEGF production and tumour angiogenesis via PI3K/AKT signalling. *J. Pathol.* **2011**, *224*, 344–354. [CrossRef] [PubMed]
113. Graham, G.J. D6 and the atypical chemokine receptor family: Novel regulators of immune and inflammatory processes. *Eur. J. Immunol.* **2009**, *39*, 342–351. [CrossRef] [PubMed]
114. Shenoy, S.K.; Lefkowitz, R.J. Multifaceted roles of β-arrestins in the regulation of seven-membrane-spanning receptor trafficking and signalling. *Biochem. J.* **2003**, *375*, 503–515. [CrossRef] [PubMed]
115. Chen, Q.; Zhang, M.; Li, Y.; Xu, D.; Wang, Y.; Song, A.; Zhu, B.; Huang, Y.; Zheng, J.C. CXCR7 Mediates Neural Progenitor Cells Migration to CXCL12 Independent of CXCR4. *Stem Cells* **2015**, *33*, 2574–2585. [CrossRef] [PubMed]
116. Walters, M.J.; Ebsworth, K.; Berahovich, R.D.; Penfold, M.E.T.; Liu, S.-C.; Al Omran, R.; Kioi, M.; Chernikova, S.B.; Tseng, D.; Mulkearns-Hubert, E.E.; et al. Inhibition of CXCR7 extends survival following irradiation of brain tumours in mice and rats. *Br. J. Cancer* **2014**, *110*, 1179–1188. [CrossRef]
117. Orsini, M.J.; Parent, J.-L.; Mundell, S.J.; Benovic, J.L. Trafficking of the HIV coreceptor CXCR4: Role of arrestins and identification of residues in the C-terminal tail that mediate receptor internalization. *J. Biol. Chem.* **1999**, *274*, 31076–31086. [CrossRef]
118. Haribabu, B.; Richardson, R.M.; Fisher, I.; Sozzani, S.; Peiper, S.C.; Horuk, R.; Ali, H.; Snyderman, R. Regulation of human chemokine receptors CXCR4: Role of phosphorylation in desensitization and internalization. *J. Biol. Chem.* **1997**, *272*, 28726–28731. [CrossRef]
119. Mousavi, A. CXCL12/CXCR4 signal transduction in diseases and its molecular approaches in targeted-therapy. *Immunol. Lett.* **2020**, *217*, 91–115. [CrossRef]
120. Urbantat, R.M.; Vajkoczy, P.; Brandenburg, S. Advances in Chemokine Signaling Pathways as Therapeutic Targets in Glioblastoma. *Cancers* **2021**, *13*, 2983. [CrossRef]
121. Fricker, S.P. Physiology and pharmacology of plerixafor. *Transfus. Med. Hemother.* **2013**, *40*, 237–245. [CrossRef]
122. Hartmann, T.N.; Burger, J.A.; Glodek, A.; Fujii, N.; Burger, M. CXCR4 chemokine receptor and integrin signaling co-operate in mediating adhesion and chemoresistance in small cell lung cancer (SCLC) cells. *Oncogene* **2005**, *24*, 4462–4471. [CrossRef]
123. Engl, T.; Relja, B.; Marian, D.; Blumenberg, C.; Müller, I.; Beecken, W.-D.; Jones, J.; Ringel, E.M.; Bereiter-Hahn, J.; Jonas, D.; et al. CXCR4 Chemokine Receptor Mediates Prostate Tumor Cell Adhesion through α5 and β3 Integrins. *Neoplasia* **2006**, *8*, 290–301. [CrossRef]
124. Maurer, G.D.; Tritschler, I.; Adams, B.; Tabatabai, G.; Wick, W.; Stupp, R.; Weller, M. Cilengitide modulates attachment and viability of human glioma cells, but not sensitivity to irradiation or temozolomide in vitro. *Neuro-Oncology* **2009**, *11*, 747–756. [CrossRef]
125. Kingsmore, K.M.; Logsdon, D.K.; Floyd, D.H.; Peirce, S.M.; Purow, B.W.; Munson, J.M. Interstitial flow differentially increases patient-derived glioblastoma stem cell invasion: Via CXCR4, CXCL12, and CD44-mediated mechanisms. *Integr. Biol.* **2016**, *8*, 1246–1260. [CrossRef]
126. Lei, Y.; Han, H.; Yuan, F.; Javeed, A.; Zhao, Y. The brain interstitial system: Anatomy, modeling, in vivo measurement, and applications. *Prog. Neurobiol.* **2017**, *157*, 230–246. [CrossRef]

127. Abbott, N.J. Evidence for bulk flow of brain interstitial fluid: Significance for physiology and pathology. *Neurochem. Int.* **2004**, *45*, 545–552. [CrossRef]
128. Munson, J.M. Interstitial fluid flow under the microscope: Is it a future drug target for high grade brain tumours such as glioblastoma? *Expert Opin. Ther. Targets* **2019**, *23*, 725–728. [CrossRef]
129. Boucher, Y.; Salehi, H.; Witwer, B.; Harsh, G.R.; Jain, R.K. Interstitial fluid pressure in intracranial tumours in patients and in rodents. *Br. J. Cancer* **1997**, *75*, 829–836. [CrossRef]
130. Zagzag, D.; Lukyanov, Y.; Lan, L.; Ali, M.A.; Esencay, M.; Mendez, O.; Yee, H.; Voura, E.B.; Newcomb, E.W. Hypoxia-inducible factor 1 and VEGF upregulate CXCR4 in glioblastoma: Implications for angiogenesis and glioma cell invasion. *Lab. Investig.* **2006**, *86*, 1221–1232. [CrossRef]
131. Burridge, K.; Monaghan-Benson, E.; Graham, D.M. Mechanotransduction: From the cell surface to the nucleus via RhoA. *Philos. Trans. R. Soc. B Biol. Sci.* **2019**, *374*, 20180229. [CrossRef] [PubMed]
132. Qazi, H.; Shi, Z.-D.D.; Tarbell, J.M. Fluid shear stress regulates the invasive potential of glioma cells via modulation of migratory activity and matrix metalloproteinase expression. *PLoS ONE* **2011**, *6*, e20348. [CrossRef] [PubMed]
133. Friedl, P.; Wolf, K. Tumour-cell invasion and migration: Diversity and escape mechanisms. *Nat. Rev. Cancer* **2003**, *3*, 362–374. [CrossRef] [PubMed]
134. O'Neill, G.M.; Zhong, J.; Paul, A.; Kellie, S.J. Mesenchymal migration as a therapeutic target in glioblastoma. *J. Oncol.* **2010**, *2010*, 430142.
135. Vollmann-Zwerenz, A.; Leidgens, V.; Feliciello, G.; Klein, C.A.; Hau, P. Tumor Cell Invasion in Glioblastoma. *Int. J. Mol. Sci.* **2020**, *21*, 1932. [CrossRef]
136. Liu, P.; Griffiths, S.; Veljanoski, D.; Vaughn-Beaucaire, P.; Speirs, V.; Brüning-Richardson, A. Preclinical models of glioblastoma: Limitations of current models and the promise of new developments. *Expert Rev. Mol. Med.* **2021**, *23*, e20. [CrossRef]
137. Paolillo, M.; Comincini, S.; Schinelli, S. In vitro glioblastoma models: A journey into the third dimension. *Cancers* **2021**, *13*, 2449. [CrossRef]
138. Heffernan, J.M.; Overstreet, D.J.; Le, L.D.; Vernon, B.L.; Sirianni, R.W. Bioengineered scaffolds for 3D analysis of glioblastoma proliferation and invasion. *Ann. Biomed. Eng.* **2015**, *43*, 1965–1977. [CrossRef]
139. Cai, X.; Briggs, R.G.; Homburg, H.B.; Young, I.M.; Davis, E.J.; Lin, Y.-H.; Battiste, J.D.; Sughrue, M.E. Application of microfluidic devices for glioblastoma study: Current status and future directions. *Biomed. Microdevices* **2020**, *22*, 60. [CrossRef]
140. Hutter-Schmid, B.; Kniewallner, K.; Humpel, C. Organotypic brain slice cultures as a model to study angiogenesis of brain vessels. *Front. Cell Dev. Biol.* **2015**, *3*, 52. [CrossRef]
141. Haddad, A.F.; Young, J.S.; Amara, D.; Berger, M.S.; Raleigh, D.R.; Aghi, M.K.; Butowski, N.A. Mouse models of glioblastoma for the evaluation of novel therapeutic strategies. *Neuro-oncology Adv.* **2021**, *3*, vdab100. [CrossRef]
142. Rao, S.S.; Lannutti, J.J.; Viapiano, M.S.; Sarkar, A.; Winter, J.O. Toward 3D Biomimetic Models to Understand the Behavior of Glioblastoma Multiforme Cells. *Tissue Eng. Part B Rev.* **2014**, *20*, 314–327. [CrossRef]
143. Fernandes, J.T.S.; Chutna, O.; Chu, V.; Conde, J.P.; Outeiro, T.F. A Novel Microfluidic Cell Co-culture Platform for the Study of the Molecular Mechanisms of Parkinson's Disease and Other Synucleinopathies. *Front. Neurosci.* **2016**, *10*, 511. [CrossRef]
144. Ogawa, J.; Pao, G.M.; Shokhirev, M.N.; Verma, I.M. Glioblastoma Model Using Human Cerebral Organoids. *Cell Rep.* **2018**, *23*, 1220–1229. [CrossRef]
145. Holtkamp, N.; Afanasieva, A.; Elstner, A.; van Landeghem, F.K.H.; Könneker, M.; Kuhn, S.A.; Kettenmann, H.; Deimling, A. von Brain slice invasion model reveals genes differentially regulated in glioma invasion. *Biochem. Biophys. Res. Commun.* **2005**, *336*, 1227–1233. [CrossRef]
146. Kwiatkowska, A.; Nandhu, M.S.; Behera, P.; Chiocca, E.A.; Viapiano, M.S. Strategies in gene therapy for glioblastoma. *Cancers* **2013**, *5*, 1271–1305. [CrossRef]
147. Zanders, E.D.; Svensson, F.; Bailey, D.S. Therapy for glioblastoma: Is it working? *Drug Discov. Today* **2019**, *24*, 1193–1201. [CrossRef]
148. Yamamoto, M.; Curiel, D.T.T.; Ph, D.; South, S.; South, S. Cancer gene therapy. *Technol. Cancer Res. Treat.* **2005**, *4*, 315–330. [CrossRef]
149. Oka, N.; Soeda, A.; Inagaki, A.; Onodera, M.; Maruyama, H.; Hara, A.; Kunisada, T.; Mori, H.; Iwama, T. VEGF promotes tumorigenesis and angiogenesis of human glioblastoma stem cells. *Biochem. Biophys. Res. Commun.* **2007**, *360*, 553–559. [CrossRef]
150. Triozzi, P.L.; Borden, E.C. VB-111 for cancer. *Expert Opin. Biol. Ther.* **2011**, *11*, 1669–1676. [CrossRef]
151. Arend, R.C.; Beer, H.M.; Cohen, Y.C.; Berlin, S.; Birrer, M.J.; Campos, S.M.; Rachmilewitz Minei, T.; Harats, D.; Wall, J.A.; Foxall, M.E.; et al. Ofranergene obadenovec (VB-111) in platinum-resistant ovarian cancer; favorable response rates in a phase I/II study are associated with an immunotherapeutic effect. *Gynecol. Oncol.* **2020**, *157*, 578–584. [CrossRef] [PubMed]
152. Cloughesy, T.F.; Brenner, A.; De Groot, J.F.; Butowski, N.A.; Zach, L.; Campian, J.L.; Ellingson, B.M.; Freedman, L.S.; Cohen, Y.C.; Lowenton-Spier, N. A randomized controlled phase III study of VB-111 combined with bevacizumab vs bevacizumab monotherapy in patients with recurrent glioblastoma (GLOBE). *Neuro-Oncology* **2020**, *22*, 705–717. [CrossRef]
153. Friedman, H.S.; Prados, M.D.; Wen, P.Y.; Mikkelsen, T.; Schiff, D.; Abrey, L.E.; Yung, W.K.A.; Paleologos, N.; Nicholas, M.K.; Jensen, R. Bevacizumab alone and in combination with irinotecan in recurrent glioblastoma. *J. Clin. Oncol.* **2009**, *27*, 4733–4740. [CrossRef] [PubMed]
154. Jiang, G.; Wei, Z.-P.; Pei, D.-S.; Xin, Y.; Liu, Y.-Q.; Zheng, J.-N. A novel approach to overcome temozolomide resistance in glioma and melanoma: Inactivation of MGMT by gene therapy. *Biochem. Biophys. Res. Commun.* **2011**, *406*, 311–314. [CrossRef] [PubMed]

155. Przystal, J.M.; Waramit, S.; Pranjol, M.Z.I.; Yan, W.; Chu, G.; Chongchai, A.; Samarth, G.; Olaciregui, N.G.; Tabatabai, G.; Carcaboso, A.M. Efficacy of systemic temozolomide-activated phage-targeted gene therapy in human glioblastoma. *EMBO Mol. Med.* **2019**, *11*, e8492. [CrossRef] [PubMed]
156. Kim, S.M.; Woo, J.S.; Jeong, C.H.; Ryu, C.H.; Jang, J.-D.; Jeun, S.-S. Potential application of temozolomide in mesenchymal stem cell-based TRAIL gene therapy against malignant glioma. *Stem Cells Transl. Med.* **2014**, *3*, 172–182. [CrossRef] [PubMed]
157. Tang, X.; Peng, H.; Xu, P.; Zhang, L.; Fu, R.; Tu, H.; Guo, X.; Huang, K.; Lu, J.; Chen, H. Synthetic mRNA-based gene therapy for glioblastoma: TRAIL-mRNA synergistically enhances PTEN-mRNA-based therapy. *Mol. Ther.* **2022**, *24*, 707–718. [CrossRef]
158. Tang, X.; Zhang, S.; Fu, R.; Zhang, L.; Huang, K.; Peng, H.; Dai, L.; Chen, Q. Therapeutic prospects of mRNA-based gene therapy for glioblastoma. *Front. Oncol.* **2019**, *9*, 1208. [CrossRef]
159. Long, Y.; Tao, H.; Karachi, A.; Grippin, A.J.; Jin, L.; Chang, Y.E.; Zhang, W.; Dyson, K.A.; Hou, A.Y.; Na, M. Dysregulation of glutamate transport enhances treg function that promotes VEGF blockade resistance in glioblastoma. *Cancer Res.* **2020**, *80*, 499–509. [CrossRef]
160. Tian, R.-F.; Li, X.-F.; Xu, C.; Wu, H.; Liu, L.; Wang, L.-H.; He, D.; Cao, K.; Cao, P.-G.; Ma, J.K. SiRNA targeting PFK1 inhibits proliferation and migration and enhances radiosensitivity by suppressing glycolysis in colorectal cancer. *Am. J. Transl. Res.* **2020**, *12*, 4923.
161. Yang, B.; Hao, A.; Chen, L. Mirror siRNAs loading for dual delivery of doxorubicin and autophagy regulation siRNA for multidrug reversing chemotherapy. *Biomed. Pharmacother.* **2020**, *130*, 110490. [CrossRef]
162. Önay Uçar, E.; Şengelen, A. Resveratrol and siRNA in combination reduces Hsp27 expression and induces caspase-3 activity in human glioblastoma cells. *Cell Stress Chaperones* **2019**, *24*, 763–775. [CrossRef]
163. Zhang, C.; Yuan, W.; Wu, Y.; Wan, X.; Gong, Y. Co-delivery of EGFR and BRD4 siRNA by cell-penetrating peptides-modified redox-responsive complex in triple negative breast cancer cells. *Life Sci.* **2021**, *266*, 118886. [CrossRef]
164. Mirzaei, S.; Mahabady, M.K.; Zabolian, A.; Abbaspour, A.; Fallahzadeh, P.; Noori, M.; Hashemi, F.; Hushmandi, K.; Daneshi, S.; Kumar, A.P.; et al. Small interfering RNA (siRNA) to target genes and molecular pathways in glioblastoma therapy: Current status with an emphasis on delivery systems. *Life Sci.* **2021**, *275*, 119368. [CrossRef]
165. Huang, W.; Liang, Y.; Sang, C.; Mei, C.; Li, X.; Chen, T. Therapeutic nanosystems co-deliver anticancer drugs and oncogene SiRNA to achieve synergetic precise cancer chemo-gene therapy. *J. Mater. Chem. B* **2018**, *6*, 3013–3022. [CrossRef]
166. Danhier, F.; Messaoudi, K.; Lemaire, L.; Benoit, J.-P.; Lagarce, F. Combined anti-Galectin-1 and anti-EGFR siRNA-loaded chitosan-lipid nanocapsules decrease temozolomide resistance in glioblastoma: In vivo evaluation. *Int. J. Pharm.* **2015**, *481*, 154–161. [CrossRef]
167. Egorova, A.; Shubina, A.; Sokolov, D.; Selkov, S.; Baranov, V.; Kiselev, A. CXCR4-targeted modular peptide carriers for efficient anti-VEGF siRNA delivery. *Int. J. Pharm.* **2016**, *515*, 431–440. [CrossRef]
168. Liu, E.K.; Sulman, E.P.; Wen, P.Y.; Kurz, S.C. Novel Therapies for Glioblastoma. *Curr. Neurol. Neurosci. Rep.* **2020**, *20*, 19. [CrossRef]
169. Bagchi, S.; Yuan, R.; Engleman, E.G. Immune Checkpoint Inhibitors for the Treatment of Cancer: Clinical Impact and Mechanisms of Response and Resistance. *Annu. Rev. Pathol.* **2021**, *16*, 223–249. [CrossRef]
170. Maxwell, R.; Jackson, C.M.; Lim, M. Clinical Trials Investigating Immune Checkpoint Blockade in Glioblastoma. *Curr. Treat. Options Oncol.* **2017**, *18*, 51. [CrossRef]
171. Romani, M.; Pistillo, M.P.; Carosio, R.; Morabito, A.; Banelli, B. Immune Checkpoints and Innovative Therapies in Glioblastoma. *Front. Oncol.* **2018**, *8*, 464. [CrossRef] [PubMed]
172. Lukas, R.V.; Rodon, J.; Becker, K.; Wong, E.T.; Shih, K.; Touat, M.; Fassò, M.; Osborne, S.; Molinero, L.; O'Hear, C. Clinical activity and safety of atezolizumab in patients with recurrent glioblastoma. *J. Neuro-Oncol.* **2018**, *140*, 317–328. [CrossRef] [PubMed]
173. Gardell, J.L.; Matsumoto, L.R.; Chinn, H.; DeGolier, K.R.; Kreuser, S.A.; Prieskorn, B.; Balcaitis, S.; Davis, A.; Ellenbogen, R.G.; Crane, C.A. Human macrophages engineered to secrete a bispecific T cell engager support antigen-dependent T cell responses to glioblastoma. *J. Immunother. Cancer* **2020**, *8*, e001202. [CrossRef] [PubMed]
174. Newick, K.; O'Brien, S.; Moon, E.; Albelda, S.M. CAR T cell therapy for solid tumors. *Annu. Rev. Med.* **2017**, *68*, 139–152. [CrossRef]
175. O'Rourke, D.M.; Nasrallah, M.P.; Desai, A.; Melenhorst, J.J.; Mansfield, K.; Morrissette, J.J.D.; Martinez-Lage, M.; Brem, S.; Maloney, E.; Shen, A.; et al. A single dose of peripherally infused EGFRvIII-directed CAR T cells mediates antigen loss and induces adaptive resistance in patients with recurrent glioblastoma. *Sci. Transl. Med.* **2017**, *9*, eaaa0984. [CrossRef]
176. Polyzoidis, S.; Ashkan, K. DCVax®-L—Developed by northwest biotherapeutics. *Hum. Vaccin. Immunother.* **2014**, *10*, 3139–3145. [CrossRef]
177. Liau, L.M.; Ashkan, K.; Tran, D.D.; Campian, J.L.; Trusheim, J.E.; Cobbs, C.S.; Heth, J.A.; Salacz, M.; Taylor, S.; D'Andre, S.D. First results on survival from a large Phase 3 clinical trial of an autologous dendritic cell vaccine in newly diagnosed glioblastoma. *J. Transl. Med.* **2018**, *16*, 142.
178. Jain, K.K. A critical overview of targeted therapies for glioblastoma. *Front. Oncol.* **2018**, *8*, 419. [CrossRef]
179. Desjardins, A.; Gromeier, M.; Herndon, J.E., 2nd; Beaubier, N.; Bolognesi, D.P.; Friedman, A.H.; Friedman, H.S.; McSherry, F.; Muscat, A.M.; Nair, S.; et al. Recurrent Glioblastoma Treated with Recombinant Poliovirus. *N. Engl. J. Med.* **2018**, *379*, 150–161. [CrossRef]
180. Gopalan, D.; Pandey, A.; Udupa, N.; Mutalik, S. Receptor specific, stimuli responsive and subcellular targeted approaches for effective therapy of Alzheimer: Role of surface engineered nanocarriers. *J. Control Release* **2020**, *319*, 183–200. [CrossRef]
181. Angeli, E.; Nguyen, T.T.; Janin, A.; Bousquet, G. How to make anticancer drugs cross the blood–brain barrier to treat brain metastases. *Int. J. Mol. Sci.* **2019**, *21*, 22. [CrossRef]

182. Wang, C.; Li, K.; Li, T.; Chen, Z.; Wen, Y.; Liu, X.; Jia, X.; Zhang, Y.; Xu, Y.; Han, M.; et al. Monocyte-mediated chemotherapy drug delivery in glioblastoma. *Nanomedicine* **2017**, *13*, 157–178. [CrossRef]
183. Anselmo, A.C.; Mitragotri, S. Cell-mediated delivery of nanoparticles: Taking advantage of circulatory cells to target nanoparticles. *J. Control. Release* **2014**, *190*, 531–541. [CrossRef]
184. Su, Y.; Xie, Z.; Kim, G.B.; Dong, C.; Yang, J. Design strategies and applications of circulating cell-mediated drug delivery systems. *ACS Biomater. Sci. Eng.* **2015**, *1*, 201–217. [CrossRef]
185. Ehtesham, M.; Kabos, P.; Gutierrez, M.A.R.; Chung, N.H.C.; Griffith, T.S.; Black, K.L.; Yu, J.S. Induction of Glioblastoma Apoptosis Using Neural Stem Cell-mediated Delivery of Tumor Necrosis Factor-related Apoptosis-inducing Ligand1. *Cancer Res.* **2002**, *62*, 7170–7174.
186. Pang, L.; Qin, J.; Han, L.; Zhao, W.; Liang, J.; Xie, Z.; Yang, P.; Wang, J. Exploiting macrophages as targeted carrier to guide nanoparticles into glioma. *Oncotarget* **2016**, *7*, 37081–37091. [CrossRef]
187. Liao, W.; Fan, S.; Zheng, Y.; Liao, S.; Xiong, Y.; Li, Y.; Liu, J. Recent advances on glioblastoma multiforme and nano-drug carriers: A review. *Curr. Med. Chem.* **2019**, *26*, 5862–5874. [CrossRef]
188. Reis, C.P.; Neufeld, R.J.; Ribeiro, A.J.; Veiga, F. Nanoencapsulation I. Methods for preparation of drug-loaded polymeric nanoparticles. *Nanomed. Nanotechnol. Biol. Med.* **2006**, *2*, 8–21. [CrossRef]
189. Frellsen, A.F.; Hansen, A.E.; Jølck, R.I.; Kempen, P.J.; Severin, G.W.; Rasmussen, P.H.; Kjær, A.; Jensen, A.T.I.; Andresen, T.L. Mouse Positron Emission Tomography Study of the Biodistribution of Gold Nanoparticles with Different Surface Coatings Using Embedded Copper-64. *ACS Nano* **2016**, *10*, 9887–9898. [CrossRef]
190. Malikmammadov, E.; Tanir, T.E.; Kiziltay, A.; Hasirci, V.; Hasirci, N. PCL and PCL-based materials in biomedical applications. *J. Biomater. Sci. Polym. Ed.* **2018**, *29*, 863–893. [CrossRef]
191. Bregoli, L.; Movia, D.; Gavigan-Imedio, J.D.; Lysaght, J.; Reynolds, J.; Prina-Mello, A. Nanomedicine applied to translational oncology: A future perspective on cancer treatment. *Nanomed. Nanotechnol. Biol. Med.* **2016**, *12*, 81–103. [CrossRef]
192. Rejman, J.; Oberle, V.; Zuhorn, I.S.; Hoekstra, D. Size-dependent internalization of particles via the pathways of clathrin- and caveolae-mediated endocytosis. *Biochem. J.* **2004**, *377*, 159–169. [CrossRef] [PubMed]
193. Shu, X.Z.; Zhu, K.J. A novel approach to prepare tripolyphosphate/chitosan complex beads for controlled release drug delivery. *Int. J. Pharm.* **2000**, *201*, 51–58. [CrossRef]
194. Jo, D.H.; Kim, J.H.J.H.; Lee, T.G.; Kim, J.H.J.H. Size, surface charge, and shape determine therapeutic effects of nanoparticles on brain and retinal diseases. *Nanomed. Nanotechnol. Biol. Med.* **2015**, *11*, 1603–1611. [CrossRef] [PubMed]
195. Truong, N.P.; Whittaker, M.R.; Mak, C.W.; Davis, T.P. The importance of nanoparticle shape in cancer drug delivery. *Expert Opin. Drug Deliv.* **2015**, *12*, 129–142. [CrossRef] [PubMed]
196. Hsu, J.-F.; Chu, S.-M.; Liao, C.-C.; Wang, C.-J.; Wang, Y.-S.; Lai, M.-Y.; Wang, H.-C.; Huang, H.-R.; Tsai, M.-H. Nanotechnology and nanocarrier-based drug delivery as the potential therapeutic strategy for glioblastoma multiforme: An update. *Cancers* **2021**, *13*, 195. [CrossRef] [PubMed]
197. Paroha, S.; Chandel, A.K.S.; Dubey, R.D. Nanosystems for drug delivery of coenzyme Q10. *Environ. Chem. Lett.* **2018**, *16*, 71–77. [CrossRef]
198. Paroha, S.; Chandel, A.K.S.; Dubey, R.D. Nanotechnology delivery systems of coenzyme Q10: Pharmacokinetic and clinical implications. In *Nanoscience in Food and Agriculture 4*; Springer: Cham, Switzerland, 2017; pp. 213–228.
199. Glaser, T.; Han, I.; Wu, L.; Zeng, X. Targeted nanotechnology in glioblastoma multiforme. *Front. Pharmacol.* **2017**, *8*, 166. [CrossRef]
200. Hosseini, M.; Haji-Fatahaliha, M.; Jadidi-Niaragh, F.; Majidi, J.; Yousefi, M. The use of nanoparticles as a promising therapeutic approach in cancer immunotherapy. *Artif. Cells Nanomed. Biotechnol.* **2016**, *44*, 1051–1061. [CrossRef]
201. Gonçalves, C.; Ramalho, M.J.; Silva, R.; Silva, V.; Marques-Oliveira, R.; Silva, A.C.; Pereira, M.C.; Loureiro, J.A. Lipid Nanoparticles Containing Mixtures of Antioxidants to Improve Skin Care and Cancer Prevention. *Pharmaceutics* **2021**, *13*, 2042. [CrossRef]
202. Patidar, A.; Thakur, D.S.; Kumar, P.; Verma, J. A review on novel lipid based nanocarriers. *Int. J. Pharm. Pharm. Sci.* **2010**, *2*, 30–35.
203. Jnaidi, R.; Almeida, A.J.; Gonçalves, L.M. Solid Lipid Nanoparticles and Nanostructured Lipid Carriers as Smart Drug Delivery Systems in the Treatment of Glioblastoma Multiforme. *Pharmaceutics* **2020**, *12*, 860. [CrossRef]
204. Shevtsov, M.A.; Nikolaev, B.P.; Yakovleva, L.Y.; Marchenko, Y.Y.; Dobrodumov, A.V.; Mikhrina, A.L.; Martynova, M.G.; Bystrova, O.A.; Yakovenko, I.V.; Ischenko, A.M. Superparamagnetic iron oxide nanoparticles conjugated with epidermal growth factor (SPION-EGF) for targeting brain tumors. *Int. J. Nanomedicine* **2014**, *9*, 273–287. [CrossRef]
205. Shi, Y. Self-Assembled Gold Nanoplexes for Cancer-Targeted SiRNA Delivery. Master's Thesis, University of Southern Mississippi, Hattiesburg, MS, USA, 2014. Available online: https://aquila.usm.edu/cgi/viewcontent.cgi?article=1052&context=masters_theses (accessed on 30 April 2022).
206. Guglielmelli, A.; Rosa, P.; Contardi, M.; Prato, M.; Mangino, G.; Miglietta, S.; Petrozza, V.; Pani, R.; Calogero, A.; Athanassiou, A. Biomimetic keratin gold nanoparticle-mediated in vitro photothermal therapy on glioblastoma multiforme. *Nanomedicine* **2020**, *16*, 121–138. [CrossRef]
207. Liu, D.; Cheng, Y.; Cai, R.; Wang, W.; Cui, H.; Liu, M.; Mei, Q.; Zhou, S. The enhancement of siPLK1 penetration across BBB and its anti glioblastoma activity in vivo by magnet and transferrin co-modified nanoparticle. *Nanomed. Nanotechnol. Biol. Med.* **2018**, *14*, 991–1003. [CrossRef] [PubMed]
208. Zhu, X.; Zhou, H.; Liu, Y.; Wen, Y.; Wei, C.; Yu, Q.; Liu, J. Transferrin/aptamer conjugated mesoporous ruthenium nanosystem for redox-controlled and targeted chemo-photodynamic therapy of glioma. *Acta Biomater.* **2018**, *82*, 143–157. [CrossRef]

209. Taghipour-Sabzevar, V.; Sharifi, T.; Moghaddam, M.M. Polymeric nanoparticles as carrier for targeted and controlled delivery of anticancer agents. *Ther. Deliv.* **2019**, *10*, 527–550. [CrossRef]
210. Shi, J.; Xiao, Z.; Kamaly, N.; Farokhzad, O.C. Self-assembled targeted nanoparticles: Evolution of technologies and bench to bedside translation. *Acc. Chem. Res.* **2011**, *44*, 1123–1134. [CrossRef]
211. Chenthamara, D.; Subramaniam, S.; Ramakrishnan, S.G.; Krishnaswamy, S.; Essa, M.M.; Lin, F.-H.; Qoronfleh, M.W. Therapeutic efficacy of nanoparticles and routes of administration. *Biomater. Res.* **2019**, *23*, 1–29. [CrossRef]
212. Owens, D.E., III; Peppas, N.A. Opsonization, biodistribution, and pharmacokinetics of polymeric nanoparticles. *Int. J. Pharm.* **2006**, *307*, 93–102. [CrossRef]
213. Haji Mansor, M.; Najberg, M.; Contini, A.; Alvarez-Lorenzo, C.; Garcion, E.; Jérôme, C.; Boury, F. Development of a non-toxic and non-denaturing formulation process for encapsulation of SDF-1α into PLGA/PEG-PLGA nanoparticles to achieve sustained release. *Eur. J. Pharm. Biopharm.* **2018**, *125*, 38–50. [CrossRef] [PubMed]
214. Pourgholi, F.; Hajivalili, M.; Farhad, J.-N.; Kafil, H.S.; Yousefi, M. Nanoparticles: Novel vehicles in treatment of Glioblastoma. *Biomed. Pharmacother.* **2016**, *77*, 98–107. [CrossRef] [PubMed]
215. Couvreur, P.; Vauthier, C. Nanotechnology: Intelligent design to treat complex disease. *Pharm. Res.* **2006**, *23*, 1417–1450. [CrossRef]
216. Rescignano, N.; Fortunati, E.; Armentano, I.; Hernandez, R.; Mijangos, C.; Pasquino, R.; Kenny, J.M. Use of alginate, chitosan and cellulose nanocrystals as emulsion stabilizers in the synthesis of biodegradable polymeric nanoparticles. *J. Colloid Interface Sci.* **2015**, *445*, 31–39. [CrossRef]
217. Allouss, D.; Makhado, E.; Zahouily, M. Recent Progress in Polysaccharide-Based Hydrogel Beads as Adsorbent for Water Pollution Remediation. *Funct. Polym. Nanocomposites Wastewater Treat.* **2022**, *323*, 55–88.
218. He, W.; Hosseinkhani, H.; Mohammadinejad, R.; Roveimiab, Z.; Hueng, D.; Ou, K.; Domb, A.J. Polymeric nanoparticles for therapy and imaging. *Polym. Adv. Technol.* **2014**, *25*, 1216–1225. [CrossRef]
219. Elzoghby, A.O.; Abd-Elwakil, M.M.; Abd-Elsalam, K.; Elsayed, M.T.; Hashem, Y.; Mohamed, O. Natural polymeric nanoparticles for brain-targeting: Implications on drug and gene delivery. *Curr. Pharm. Des.* **2016**, *22*, 3305–3323. [CrossRef]
220. Morshed, R.; Cheng, Y.; Auffinger, B.; Wegscheid, M.; Lesniak, M.S. The potential of polymeric micelles in the context of glioblastoma therapy. *Front. Pharmacol.* **2013**, *4*, 157. [CrossRef]
221. Nishiyama, N.; Matsumura, Y.; Kataoka, K. Development of polymeric micelles for targeting intractable cancers. *Cancer Sci.* **2016**, *107*, 867–874. [CrossRef]
222. Saxena, V.; Hussain, M.D. Formulation and in vitro evaluation of 17-allyamino-17-demethoxygeldanamycin (17-AAG) loaded polymeric mixed micelles for glioblastoma multiforme. *Colloids Surf. B Biointerfaces* **2013**, *112*, 350–355. [CrossRef]
223. Fu, Z.; Xiang, J. Aptamer-functionalized nanoparticles in targeted delivery and cancer therapy. *Int. J. Mol. Sci.* **2020**, *21*, 9123. [CrossRef] [PubMed]
224. Stenström, P.; Manzanares, D.; Zhang, Y.; Ceña, V.; Malkoch, M. Evaluation of amino-functional polyester dendrimers based on Bis-MPA as nonviral vectors for siRNA delivery. *Molecules* **2018**, *23*, 2028. [CrossRef] [PubMed]
225. Torchilin, V.P. Nanocarriers. *Pharm. Res.* **2007**, *24*, 2333–2334. [CrossRef] [PubMed]
226. Zhang, Y.; Qu, H.; Xue, X. Blood–brain barrier penetrating liposomes with synergistic chemotherapy for glioblastoma treatment. *Biomater. Sci.* **2022**, *10*, 423–434. [CrossRef]
227. Papachristodoulou, A.; Signorell, R.D.; Werner, B.; Brambilla, D.; Luciani, P.; Cavusoglu, M.; Grandjean, J.; Silginer, M.; Rudin, M.; Martin, E.; et al. Chemotherapy sensitization of glioblastoma by focused ultrasound-mediated delivery of therapeutic liposomes. *J. Control. Release* **2019**, *295*, 130–139. [CrossRef]
228. Jhaveri, A.; Deshpande, P.; Pattni, B.; Torchilin, V. Transferrin-targeted, resveratrol-loaded liposomes for the treatment of glioblastoma. *J. Control. Release* **2018**, *277*, 89–101. [CrossRef]
229. Shirazi, A.S.; Varshochian, R.; Rezaei, M.; Ardakani, Y.H.; Dinarvand, R. SN38 loaded nanostructured lipid carriers (NLCs); preparation and in vitro evaluations against glioblastoma. *J. Mater. Sci. Mater. Med.* **2021**, *32*, 78. [CrossRef]
230. Paraiso, W.K.D.; Garcia-Chica, J.; Ariza, X.; Zagmutt, S.; Fukushima, S.; Garcia, J.; Mochida, Y.; Serra, D.; Herrero, L.; Kinoh, H. Poly-ion complex micelles effectively deliver CoA-conjugated CPT1A inhibitors to modulate lipid metabolism in brain cells. *Biomater. Sci.* **2021**, *9*, 7076–7091. [CrossRef]
231. Song, S.; Mao, G.; Du, J.; Zhu, X. Novel RGD containing, temozolomide-loading nanostructured lipid carriers for glioblastoma multiforme chemotherapy. *Drug Deliv.* **2016**, *23*, 1404–1408. [CrossRef]
232. Zwain, T.; Alder, J.E.; Sabagh, B.; Shaw, A.; Burrow, A.J.; Singh, K.K. Tailoring functional nanostructured lipid carriers for glioblastoma treatment with enhanced permeability through in-vitro 3D BBB/BBTB models. *Mater. Sci. Eng. C* **2021**, *121*, 111774. [CrossRef]
233. Kuo, Y.-C.; Liang, C.-T. Inhibition of human brain malignant glioblastoma cells using carmustine-loaded catanionic solid lipid nanoparticles with surface anti-epithelial growth factor receptor. *Biomaterials* **2011**, *32*, 3340–3350. [CrossRef]
234. Sun, Y.; Wang, Y.; Liu, Y.; Zou, Y.; Zheng, M.; Shi, B. Recent advances in polymeric nanomedicines for glioblastoma therapy. *Sci. Sin. Vitae* **2021**, *51*, 819–835. [CrossRef]
235. Han, H.; Zhang, Y.; Jin, S.; Chen, P.; Liu, X.; Xie, Z.; Jing, X.; Wang, Z. Paclitaxel-loaded dextran nanoparticles decorated with RVG29 peptide for targeted chemotherapy of glioma: An in vivo study. *New J. Chem.* **2020**, *44*, 5692–5701. [CrossRef]
236. Esfandiarpour-Boroujeni, S.; Bagheri-Khoulenjani, S.; Mirzadeh, H.; Amanpour, S. Fabrication and study of curcumin loaded nanoparticles based on folate-chitosan for breast cancer therapy application. *Carbohydr. Polym.* **2017**, *168*, 14–21. [CrossRef]

237. Sekar, V.; Rajendran, K.; Vallinayagam, S.; Deepak, V.; Mahadevan, S. Synthesis and characterization of chitosan ascorbate nanoparticles for therapeutic inhibition for cervical cancer and their in silico modeling. *J. Ind. Eng. Chem.* **2018**, *62*, 239–249. [CrossRef]
238. Yin, T.; Bader, A.R.; Hou, T.K.; Maron, B.A.; Kao, D.D.; Qian, R.; Kohane, D.S.; Handy, D.E.; Loscalzo, J.; Zhang, Y.-Y. SDF-1α in glycan nanoparticles exhibits full activity and reduces pulmonary hypertension in rats. *Biomacromolecules* **2013**, *14*, 4009–4020. [CrossRef]
239. Saulnier, P.; Benoit, J. Active targeting of brain tumors using nanocarriers. *Biomaterials* **2007**, *28*, 4947–4967.
240. Geldenhuys, W.; Wehrung, D.; Groshev, A.; Hirani, A.; Sutariya, V. Brain-targeted delivery of doxorubicin using glutathione-coated nanoparticles for brain cancers. *Pharm. Dev. Technol.* **2015**, *20*, 497–506. [CrossRef]
241. Ramalho, M.J.; Sevin, E.; Gosselet, F.; Lima, J.; Coelho, M.A.N.; Loureiro, J.A.; Pereira, M.C. Receptor-mediated PLGA nanoparticles for glioblastoma multiforme treatment. *Int. J. Pharm.* **2018**, *545*, 84–92. [CrossRef]
242. Caban-Toktas, S.; Sahin, A.; Lule, S.; Esendagli, G.; Vural, I.; Oguz, K.K.; Soylemezoglu, F.; Mut, M.; Dalkara, T.; Khan, M. Combination of Paclitaxel and R-flurbiprofen loaded PLGA nanoparticles suppresses glioblastoma growth on systemic administration. *Int. J. Pharm.* **2020**, *578*, 119076. [CrossRef]
243. Gascon, S.; Solano, A.G.; El Kheir, W.; Therriault, H.; Berthelin, P.; Cattier, B.; Marcos, B.; Virgilio, N.; Paquette, B.; Faucheux, N.; et al. Characterization and mathematical modeling of alginate/chitosan-based nanoparticles releasing the chemokine cxcl12 to attract glioblastoma cells. *Pharmaceutics* **2020**, *12*, 356. [CrossRef] [PubMed]
244. Alghamri, M.S.; Banerjee, K.; Mujeeb, A.A.; Mauser, A.; Taher, A.; Thalla, R.; McClellan, B.L.; Varela, M.L.; Stamatovic, S.M.; Martinez-Revollar, G.; et al. Systemic Delivery of an Adjuvant CXCR4-CXCL12 Signaling Inhibitor Encapsulated in Synthetic Protein Nanoparticles for Glioma Immunotherapy. *ACS Nano* **2022**. [CrossRef] [PubMed]
245. Malinovskaya, Y.; Melnikov, P.; Baklaushev, V.; Gabashvili, A.; Osipova, N.; Mantrov, S.; Ermolenko, Y.; Maksimenko, O.; Gorshkova, M.; Balabanyan, V. Delivery of doxorubicin-loaded PLGA nanoparticles into U87 human glioblastoma cells. *Int. J. Pharm.* **2017**, *524*, 77–90. [CrossRef] [PubMed]
246. Hao, Y.; Wang, L.; Zhao, Y.; Meng, D.; Li, D.; Li, H.; Zhang, B.; Shi, J.; Zhang, H.; Zhang, Z. Targeted imaging and chemo-phototherapy of brain cancer by a multifunctional drug delivery system. *Macromol. Biosci.* **2015**, *15*, 1571–1585. [CrossRef]
247. Xu, H.-L.; ZhuGe, D.-L.; Chen, P.-P.; Tong, M.-Q.; Lin, M.-T.; Jiang, X.; Zheng, Y.-W.; Chen, B.; Li, X.-K.; Zhao, Y.-Z. Silk fibroin nanoparticles dyeing indocyanine green for imaging-guided photo-thermal therapy of glioblastoma. *Drug Deliv.* **2018**, *25*, 364–375. [CrossRef]
248. Bastiancich, C.; Bozzato, E.; Henley, I.; Newland, B. Does local drug delivery still hold therapeutic promise for brain cancer? A systematic review. *J. Control. Release* **2021**, *337*, 296–305. [CrossRef]
249. Bregy, A.; Shah, A.H.; Diaz, M.V.; Pierce, H.E.; Ames, P.L.; Diaz, D.; Komotar, R.J. The role of Gliadel wafers in the treatment of high-grade gliomas. *Expert Rev. Anticancer Ther.* **2013**, *13*, 1453–1461. [CrossRef]
250. Alghamdi, M.; Gumbleton, M.; Newland, B. Local delivery to malignant brain tumors: Potential biomaterial-based therapeutic/adjuvant strategies. *Biomater. Sci.* **2021**, *9*, 6037–6051. [CrossRef]
251. Bruinsmann, F.A.; Richter Vaz, G.; de Cristo Soares Alves, A.; Aguirre, T.; Raffin Pohlmann, A.; Stanisçuaski Guterres, S.; Sonvico, F. Nasal Drug Delivery of Anticancer Drugs for the Treatment of Glioblastoma: Preclinical and Clinical Trials. *Molecules* **2019**, *24*, 4312. [CrossRef]
252. Blacher, E.; Ben Baruch, B.; Levy, A.; Geva, N.; Green, K.D.; Garneau-Tsodikova, S.; Fridman, M.; Stein, R. Inhibition of glioma progression by a newly discovered CD38 inhibitor. *Int. J. Cancer* **2015**, *136*, 1422–1433. [CrossRef]
253. Levy, A.; Blacher, E.; Vaknine, H.; Lund, F.E.; Stein, R.; Mayo, L. CD38 deficiency in the tumor microenvironment attenuates glioma progression and modulates features of tumor-associated microglia/macrophages. *Neuro-Oncology* **2012**, *14*, 1037–1049. [CrossRef]
254. Mayo, L.; Jacob-Hirsch, J.; Amariglio, N.; Rechavi, G.; Moutin, M.-J.; Lund, F.E.; Stein, R. Dual role of CD38 in microglial activation and activation-induced cell death. *J. Immunol.* **2008**, *181*, 92–103. [CrossRef]
255. Li, Y.; Gao, Y.; Liu, G.; Zhou, X.; Wang, Y.; Ma, L. Intranasal administration of temozolomide for brain-targeting delivery: Therapeutic effect on glioma in rats. *J. South. Med. Univ.* **2014**, *34*, 631–635.
256. Ferreira, N.N.; Granja, S.; Boni, F.I.; Prezotti, F.G.; Ferreira, L.M.B.; Cury, B.S.F.; Reis, R.M.; Baltazar, F.; Gremião, M.P.D. Modulating chitosan-PLGA nanoparticle properties to design a co-delivery platform for glioblastoma therapy intended for nose-to-brain route. *Drug Deliv. Transl. Res.* **2020**, *10*, 1729–1747. [CrossRef]
257. Alex, A.T.; Joseph, A.; Shavi, G.; Rao, J.V.; Udupa, N. Development and evaluation of carboplatin-loaded PCL nanoparticles for intranasal delivery. *Drug Deliv.* **2016**, *23*, 2144–2153. [CrossRef]
258. de Oliveira Junior, E.R.; Nascimento, T.L.; Salomão, M.A.; da Silva, A.C.G.; Valadares, M.C.; Lima, E.M. Increased nose-to-brain delivery of melatonin mediated by polycaprolactone nanoparticles for the treatment of glioblastoma. *Pharm. Res.* **2019**, *36*, 131. [CrossRef]
259. Madane, R.G.; Mahajan, H.S. Curcumin-loaded nanostructured lipid carriers (NLCs) for nasal administration: Design, characterization, and in vivo study. *Drug Deliv.* **2016**, *23*, 1326–1334. [CrossRef]
260. Ferreira, N.N.; de Oliveira Junior, E.; Granja, S.; Boni, F.I.; Ferreira, L.M.B.; Cury, B.S.F.; Santos, L.C.R.; Reis, R.M.; Lima, E.M.; Baltazar, F.; et al. Nose-to-brain co-delivery of drugs for glioblastoma treatment using nanostructured system. *Int. J. Pharm.* **2021**, *603*, 120714. [CrossRef]

261. Sousa, F.; Dhaliwal, H.K.; Gattacceca, F.; Sarmento, B.; Amiji, M.M. Enhanced anti-angiogenic effects of bevacizumab in glioblastoma treatment upon intranasal administration in polymeric nanoparticles. *J. Control. Release* **2019**, *309*, 37–47. [CrossRef]
262. D'Amico, R.S.; Aghi, M.K.; Vogelbaum, M.A.; Bruce, J.N. Convection-enhanced drug delivery for glioblastoma: A review. *J. Neuro-Oncol.* **2021**, *151*, 415–427. [CrossRef]
263. Ung, T.H.; Malone, H.; Canoll, P.; Bruce, J.N. Convection-enhanced delivery for glioblastoma: Targeted delivery of antitumor therapeutics. *CNS Oncol.* **2015**, *4*, 225–234. [CrossRef] [PubMed]
264. Chakroun, R.W.; Zhang, P.; Lin, R.; Schiapparelli, P.; Quinones-Hinojosa, A.; Cui, H. Nanotherapeutic systems for local treatment of brain tumors. *Wiley Interdiscip. Rev. Nanomed. Nanobiotechnol.* **2018**, *10*, e1479. [CrossRef] [PubMed]
265. Debinski, W.; Tatter, S.B. Convection-enhanced delivery for the treatment of brain tumors. *Expert Rev. Neurother.* **2009**, *9*, 1519–1527. [CrossRef] [PubMed]
266. Bobo, R.H.; Laske, D.W.; Akbasak, A.; Morrison, P.F.; Dedrick, R.L.; Oldfield, E.H. Convection-enhanced delivery of macromolecules in the brain. *Proc. Natl. Acad. Sci. USA* **1994**, *91*, 2076–2080. [CrossRef]
267. Lidar, Z.; Mardor, Y.; Jonas, T.; Pfeffer, R.; Faibel, M.; Nass, D.; Hadani, M.; Ram, Z. Convection-enhanced delivery of paclitaxel for the treatment of recurrent malignant glioma: A Phase I/II clinical study. *J. Neurosurg.* **2004**, *100*, 472–479. [CrossRef]
268. Séhédic, D.; Chourpa, I.; Tétaud, C.; Griveau, A.; Loussouarn, C.; Avril, S.; Legendre, C.; Lepareur, N.; Wion, D.; Hindré, F.; et al. Locoregional Confinement and Major Clinical Benefit of (188)Re-Loaded CXCR4-Targeted Nanocarriers in an Orthotopic Human to Mouse Model of Glioblastoma. *Theranostics* **2017**, *7*, 4517–4536. [CrossRef]
269. Zhang, C.; Nance, E.A.; Mastorakos, P.; Chisholm, J.; Berry, S.; Eberhart, C.; Tyler, B.; Brem, H.; Suk, J.S.; Hanes, J. Convection enhanced delivery of cisplatin-loaded brain penetrating nanoparticles cures malignant glioma in rats. *J. Control. Release* **2017**, *263*, 112–119. [CrossRef]
270. Stephen, Z.R.; Kievit, F.M.; Veiseh, O.; Chiarelli, P.A.; Fang, C.; Wang, K.; Hatzinger, S.J.; Ellenbogen, R.G.; Silber, J.R.; Zhang, M. Redox-responsive magnetic nanoparticle for targeted convection-enhanced delivery of O 6-benzylguanine to brain tumors. *ACS Nano* **2014**, *8*, 10383–10395. [CrossRef]
271. Chen, P.-Y.; Ozawa, T.; Drummond, D.C.; Kalra, A.; Fitzgerald, J.B.; Kirpotin, D.B.; Wei, K.-C.; Butowski, N.; Prados, M.D.; Berger, M.S.; et al. Comparing routes of delivery for nanoliposomal irinotecan shows superior anti-tumor activity of local administration in treating intracranial glioblastoma xenografts. *Neuro-Oncology* **2013**, *15*, 189–197. [CrossRef]
272. Cruickshank, G.; Fayeye, O.; Ngoga, D.; Connor, J.; Detta, A. ATNT-05: Intraoperative Intraparenchymal Injection of Irinotecan Drug Loaded Beads in Patients with Recurrent Glioblastoma (Gbm): A Safe New Depot Approach for Loco-Regional Therapy (NCT02433392). *Neuro-Oncology* **2015**, *17*, v11. [CrossRef]
273. Kim, D.G.; Kim, K.H.; Seo, Y.J.; Yang, H.; Marcusson, E.G.; Son, E.; Lee, K.; Sa, J.K.; Lee, H.W.; Nam, D.-H. Anti-miR delivery strategies to bypass the blood-brain barrier in glioblastoma therapy. *Oncotarget* **2016**, *7*, 29400. [CrossRef]
274. Wait, S.D.; Prabhu, R.S.; Burri, S.H.; Atkins, T.G.; Asher, A.L. Polymeric drug delivery for the treatment of glioblastoma. *Neuro-Oncology* **2015**, *17*, ii9–ii23. [CrossRef]
275. Valtonen, S.; Timonen, U.I.; Toivanen, P.; Kalimo, H.; Kivipelto, L.; Heiskanen, O.; Unsgaard, G.; Kuurne, T. Interstitial chemotherapy with carmustine-loaded polymers for high-grade gliomas: A randomized double-blind study. *Neurosurgery* **1997**, *41*, 44–49. [CrossRef]
276. Walter, K.A.; Cahan, M.A.; Gur, A.; Tyler, B.; Hilton, J.; Colvin, O.M.; Burger, P.C.; Domb, A.; Brem, H. Interstitial taxol delivered from a biodegradable polymer implant against experimental malignant glioma. *Cancer Res.* **1994**, *54*, 2207–2212.
277. Mangraviti, A.; Raghavan, T.; Volpin, F.; Skuli, N.; Gullotti, D.; Zhou, J.; Asnaghi, L.; Sankey, E.; Liu, A.; Wang, Y. HIF-1α-targeting acriflavine provides long term survival and radiological tumor response in brain cancer therapy. *Sci. Rep.* **2017**, *7*, 14978.
278. Lesniak, M.S.; Upadhyay, U.; Goodwin, R.; Tyler, B.; Brem, H. Local delivery of doxorubicin for the treatment of malignant brain tumors in rats. *Anticancer Res.* **2005**, *25*, 3825–3831.
279. Ranganath, S.H.; Fu, Y.; Arifin, D.Y.; Kee, I.; Zheng, L.; Lee, H.-S.; Chow, P.K.-H.; Wang, C.-H. The use of submicron/nanoscale PLGA implants to deliver paclitaxel with enhanced pharmacokinetics and therapeutic efficacy in intracranial glioblastoma in mice. *Biomaterials* **2010**, *31*, 5199–5207. [CrossRef]
280. Ranganath, S.H.; Wang, C.-H. Biodegradable microfiber implants delivering paclitaxel for post-surgical chemotherapy against malignant glioma. *Biomaterials* **2008**, *29*, 2996–3003. [CrossRef]
281. Shapira-Furman, T.; Serra, R.; Gorelick, N.; Doglioli, M.; Tagliaferri, V.; Cecia, A.; Peters, M.; Kumar, A.; Rottenberg, Y.; Langer, R. Biodegradable wafers releasing Temozolomide and Carmustine for the treatment of brain cancer. *J. Control. Release* **2019**, *295*, 93–101. [CrossRef]
282. Zhang, Y.S.; Khademhosseini, A. Advances in engineering hydrogels. *Science* **2017**, *356*, eaaf3627. [CrossRef]
283. Hoffman, A.S. Hydrogels for biomedical applications. *Adv. Drug Deliv. Rev.* **2012**, *64*, 18–23. [CrossRef]
284. Peppas, N.A.; Hilt, J.Z.; Khademhosseini, A.; Langer, R. Hydrogels in biology and medicine: From molecular principles to bionanotechnology. *Adv. Mater.* **2006**, *18*, 1345–1360. [CrossRef]
285. Peppas, N.A.; Bures, P.; Leobandung, W.S.; Ichikawa, H. Hydrogels in pharmaceutical formulations. *Eur. J. Pharm. Biopharm.* **2000**, *50*, 27–46. [CrossRef]
286. Wang, C.; Tong, X.; Yang, F. Bioengineered 3D brain tumor model to elucidate the effects of matrix stiffness on glioblastoma cell behavior using PEG-based hydrogels. *Mol. Pharm.* **2014**, *11*, 2115–2125. [CrossRef]

287. Hosseinzadeh, R.; Mirani, B.; Pagan, E.; Mirzaaghaei, S.; Nasimian, A.; Kawalec, P.; da Silva Rosa, S.C.; Hamdi, D.; Fernandez, N.P.; Toyota, B.D. A drug-eluting 3D-printed mesh (GlioMesh) for management of glioblastoma. *Adv. Ther.* **2019**, *2*, 1900113. [CrossRef]
288. Schiapparelli, P.; Zhang, P.; Lara-Velazquez, M.; Guerrero-Cazares, H.; Lin, R.; Su, H.; Chakroun, R.W.; Tusa, M.; Quiñones-Hinojosa, A.; Cui, H. Self-assembling and self-formulating prodrug hydrogelator extends survival in a glioblastoma resection and recurrence model. *J. Control. Release* **2020**, *319*, 311–321. [CrossRef]
289. Turabee, M.H.; Jeong, T.H.; Ramalingam, P.; Kang, J.H.; Ko, Y.T. N, N, N-trimethyl chitosan embedded in situ Pluronic F127 hydrogel for the treatment of brain tumor. *Carbohydr. Polym.* **2019**, *203*, 302–309. [CrossRef] [PubMed]
290. Bastiancich, C.; Danhier, P.; Préat, V.; Danhier, F. Anticancer drug-loaded hydrogels as drug delivery systems for the local treatment of glioblastoma. *J. Control. Release* **2016**, *243*, 29–42. [CrossRef]
291. Akbar, U.; Jones, T.; Winestone, J.; Michael, M.; Shukla, A.; Sun, Y.; Duntsch, C. Delivery of temozolomide to the tumor bed via biodegradable gel matrices in a novel model of intracranial glioma with resection. *J. Neuro-Oncol.* **2009**, *94*, 203–212. [CrossRef] [PubMed]
292. Bouché, M.; Dong, Y.C.; Sheikh, S.; Taing, K.; Saxena, D.; Hsu, J.C.; Chen, M.H.; Salinas, R.D.; Song, H.; Burdick, J.A.; et al. Novel Treatment for Glioblastoma Delivered by a Radiation Responsive and Radiopaque Hydrogel. *ACS Biomater. Sci. Eng.* **2021**, *7*, 3209–3220. [CrossRef] [PubMed]
293. Vellimana, A.K.; Recinos, V.R.; Hwang, L.; Fowers, K.D.; Li, K.W.; Zhang, Y.; Okonma, S.; Eberhart, C.G.; Brem, H.; Tyler, B.M. Combination of paclitaxel thermal gel depot with temozolomide and radiotherapy significantly prolongs survival in an experimental rodent glioma model. *J. Neuro-Oncol.* **2013**, *111*, 229–236. [CrossRef]
294. Zentner, G.M.; Rathi, R.; Shih, C.; McRea, J.C.; Seo, M.-H.; Oh, H.; Rhee, B.G.; Mestecky, J.; Moldoveanu, Z.; Morgan, M. Biodegradable block copolymers for delivery of proteins and water-insoluble drugs. *J. Control. Release* **2001**, *72*, 203–215. [CrossRef]
295. Déry, L.; Charest, G.; Guérin, B.; Akbari, M.; Fortin, D. Chemoattraction of Neoplastic Glial Cells with CXCL10, CCL2 and CCL11 as a Paradigm for a Promising Therapeutic Approach for Primary Brain Tumors. *Int. J. Mol. Sci.* **2021**, *22*, 12150. [CrossRef]
296. Ye, E.; Loh, X.J. Polymeric hydrogels and nanoparticles: A merging and emerging field. *Aust. J. Chem.* **2013**, *66*, 997–1007. [CrossRef]
297. Najberg, M.; Mansor, M.H.; Boury, F.; Alvarez-Lorenzo, C.; Garcion, E. Reversing the Tumor Target: Establishment of a Tumor Trap. *Front. Pharmacol.* **2019**, *10*, 887. [CrossRef]
298. Brachi, G.; Ruiz-Ramírez, J.; Dogra, P.; Wang, Z.; Cristini, V.; Ciardelli, G.; Rostomily, R.C.; Ferrari, M.; Mikheev, A.M.; Blanco, E. Intratumoral injection of hydrogel-embedded nanoparticles enhances retention in glioblastoma. *Nanoscale* **2020**, *12*, 23838–23850. [CrossRef]
299. Zhao, M.; Danhier, F.; Bastiancich, C.; Joudiou, N.; Ganipineni, L.P.; Tsakiris, N.; Gallez, B.; des Rieux, A.; Jankovski, A.; Bianco, J.; et al. Post-resection treatment of glioblastoma with an injectable nanomedicine-loaded photopolymerizable hydrogel induces long-term survival. *Int. J. Pharm.* **2018**, *548*, 522–529. [CrossRef]
300. Nutan, B.; Chandel, A.K.S.; Jewrajka, S.K. Liquid prepolymer-based in situ formation of degradable poly (ethylene glycol)-linked-poly (caprolactone)-linked-poly (2-dimethylaminoethyl) methacrylate amphiphilic conetwork gels showing polarity driven gelation and bioadhesion. *ACS Appl. Bio Mater.* **2018**, *1*, 1606–1619. [CrossRef]
301. Chandel, A.K.S.; Kannan, D.; Nutan, B.; Singh, S.; Jewrajka, S.K. Dually crosslinked injectable hydrogels of poly (ethylene glycol) and poly [(2-dimethylamino) ethyl methacrylate]-b-poly (N-isopropyl acrylamide) as a wound healing promoter. *J. Mater. Chem. B* **2017**, *5*, 4955–4965. [CrossRef]
302. Chandel, A.K.S.; Nutan, B.; Raval, I.H.; Jewrajka, S.K. Self-Assembly of Partially Alkylated Dextran- graft -poly[(2-dimethylamino)ethyl methacrylate] Copolymer Facilitating Hydrophobic/Hydrophilic Drug Delivery and Improving Conetwork Hydrogel Properties. *Biomacromolecules* **2018**, *19*, 1142–1153. [CrossRef]
303. Giarra, S.; Ierano, C.; Biondi, M.; Napolitano, M.; Campani, V.; Pacelli, R.; Scala, S.; De Rosa, G.; Mayol, L. Engineering of thermoresponsive gels as a fake metastatic niche. *Carbohydr. Polym.* **2018**, *191*, 112–118. [CrossRef]
304. Molina-Peña, R.; Haji Mansor, M.; Najberg, M.; Thomassin, J.M.; Gueza, B.; Alvarez-Lorenzo, C.; Garcion, E.; Jérôme, C.; Boury, F. Nanoparticle-containing electrospun nanofibrous scaffolds for sustained release of SDF-1α. *Int. J. Pharm.* **2021**, *610*, 121205. [CrossRef]

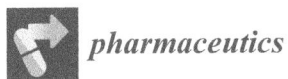

Review

Delivery of Intravenously Administered Antibodies Targeting Alzheimer's Disease-Relevant Tau Species into the Brain Based on Receptor-Mediated Transcytosis

Toshihiko Tashima

Tashima Laboratories of Arts and Sciences, 1239-5 Toriyama-cho, Kohoku-ku, Yokohama 222-0035, Japan; tashima_lab@yahoo.co.jp

Abstract: Alzheimer's disease (AD) is a neurodegenerative disease that causes memory loss, cognitive decline, and eventually dementia. The etiology of AD and its pathological mechanisms remain unclear due to its complex pathobiology. At the same time, the number of patients with AD is increasing worldwide. However, no therapeutic agents for AD are currently available for definitive care. Several phase 3 clinical trials using agents targeting amyloid β (Aβ) and its related molecules have failed, with the exception of aducanumab, an anti-Aβ monoclonal antibody (mAb), clinically approved by the US Food and Drug Administration in 2021, which could be modified for AD drug development due to controversial approval. Neurofibrillary tangles (NFTs) composed of tau rather than senile plaques composed of Aβ are correlated with AD pathogenesis. Moreover, Aβ and tau pathologies initially proceed independently. At a certain point in the progression of AD symptoms, the Aβ pathology is involved in the alteration and spreading of the tau pathology. Therefore, tau-targeting therapies have attracted the attention of pharmaceutical scientists, as well as Aβ-targeting therapies. In this review, I introduce the implementations and potential of AD immunotherapy using intravenously administered anti-tau and anti-receptor bispecific mAbs. These cross the blood-brain barrier (BBB) based on receptor-mediated transcytosis and are subsequently cleared by microglia based on Fc-mediated endocytosis after binding to tau and lysosomal degradation.

Keywords: drug delivery into the brain; transendothelium based on receptor-mediated transcytosis; immunotherapy; Alzheimer's disease; anti-tau and anti-receptor bispecific monoclonal antibodies; Alzheimer's disease-relevant tau species; temporal-spatial pathological Aβ and tau distribution; interactions between Aβ and tau; tau clearance in microglia; tau clearance in neurons

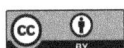

1. Introduction

Medicinal remedies provide long-term health benefits to humans. However, treatments for several important diseases have yet to be developed, including neurodegenerative diseases, such as Alzheimer's disease (AD) and Parkinson's disease (PD). Almost all clinical trials for AD, including phase 3 studies using pharmaceutical agents targeting amyloid β (Aβ) and its related molecules, such as β-secretase 1 and γ-secretase, have failed. Despite this, several approved AD drugs do not target Aβ. As a result, many pharmaceutical companies have abandoned efforts to develop AD drugs [1]. Under these circumstances, aducanumab [2], anti-insoluble Aβ fibrils, and anti-soluble Aβ oligomer monoclonal antibody (mAb), was approved by the US Food and Drug Administration (FDA) in 2021. Other existing AD drugs, such as four cholinesterase inhibitors (tacrine, donepezil, rivastigmine, and galantamine) and an N-methyl-D-aspartate (NMDA) receptor antagonist (memantine) (Figure 1) [3], have been found to transiently slow down the progression of symptoms; however, they do not lead to definitive therapy. Accordingly, innovative therapeutic agents for AD are expected to be produced as early as possible. An analysis of several clinical trial failures and AD research has suggested alternative strategies for the targeting of tau, in addition to Aβ. The so-called amyloid hypothesis, which states that the accumulation and deposition of oligomeric or fibrillar Aβ peptide are the primary cause of AD, may need to be modified in line with these novel findings. Although Aβ and tau pathologies initially proceed independently, Aβ pathology is involved in the alteration and spreading of tau pathology at a certain point of AD symptom progression [4]. Moreover, the presence of neurofibrillary tangles (NFTs) composed of tau rather than senile plaques composed of Aβ is correlated with AD pathogenesis [5]. Thus, tau clearance in the brain is a promising methodology for treating AD.

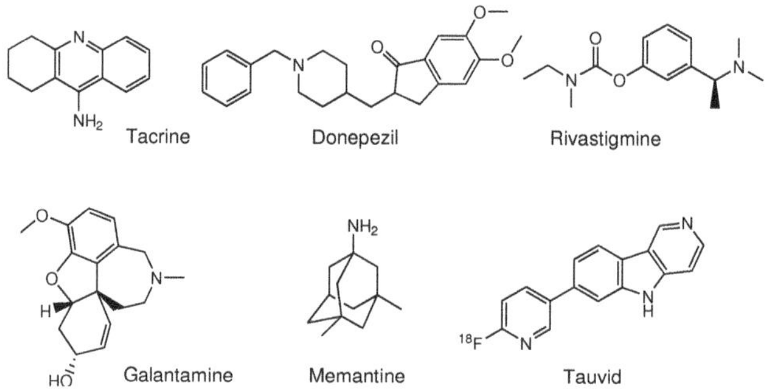

Figure 1. Structures of approved drugs and a tau imaging agent for Alzheimer's disease.

Drug membrane permeability is a serious problem that needs to be addressed in the field of drug discovery and development. The blood-brain barrier (BBB) prevents drugs that target the central nervous system (CNS) from entering the brain. The BBB consists of: (i) a biological barrier based on excretion transporters, such as multiple drug resistance 1 (MDR1), which excludes hydrophobic low-molecular compounds just passing inside the membrane; (ii) a physical barrier based on the tight junctions between the capillary endothelial cells backed by pericytes. Nonetheless, strategies that enable the delivery of substances into the brain across the BBB, based on solute carrier (SLC) transporter-mediated transport or receptor-mediated transcytosis, depending on molecular size and hydrophilicity, have been developed. Several methods for membrane substance permeation exist, including substances that (i) are subject to SLC transporter-mediated transport across the membrane [6], (ii) are transported into cells using cell penetrating peptides (CPPs) [7], (iii) specifically enter cancer cells through receptor-mediated endocytosis based on the enhanced permeability and retention (EPR) effect using nanoparticles [8], (iv) are delivered into the brain based on receptor-mediated transcytosis across the BBB after intravenous administration [9] or (v) across the olfactory epithelium after intranasal administration using insulin as a carrier [10], and (vi) deliver orally administered mAbs as cargo through neonatal Fc receptor (FcRn)-mediated transcytosis across the intestinal epithelium into systemic circulation using enteric nanoparticles [11]. These pharmacokinetic findings are also useful for the design and development of AD drugs. In response to the molecular size and hydrophobicity of drugs used in pharmacological treatment, the methodology of drug design and pharmacokinetic trajectory vary. CNS drugs, such as AD therapeutic agents, must cross the BBB to elicit their activity. It is difficult for anti-tau mAbs to cross the cell membrane, because they are large and hydrophilic molecules. In this perspective review, I introduce immunotherapy using intravenously administered anti-tau mAbs to be delivered into the brain based on receptor-mediated transcytosis, particularly using a bispecific strategy (Figure 2). Furthermore, to accomplish well-defined mAb drug design, I refer AD pathological mechanisms caused by factors such as Aβ and tau.

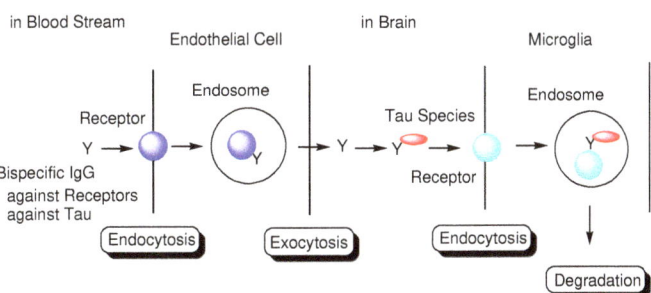

Figure 2. Strategy used to eliminate tau species using anti-receptor and anti-tau bispecific monoclonal antibodies based on receptor-mediated endocytosis and lysosomal degradation in microglia to cure Alzheimer's disease.

2. Discussion

2.1. Alzheimer's Disease

AD is a progressive neurodegenerative disorder that leads to synapse loss, neuronal cell death, and eventually dementia, first reported by Alois Alzheimer in 1906. The number of American AD patients aged 65 and older in 2021 is 6.2 million, which is estimated to rise to 13.8 million by 2060 [12]. Worldwide, approximately 50 million people were reported as having dementia in 2020, 60–70% of whom are also associated with AD. This is expected to rise to 82 million in 2030 and 152 million in 2050 [13]. The social and economic impacts of AD, including treatment by care takers and health care workers, patient dignity, and medical bills, are important issues. However, many aspects of AD, including its etiology, progression, and treatment, remain unknown due to its multifactorial and complex mechanisms. The structure of AD based on structuralism advocated by Lévi-Strauss, which systematically and comprehensively regulates AD pathogenesis and pathology based on biological and physical components, remains poorly understood.

Senile plaques composed of Aβ and NFTs comprised of hyperphosphorylated tau are widely accepted hallmarks of AD. This implies that Aβ and tau play important roles in the onset and progression of AD. Currently, AD drugs that focus on Aβ modulators or tau modulators have been developed. However, they are considered unlikely to be able to achieve the desired outcomes in many cases. Therefore, a well-defined drug design based on the biological and physical structures that result in AD pathology needs to be developed.

2.2. Amyloid Hypothesis

Although the mechanism of AD onset and progression remains unclear, the amyloid hypothesis is widely accepted to explain the primary cause of AD in drug development. According to this theory, Aβ, which is mainly divided into Aβ (1–42) and Aβ (1–40) due to amino acid sequence length, is cleaved by β-secretase (β-site APP cleaving enzyme 1 (BACE1)) and then by γ-secretase from amyloid precursor protein (APP) [14]. The population of Aβ (1–42) is less than that of Aβ (1–40). However, Aβ (1–42) is supposed to aggregates more easily than Aβ (1–40), subsequently eliciting neurotoxicity. Aβ assembly species structurally mutate from unfolded monomers, folded monomers, oligomers, and protofibrils to fibrils. The structures and locations of the deposited Aβ differ.

Senile plaques are believed to be the main factor in the pathology of AD. Although Aβ modulators, such as BACE1 inhibitors, γ-secretase inhibitors, and anti-Aβ Abs, have been developed to date, only aducanumab has been clinically approved for use by the FDA. Despite this, therapeutic approaches to AD treatment using Aβ modulators have been unsuccessful. Nonetheless, the amyloid hypothesis is believed to hold due to APP mutations causing familial AD accounts for 5 to 10% of total AD, although the involvement of tau mutations has not yet been observed in familial AD, in contrast to other tauopathies, such as frontotemporal dementia and parkinsonism linked to chromosome 17 (FTDP-17).

Three known genes with mutations associated with familial AD are *presenilin 1 (PSEN1)*, *presenilin 2 (PSEN2)*, and *APP*. Presenilin 1 (PS1) and presenilin 2 (PS2) form the catalytic core component of the γ-secretase complex. Many APP mutations have been reported. Among them, the Osaka mutation, with APP E693del, did not form Aβ protofibrils, senile plaques, and NFTs, but formed Aβ oligomers and phosphorylated tau in transgenic mice with APP E693del (Osaka). In this in vivo assay, most AD pathologies were reproduced, even without NFT formation. Moreover, Aβ oligomer accumulation, NFT formation, and AD pathologies, such as synapse loss, neuronal loss, and memory impairment, were observed in double transgenic mice with APP E693del (Osaka) and human tau [15]. These findings suggest that Aβ monomers and/or oligomers induce AD pathologies by interacting with AD-relevant tau species through direct and/or indirect interactions between Aβ and tau. Nevertheless, Aβ protofibrils and other non-oligomeric species may elicit neurotoxicity through ways other than Aβ monomers and oligomers, as the pathology of AD is known to be established via complex and intricate processes.

AN-1792 is a synthetic full-length Aβ peptide with QS-21 adjuvant as a vaccine to produce anti-Aβ Abs, which was evaluated for its efficacy in clinical trials against mild to moderate AD patients. Surprisingly, as a result, AD dementia in some patients was found to progress, although their senile plaques in the brain disappeared [16]. However, Aβ oligomers were not completely eliminated [17]. Based on these results, several conclusions were suggested: (i) factors different from Aβ, such as tau, may act as causative substances; (ii) Aβ oligomers rather than senile plaques may evoke AD pathology; (iii) treatment was delayed after the onset of AD symptoms started to appear. This suggests that AD could not be cured, even though senile plaques were eliminated. Therefore, alternative therapeutic approaches should be developed. In fact, the amyloid hypothesis was modified by considering the interaction between Aβ oligomers and tau oligomers after a certain stage of AD.

2.3. Tau Proteins

Tau protein [14,18] is encoded by the microtubule-associated protein tau (MAPT) gene on chromosome 17. According to the splicing pattern, there are six tau protein isoforms (0N3R, 0N4R, 1N3R, 1N4R, 2N3R, and 2N4R) composed of four regions: the *N*-terminal domain, proline-rich domain (PRD), microtubule-binding domain (MBD), and *C*-terminal domain. While the 3-repeat (3R tau) isoform is exclusively expressed in the fetal brain, the 4-repeat (4R tau) and 3R tau isoforms are evenly expressed in the adult brain (Figure 3).

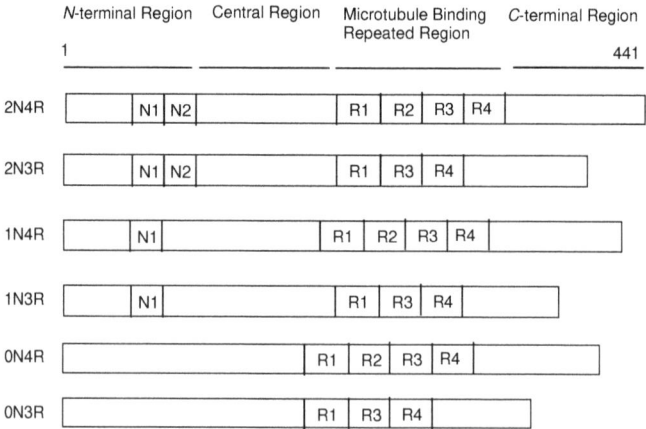

Figure 3. Schematic representation of the protein structures of tau.

Physiological tau proteins play a vital role not only in the stabilization of microtubules in axions via their MBDs, but also in other biological functions [14]. When tau is phosphorylated, tau becomes detached from the microtubules, resulting in microtubule instability. Currently, there are at least 30 phosphorylation sites among 85 residues with hydroxyl groups in a tau protein (2N4R). Mathematically, the number of multiphosphorylated tau proteins is a myriad. At least eight sites are phosphorylated in AD pathological tau, whereas 2 to 3 sites are phosphorylated in normal physiological tau [19]. Moreover, tau is involved in other post-transcriptional modifications, such as acetylation, glycosylation, ubiquitination, and truncation. Thus, a variety of tau species exist with respect to isoforms and post-transcriptional modification, which renders the pathological mechanism unclear.

Phosphorylated tau (p-tau) monomers and p-tau oligomers exhibit neurotoxicity, intercellular distribution, seeding, and aggregation, which are different from physiologically intact tau proteins. Tau assembly species structurally mutate from phosphorylated monomers, phosphorylated oligomers, and filaments, such as paired helical filaments (PHF), to tangles. It has been pointed out that the population of NFTs is correlated with the pathogenesis of AD dementia, while that of Aβ plaques is not [5]. Therefore, it is suggested that tau plays a vital role in AD pathology, although Aβ is also involved in it due to the existence of familial AD accompanied by mutations in APP, presenilin 1, or presenilin 2.

NFT formation in the neuronal cell body is thought to be associated with the progressive AD process due to detoxification [20,21]. NFTs were thoroughly inactive, such that they remained as extracellular ghost tangles, even though the host neurons died and disappeared. p-Tau oligomers were found to be the most toxic species. Thus, PHFs may also form as a result of the progressive AD process, although they elicit toxicity as physical substances. Inactive p-tau aggregates were not soluble, even with detergents. Accordingly, approaches using Abs neutralizing soluble p-tau oligomers and p-tau monomers as their composition are promising methods for AD therapy [22].

2.4. Aβ and Tau Pathologies

2.4.1. Temporal-Spatial Pathological Aβ and Tau Distribution in the Brain

In 1989, Ihara pointed out that AD progression irreversibly began when tau was distributed until the temporal lobe across the collateral sulcus via the hippocampus and the parahippocampal gyrus [23]. More recently, it was revealed that the temporal-spatial behavior of Aβ and tau proteins changes with respect to formation and distribution. Aβ pathology and tau pathology were performed independently. However, at a certain point, Aβ pathology began to assist tau pathology to enhance the pathological process of AD [4,24]. This pathophysiological hypothesis is consistent with familial AD due to APP mutations. At the onset of dementia, Aβ is already saturated in the brain. Even though Aβ was removed, dementia proceeded without Aβ, most likely due to the formation of the pathological tau seeds, which duplicated and transmitted cell-to-cell, via interactions with Aβ at that stage, propagating pathological tau as a result. As widely accepted among medicinal chemists, seed crystals initiate crystallization during organic synthesis. When washing using glass vessels is insufficient, crystallization of the same compounds proceeds by the remaining crystals without the addition of seed crystals. Therefore, the clearance of tau to avoid its propagation may be useful for the treatment of AD.

Tauvid, approved by the FDA in 2020, was the first and only agent to image tau pathology, particularly NFTs, using positron emission tomography (PET) (Figure 1). Tau imaging enables the observation of the distribution of tau in the brain of AD patients, allowing to predict AD symptom progression by comparing data on the correlation between the temporal-spatial distribution of pathological tau and the pathology of AD.

2.4.2. Cell-to-Cell Pathology Transmission

Knowledge of tau trajectory is useful for anti-tau mAb drug design. Some inspired readers should suggest better ideas. Tau pathology is thought to be template-dependent progressive cell-to-cell and occur via regional transmission in a prion-like manner. The physical and pathological properties of tau are inherited from the original tau seeds, which form disease-specific tau pathology based on tau strains in AD, Pick's disease (PiD), progressive supranuclear palsy (PSP), and corticobasal degeneration (CBD) [25], appearing to belong to unelucidated respective certain strains. It is likely that extracellular tau is released from a donor neuron into the brain interstitial fluid (ISF) and transferred into the synaptically connected recipient neurons across the plasma membrane through endocytosis rather than into neurons of spatial proximity. The precise mechanisms of such transportation processes during the development of tauopathy remain a topic of controversy [18,26–28].

Tau species enter neuronal cells either: (i) through several internalization mechanisms based on endocytosis, such as receptor-mediated endocytosis (Figure 4), or (ii) through exosome fusion to the plasma membrane of recipient cells (Figure 5). Monomeric tau, such as monomeric tau p301S covalently labeled with Dylight, a fluorescent dye, or with pHrodo, a pH-sensitive dye, was internalized into neurons through dynamin-dependent endocytosis and micropinocytosis, using human stem cell-derived neurons. On the other hand, aggregated tau, such as aggregated tau p301S covalently labeled with Dylight or pHrodo, was internalized through dynamin-dependent endocytosis. Monomeric and aggregated tau in early endosomes (pH 6.5) was degraded in lysosomes (pH 4.5) as endosome maturation via late endosomes (pH 5.5). These processes of tau entry occur not only in AD pathological neurons but also in physiologically normal neurons [29].

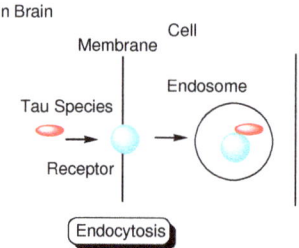

Figure 4. Tau species enter the cells based on endocytosis such as receptor-mediated endocytosis.

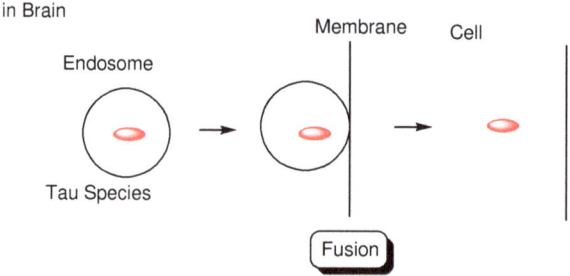

Figure 5. Tau species in endosomes enter the recipient cells based on membrane fusion.

Second, Alexa Fluor™-labeled tau oligomers derived from AD and DLB brains were transported into cortical neurons isolated from C57BL/6 mice through heparan sulfate proteoglycan (HSPG)-induced, clathrin- and caveolae-independent endocytosis, and remained in endosomes from early endosomes to lysosomes. In contrast, labeled tau oligomers derived from PSP brains were transported through other pathways [30]. Positively charged CPPs, short amino acid oligomers (5–30 residues), such as TAT and R8, electrostatically interact with negatively charged HSPGs to induce endocytosis [31]. Accordingly, this suggests that p-tau (352 residues (0N3R)–441 residues (2N4R)) is able to enter neurons through HSPG-induced endocytosis based on electrostatic interactions, since it has as many as 44 lysine residues and 14 arginine residues in the 441 amino acid sequence (Figure 6).

Tau and HSPG are able to interact due to the fact that heparin acts as a core for tau seeding and aggregation [32,33].

```
  1           11          21          31          41
MAEP QEFEV MEDHAGTYGL GD KDQGGYT MHQDQEGDTD AGLKESPLQT
 51          61          71          81          91
PTEDGSEEPG SETSDAKSTP TAEDVTAPLV DEGAPGKQAA AQPHTEIPEG
101         111         121         131         141
TTAEEAGIGD TPSLEDEAAG HVTQA MVSK SKDGTGSDDK KAKGADGKTK
151         161         171         181         191
IATP GAAPP GQKGQANAT IPAKTPPAPK TPPSSGEPPK SGD SGYSSP
201         211         221         231         241
GSPGTPGS S TPSLPTPPT EPKKVAVV TPPKSPSSAK S LQTAPVPM
251         261         271         281         291
PDLKNVKSKI GSTENLKHQP GGGKVQIINK KLDLSNVQSK CGSKDNIKHV
301         311         321         331         341
SGGGSVQIVY KPVDLSKVTS KCGSLGNIHH KPGGGQVEVK SEKLDFKD V
351         361         371         381         391
QSKIGSLDNI THVPGGGNKK IETHKLTF E NAKAKTDHGA EIVYKSPVVS
401         411         421         431         441
GDTSP HLSN VSSTGSIDMV DSPQLATLAD EVSASLAKQG L
```

Figure 6. Amino acid sequence of human tau441 (2N4R). Lysines are shown in red and arginines are shown in light blue.

Third, low-density lipoprotein receptor-related protein 1 (LRP1) is involved not only in tau endocytosis, but also in the distribution of tau in the brain. It is worth noting that this distribution was diminished in LRP1 knockout mice [34].

Fourth, M1 and M3 muscarinic receptors were correlated with tau entry into neurons. Physiologically normal tau stabilizes neurites, while pathological tau induces neurodegeneration, leading to cell death in cerebellar neuronal cultures. The uptake of tau in cerebellar neurons was inhibited by an M1 antagonist, such as pirenzepine, but not by M2 antagonists, such as AF-DX116, or an M2/M4 antagonist, such as pertussis toxin. Tau uptake was increased approximately 19-fold in CHO cells transfected with M1 or M3, and 31.5-fold in CHO cells transfected simultaneously with both M1 and M3 by immunoblot analysis using anti-human tau, compared to non-transfected CHO cells [35].

The internalization cases presented here act through the endocytosis pathway, leading to degradation in lysosomes, although some of the endocytosed tau seeds may be transported and localized in the cytoplasm by endosomal escape, or may alternatively be recycled back to the outside based on the fusion to the plasma membrane regulated by Rab7A. Accordingly, the cell-to-cell transmission of tau seeds would not be accomplished as long as tau seeds are subject to such clearance in lysosomes. Tau, which contains lysine residues that accept proton influents through vacuolar adenosine triphosphatases (V-ATPases), may be released into the cytosol from endosomes due to membrane bursting, based on the osmotic gap due to the proton sponge effect [8]. On the other hand, its direct translocation into cells across the membrane has also been suggested. In contrast to CPPs, it is difficult for tau to be internalized through direct translocation due to its size. Subsequently, tau endosomal escape into the cytosol has been found to play an important role not only in tauopathy progression, but also in physiological tau activity. Even though duplicated tau species are formed in endosomes in a prion-like manner, they are enzymatically degraded into pieces in lysosomes. In fact, tau is released from endosomes, although the mechanism by which this occurs remains unclear [36].

However, as another internalization mechanism different from endocytosis, tau in extracellular exosomes can be released into the neuronal cytoplasm after membrane fusion in recipient cells. In this case, there is no problem involved in endosomal escape because tau is not present in endosomes. In fact: (i) some tau proteins are present in exosomes secreted from cells (Figure 7) [18]. Accordingly, tau secretion mechanisms from donor cells are also important for investigating substantive tau transmission, in addition to the internalization mechanism in recipient cells. Interestingly, ectosomes (50–1000 nm in diameter) are extracellular vesicles that do not depend on the endolysosomal machinery to produce exosomes (40–100 nm in diameter) [37]. They budded out and were cut off from the plasma membrane; (ii) some tau proteins are present in these ectosomes (Figure 8). Nevertheless, it was revealed that free tau that was not in exosomes was secreted from donor neurons through (iii) endosomal fusion to the plasma membrane regulated by Rab7A (Figure 9) or (iv) direct translocation, despite its large size [38]. Surprisingly, it was reported that over 99% of tau oligomers are secreted in a membrane microdomain- and HSPG-dependent unconventional vesicular-free mechanism in mouse N2A neuroblastoma cell line, approximately 80% of which are characterized as dimers, trimers, or tetramers (Figure 10) [38]. Thus, anti-tau Abs in ISF can bind to tau to block cell-to-cell transmission. As reference examples, at the molecular level, cytoplasmic full-length TAT (101 amino acids) was attached to anionic phosphatidylinositol 4,5-bisphosphate (PI(4,5)P$_2$) in the inner leaflet of the lipid bilayer through the cationic region (residues 49–57), inserting its hydrophobic Trp11 residue for itself to be buried in the membrane, and thereby permeated to the extracellular space [39]. Moreover, cytoplasmic fibroblast growth factor 2 (FGF2) was attached to anionic PI(4,5)P$_2$ in the inner leaflet of the lipid bilayer, permeated through the membrane based on the microdomain after oligomerization, and interacted with HSPGs in the outer leaflet of the lipid bilayer to be released [40]. Similarly, cytoplasmic tau was attached to anionic PI(4,5)P$_2$ and phosphatidylserine in the inner leaflet of the lipid bilayer, went through microdomain-mediated membrane permeation after oligomerization, bound to HSPGs in the outer leaflet of the lipid bilayer, and was thereby liberated to the extracellular space in its free form [18,39]. Microdomains are composed of lipid rafts, cholesterol, and sphingomyelin.

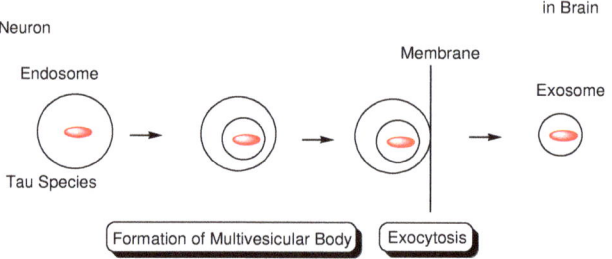

Figure 7. Tau in exosomes (40–100 nm in diameter) secreted from neurons.

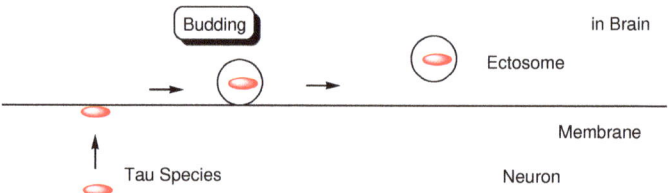

Figure 8. Tau in ectosomes (50–1000 nm in diameter) secreted from the membrane of neurons, independently on the endolysosomal machinery.

Furthermore, (v) tau may be transmitted cell-to-cell through tunneling nanotubes (50–700 nm in diameter, 20–100 μm length) (Figure 11) [41]. Although tau cannot diffuse in the extracellular space, tunneling nanotubes remain controversial in vivo, despite being recognized in cell lines [36].

mAb drugs exhibit high selectivity against antigens. Thus, conformation-selective mAbs targeting pathological tau may suppress tau toxicity and cell-to-cell pathology transmission without disturbing constitutive tau homeostasis and function due to unbinding to physiological tau.

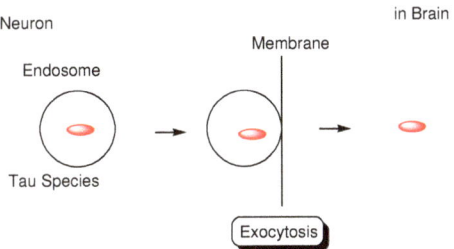

Figure 9. Tau secreted from neurons based on the endolysosomal machinery.

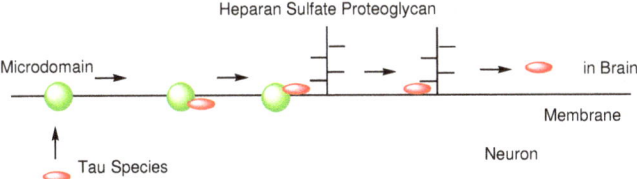

Figure 10. Tau secreted from neurons through an unconventional non-vesicular mechanism.

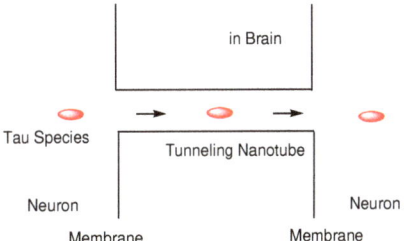

Figure 11. Tau cell-to-cell transportation through tunneling nanotubes.

2.5. Tauopathies

Tauopathy is a general term for neurodegenerative diseases with NFTs composed of tau proteins that originally spread via cell-to-cell transmission process and duplicated to tau seeds in recipient cells [25]. It is well known that disease-specific tau pathology is based on tau strains in AD, PiD, PSP, and CBD. Brain-derived tau oligomers from AD and dementia with Lewy bodies (DLB) were internalized through HSPG-mediated endocytosis using cortical neurons isolated from C57BL/6 mice, while those from PSP were internalized through not only HSPG-mediated endocytosis but also through alternative mechanisms [30]. Some tauopathies are associated with tau gene mutations. Thus, it is thought that arbitrary tau strains are doomed to induce the corresponding tauopathy-based structuralism by Lévi-Strauss. Tau oligomers composed of 3R and 4R isoforms were aggregated through the seeding of PSP brain-derived tau oligomers with 3R and 4R monomers after the addition of monomeric 3R and 4R tau in phosphate-buffered saline. However, pathologically, only NFT composed of 4R tau was formed in the PSP. It has been suggested that 4R tau is more toxic than 3R tau in PSP. Toxic 4R tau isoforms may be selectively packed into NFTs as inclusion bodies in the detoxifying process [42]. NFTs in AD are composed of 3R and 4R tau. 4R tau may be as toxic as 3R tau, particularly in oligomeric forms, in AD. Moreover, 2N4R tau is more toxic than 1N4R tau in neurons [43].

2.6. Interactions between Aβ and Tau That Induce Neurotoxicity

Aβ and tau are recognized as the major factors driving the pathology of AD. They are thought to interact with each other during pathological processes. After incubating Aβ monomers for 5 days in 10-day-old organotypic hippocampal slices prepared from rat pups, Aβ oligomers were formed. Interestingly, the phosphorylation of tau at Ser396/Ser404 binding to PHF-1 Ab and at Thr231/Ser235 binding to AT180 Ab were augmented by more than two-fold after Aβ incubation, compared to no Aβ incubation as the control, while those at Ser199/Ser202 binding to AT-8 Ab and at Thr212/Thr217/Ser214 binding to AT100 Ab did not change [44]. This result indicates that Aβ affects the profiles and levels of tau phosphorylation.

2.6.1. Cyclin-Dependent Kinase 5 (CDK5) as a Matchmaker between Aβ and Tau

Glutamatergic tripartite synapses, composed of presynaptic neurons, postsynaptic neurons, and astrocytes, play an integrative role not only in neural networks for learning and memory, but also in AD pathogenesis and pathology [45]. Synaptic N-methyl-D-aspartate receptors (sNMDARs), constituted of GluN1/GluN1/GluN2A/GluN2A subunits as major [46,47] or GluN1/GluN1/GluN2A/GluN2B subunits as minor [48], are located inside the synapse of the postsynaptic neuron and exhibit neuroprotective activity, whereas extrasynaptic N-methyl-D-aspartate receptors (eNMDARs) consisting of GluN1/GluN1/GluN2B/GluN2B subunits [46,47] are located outside the synapses of postsynaptic neurons and exhibit neurotoxic activity.

Excess Glu molecules in the synaptic cleft were sufficient to activate the eNMDARs. Aβ induces eNMDARs to influx calcium ions into neurons. Calcium ions that flow through activated eNMDARs cleave p35 into p25 and p10 by calpain. The resultant p25/CDK5 complex mediates tau phosphorylation [49].

2.6.2. Fyn as a Matchmaker

At the postsynaptic site of the glutamatergic tripartite synapse, NMDAR with GluN2B is involved in tau phosphorylation via Fyn [50], which is a cytoplasmic tyrosine kinase. Aβ oligomers bind to cellular prion protein (PrPc) and subsequently activate Fyn in the NMDAR-postsynaptic density protein-95 (PSD95)-Fyn complex at the postsynaptic site [51]. The resulting activated Fyn phosphorylates the GluN2B of sNMDAR at Tyr1472 and GluN2B of eNMDAR at Tyr1336 [52] to stabilize the NMDAR-PSD95-Fyn complex location at the membrane, which enhances glutamatergic excitotoxicity by Aβ oligomers. Moreover, p-tau bound to Fyn and/or physiological tau bound to it carried it to dendritic spines [53], and formed the NMDAR-PSD95-Fyn-p-tau complex to enhance glutamatergic excitotoxicity due to alteration of complex conformation by tau. Intriguingly, Fyn did not form a complex with NMDAR in transgenic mice expressing truncated tau and tau-/- mice [53,54]. Tau can be phosphorylated in such complexes. In particular, the Fyn-tau interaction was increased by phosphorylation at serines where AT8 Abs bind. AT8 Ab-binding phosphorylated tau was localized postsynaptically 7-fold greater than before NMDAR activation via Aβ oligomer formation in an in vitro assay detected by electron microscopy using embryonic day 18 rat hippocampal slices. By contrast, tau was phosphorylated at the sites where PHF-1 Ab (against p-Ser396/p-Ser404) or AT180 Ab (against p-Thr231/p-Ser235) bind after Aβ oligomer formation, and tau was phosphorylated at the sites where AT8 Ab (against p-Ser199/p-Ser202) or AT100 Ab (against p-Thr217/p-Ser214) bind after NMDAR activation [44]. As a result, p-tau and Aβ oligomers synergistically exacerbate AD pathology. On the other hand, Fyn activated via phosphorylation at Tyr416 by Pyk2 phosphorylated tau at Tyr18 [51]. It has been suggested that the phosphorylation of tau at Tyr18 is necessary for NMDAR-mediated excitotoxicity [55]. However, the mechanisms underlying this action remain elusive, and must be clarified in future studies. Although p-tau binding to AT8 and AT100 was not increased by the addition of Aβ, it is known that such sites are phosphorylated in the late stage of AD [44]. Therefore, the pathological mechanisms in the late stage were assumed to be different from those in the early stage.

Physiological tau monomers exist in the dendritic cytoplasm, as well as in the microtubules. Dendritic tau recruits Fyn to the NMDAR-PSD95 complex. Thus, the source of such dendritic tau is not found in the extracellular region but in the intracellular region due to local tau mRNA translation or dissociation from microtubules. Moreover, it was revealed that p-tau constitutively present in normal neurons was located in dendrites and near synapses rather than in axons. While p-tau binding to PHF-1 posed somatodendric localization in primary neurons isolated from embryonic day 18 rats, p-tau binding to AT180 and AT8 posed dendric localization [44].

2.6.3. Ca^{2+}-Dependent Calmodulin Kinase IIα (CaMKIIα) as a Matchmaker

The Aβ*56 oligomer (4.8–5.7 nm; diameter, 56 kDa) enhanced Ca^{2+} inflow by binding to sNMDAR. An increase in the intracellular Ca^{2+} concentration activated CaMKIIα and subsequently induced approximately 2.7-fold higher tau phosphorylation at Ser202 and Ser416 in 7-month-old Tg2576 mouse forebrains compared to non-transgenic littermates. Aβ dimers and trimers do not exhibit this tau phosphorylation pathway. In addition, Aβ*56 does not activate Fyn [56,57].

2.6.4. GSK3β as a Matchmaker

In terms of post-synaptic density, Aβ induces sNMDAR-mediated tau phosphorylation at Ser396 by GSK3β [58]. In contrast, the eNMDAR-PSD95-Fyn-p-tau complex involved in Aβ oligomers activates GSK3β and CDK5 [44]. Aβ oligomers bind to α2A adrenergic receptors and enhance GSK3β-mediated tau phosphorylation in mice [59].

2.6.5. c-Jun N-Terminal Kinase (JNK) as a Matchmaker

Soluble Aβ (1–42) monomers bind to β2 adrenergic receptors that belong to G protein-coupled receptors and induce JNK tau phosphorylation at Ser214 [60].

2.7. Implementation of mAbs Targeting AD-Relevant Tau Species

2.7.1. Conformation-Selective Anti-Tau mAbs Block Cell-to-Cell Transmission of Tau Pathological Seeds

It has been suggested that tau seeds drive the interneuronal propagation of tau from one area of the brain to another in AD patients over time via prion-like mechanisms. Eliminating arbitrary tau species that become seeds is a strategy to inhibit AD progression using mAbs. Several mAbs against p-tau species, particularly monomers and oligomers, have been developed [22]. Furthermore, a number of mAbs selective to tau forms and/or conformations have been developed. DMR7 and SKT82 are mAbs that selectively bind to the misfolded pathological conformation of tau. DMR7 showed EC_{50} values of 0.10 ± 0.01 nM for AD-tau extracted from postmortem human brain tissue, 0.46 ± 0.32 nM for AD-tau seeded recombinant tau preformed fibrils (AD-P1 PFFs) expressed in BL21(DE3)RIL Escherichia coli, and 12.0 ± 7.9 nM for tau monomer through sandwich ELISA measures. On the other hand, SKT82 showed those of 0.17 ± 0.03 nM for AD-tau, 2.38 ± 1.12 nM for AD-P1 PFFs, and 4.13 ± 3.74 nM for tau monomer. These two mAbs bound extracellularly to tau seeds, such as AD-P1 PFFs, and inhibited their uptake into cells and subsequent seeded fibrillization or aggregation based on internalized seeds in in vitro tests using primary neurons. This may be due to blocking of tau binding to receptors, such as LRP1, M1 and M3 muscarinic receptors, or heparan sulfate proteoglycans. Furthermore, SKT82 induced more effective tau pathology inhibition than DMR7 in slice cultures and the ipsilateral hippocampus in vivo. SKT82 (mouse IgG2b isotype) binding to AD-tau interacted with FcR on the membrane of microglia and was cleared greater than DMR7 (mouse IgG1 isotype) binding to AD-tau in a murine model. DMR7 does not interact with microglia [61].

Tau clearance in lysosomes was conducted through FcγR-mediated endocytosis after binding to the corresponding Abs in primary mouse microglial cultures [62]. FcγRI, FcγRIIa, FcγRIIb, and FcγRIIIa are upregulated in AD microglia [63]. It has been reported that human microglia do not induce an increase in inflammation by the tau-Ab complex [64], although reactive microgliosis (a particular state of inflammatory microglia) is suggested to be one of the primary causes of neurodegenerative diseases. Thus, FcR-mediated endocytosis, particularly in microglia, is a promising strategy for tau clearance using anti-tau antibodies.

2.7.2. Clinical Trial for Anti-Tau mAbs

Many clinical trials for Abs targeting Aβ and pharmaceutical agents modulating molecules related to Aβ have been unsuccessful, except for aducanumab as an anti-Aβ Ab. Accordingly, tau, instead of Aβ, has been investigated clinically (Table 1).

Active immunotherapy will result in the development of Abs based on the immune system. AADvac1 (tau 294-305; KDNIKHVPGGGS) or ACI-35 (pSer396 and 404) as active tau vaccines could neutralize tau species. Phase 1 (NCT02031198) [65] and phase 2 (NCT02579252) [66] clinical trials using AADvac1 have been completed, wherein AADvac1 exhibited a safety profile in patients with mild-to-moderate AD and induced Ab titers. Phase 1 and 2 clinical trials for AD (NCT04445831) using ACI-35 are currently ongoing.

For passive immunotherapy, LY3303560 (zagotenemab, a humanized anti-tau Ab) and BIIB076 (a human IgG1 Ab against tau), were tested in phase 1 clinical trials for AD (NCT03019536 and NCT03056729, respectively). Lu AF87908 is a humanized IgG1 Ab against tau and is currently in a phase 1 clinical trial for AD (NCT04149860).

BIIB092 (gosuranemab, a humanized IgG4 Ab against tau) was evaluated for AD in a phase 2 trial (NCT03352557). Moreover, ABBV-8E12 (tilavonemab), a humanized IgG4 Ab against tau aggregates, has been developed for the treatment of PSP and AD. Intravenously administered ABBV-8E12 has been investigated in a phase 2 clinical trial for AD (NCT03712787).

E2814, a humanized IgG1 Ab against tau, has been conducted in phases 1 and 2 for AD (NCT04971733). Phase 2 clinical trials using JNJ-63733657 (a humanized anti-tau Ab) for cognitive dysfunction (NCT04619420) and UCB0107 (Bepranemab, a humanized IgG4 Ab against tau 235-250) for AD (NCT04867616) are currently being conducted.

RO7105705 (semorinemab) is an IgG4 antibody against tau. Semorinemab was evaluated in a phase 2 clinical trial in prodromal to mild AD and was found to surprisingly not be likely to improve outcomes (NCT03289143) [67]. Nonetheless, phase 2 tests have been performed for moderate AD (NCT03828747).

No clinical trials using anti-tau antibodies in AD have led to phase 3 trials. Thus, alternative approaches using anti-tau Abs should be conducted using a well-designed strategy based on absorption, distribution, metabolism, and excretion (ADME). Intravenously administered Abs must cross the BBB and be metabolized together with the captured tau species. Clinically approved anti-Aβ Ab, aducanumab, has been shown to cross the BBB.

Table 1. Summary of clinical trials focusing on anti-tau Abs described in this review.

#	Administrated Drug	Formulation /Co-Administrated Drug	Disease	Sponsor	Phase	Study Start Date	Study Completion Date	ClinicalTrials.gov Identifier (Accessed on 25 December 2021)	Status	References
(i)	AADvac1	An active tau vaccine (tau294–305)	AD	Axon Neuroscience SE	Phase 1	January 2014	December 2016	NCT02031198	Completed	[68]
(ii)	RG7345	A humanized Ab against tau pS422	Healthy Volunteer	Hoffmann-La Roche	Phase 1	January 2015	October 2015	NCT02281786	Completed	–
(iii)	RO7105705 (Semorinemab)	An IgG4 Ab against tau	Mild-to-Moderate AD	Genentech, Inc.	Phase 1	June 2016	June 2017	NCT02820896	Completed	–
(iv)	LY3303560 (Zagotenemab)	A humanized Ab against tau/Florbetapir F18	AD	Eli Lilly and Company	Phase 1	January 2017	June 2019	NCT03019536	Completed	–
(v)	BIIB076	A human IgG1 Ab against tau	AD	Biogen	Phase 1	February 2017	March 2020	NCT03056729	Completed	–
(vi)	Lu AF87908	A humanized IgG1 Ab against tau	AD	H. Lundbeck A/S	Phase 1	September 2019	May 2021	NCT04149860	Recruiting	–
(vii)	AADvac1	An active tau vaccine (tau294–305)	Mild AD	Axon Neuroscience SE	Phase 2	March 2016	June 2019	NCT02579252	Completed	[69]
(viii)	ACI-35	An active tau vaccine (pSer396 and 404)	AD	AC Immune SA	Phase 1/2	July 2019	October 2023	NCT04445831	Recruiting	–

Table 1. Cont.

#	Administered Drug	Formulation /Co-Administered Drug	Disease	Sponsor	Phase	Study Start Date	Study Completion Date	ClinicalTrials.gov Identifier (Accessed on 25 December 2021)	Status	References
(ix)	E2814	A humanized IgG1 Ab against tau	AD	Eisai Inc.	Phase 1/2	June 2021	April 2024	NCT04971733	Recruiting	-
(x)	RO7105705 (Semorinemab)	An IgG4 Ab against tau	Prodromal to Mild AD	Genentech, Inc.	Phase 2	October 2017	January 2021	NCT03289143	Completed	[70]
(xi)	BIIB092 (Gosuranemab)	A humanized IgG4 Ab against tau	AD	Biogen	Phase 2	May 2018	August 2021	NCT03352557	Active, not recruiting	-
(xii)	RO7105705 (Semorinemab)	An IgG4 Ab against tau	Moderate AD	Genentech, Inc.	Phase 2	January 2019	October 2023	NCT03828747	Active, not recruiting	-
(xiii)	ABBV-8E12	A humanized IgG4 Ab against tau aggregates	Early AD	AbbVie	Phase 2	March 2019	July 2021	NCT03712787	Active, not recruiting	-
(xiv)	JNJ-63733657	A humanized Ab against tau	Cognitive dysfunction	Janssen Research & Development, LLC	Phase 2	January 2021	March 2025	NCT04619420	Recruiting	-
(xv)	UCB0107 (Bepranemab)	A humanized IgG4 Ab against tau235–250	AD	UCB Biopharma SRL	Phase 2	June 2021	November 2025	NCT04867616	Recruiting	-
(xvi)	intravenous mAbs	Bispecific mAbs against tau and TrR	AD						Under analysis in Tashima lab	-

2.8. Possibility and Effective Use of mAbs Targeting AD-Relevant Tau Species

2.8.1. Lymphatic and Immune System in the Brain

The brain lacks a lymphatic system. Instead, a glymphatic system based on cerebral small blood vessels, perivascular cavity, and glial cells develops and eliminates Aβ from the CNS via the bulk flow of cerebrospinal fluid (CSF) from the periarterial cavity to the perivenous cavity via intercellular space, caused by blood vessel pulsation and aquaporin-4 (AQP4) [68]. Sleep disruption promotes tau pathology [69].

Nevertheless, clearance mechanisms are assumed to be performed by brain cells, similar to phagocytosis by immune cell macrophages. Microglia play an important role in the brain. In fact, tau degradation in microglia was found to be enhanced by MC1 (anti-tau mAb) in an Fc-dependent manner [70]. Therefore, FcR-mediated endocytosis by microglia and successive lysosomal degradation may be a promising strategy for extraneuronal tau clearance using anti-tau Abs.

It has been shown that tau-Ab complexes enter neurons. MAb86 (anti-tau/pS422 Ab) bound to lipid raft-associated tau/pS422 on the surface of neurons was reported to be likely to be endocytosed and degraded in lysosomes in AD model TauPS2APP mice [71]. In addition, Dylight-labeled aggregated tau-Ab complexes were internalized to be detected in iPSC-derived human neurons, although its entry mechanism remains unknown [29]. Furthermore, 4E6G7 (anti-tau/pSer396/pSer404 Ab) labeled with ^{125}I or Alexa Fluor 568 has been reported to enter neurons in brain slice cultures from hTau/PS1 transgenic mice via clathrin-dependent FcγII/IIIR-mediated endocytosis or fluid phase endocytosis in the presence of both intracellular and extracellular tau aggregates. Ab internalization is likely to be necessary for tau reduction in primary neurons [72]. Unknown Ab endosomal escape mechanisms for the clearance of tau after endocytosis may exist, as the receptor-mediated endocytosis of Ab was found to be enhanced in the presence of tau aggregates in neurons. Moreover, after anti-tau Abs were internalized through certain mechanisms and were bound to cytosolic tau, the resultant complexes bound to TRIM21, known as not only E3 ubiquitin ligase but also as FcR, via the Fc domain, were subjected to ubiquitin-mediated degradation [73]. Therefore, the internalization or formation of tau-Ab complexes in the neuronal cytosol and successive ubiquitin degradation via TRIM21 as FcR can also be a promising strategy for intraneuronal tau clearance using anti-tau Abs. Modes of Fc-FcR interactions depend on Ab features, FcR types, and binding tau species.

2.8.2. Transportation across the BBB

Several Abs, such as DMR7, SKT82, and other anti-tau IgG molecules, have been reported to be successfully transported across the BBB in in vivo tests [61]. However, in general, Abs are unable to cross the BBB due to their large size and hydrophilic features. Interestingly, although RmAb158, a mAb against the soluble Aβ protofibrils, was reported to be transported into the central periventricular area across the blood-CSF barrier, some were transported into the cortex through damaged BBB, as a result of leakage [62]. BBB dysfunction is known to occur in AD [74]. mAbs in the bloodstream have a long half-life due to salvation based on FcRn-mediated endocytosis and successive recycling back to the blood stream at the endothelial cells without lysosomal degradation. They may be leaked gradually and specifically into the brain through the injured tight junction of the capillary endothelial cells at the BBB due to their high molecular size, similar to how nanoparticles with payloads accumulate in cancer tissues through the loose tight junctions of endothelial cells via the EPR effect [8]. However, delivery based on Ab leakage at a disordered BBB depends on the conditions of dysfunction, and may not be effective or appropriate for prophylactic use before AD pathogenesis. Therefore, more strategic approaches need to be developed. Potential methodologies are reviewed below. In addition, aducanumab has been reported to dose-dependently lower Aβ plaques in AD and evoke BBB disruption. By contrast, anti-Aβ mAbs that did not evoke BBB disruption did not lower Aβ plaques. Thus, the transendothelial mechanism of aducanumab is thought to be leakage through BBB disruption, most likely due to vasogenic edema or cerebral microhemorrhage [2]. In general, mAbs cannot cross the BBB, and aducanumab has the unique ability to cross the BBB by inducing BBB disruption.

Role of FcRn of the Endothelium at the BBB

FcRn [11] plays a vital role in transferring Abs across enterocytes in the small intestine, podocytes, renal proximal tubular cells of the kidney, and syncytiotrophoblasts of the placenta. In contrast, FcRn endocytoses Abs and recycle them back, via a process known as salvation, in the vascular endothelial cells and hepatocytes of the liver. When IgG Abs are transported to the brain across the endothelium through injured tight junctions, they are likely to be delivered from the brain to the systemic circulation through reverse transcytosis based on FcRn of the endothelial cells at the BBB [75]. This is consistent with the features of general endothelial cells that recycle back IgG molecules in endosomes to the systemic circulation based on FcRn, which results in extending the IgG half-life without being degraded in lysosomes. Furthermore, bystander Abs are internalized into endosomes based on pinocytosis, subsequently bind to FcRn via acidification and are recycled back into the bloodstream. As a result, a delivery strategy using FcRn did not achieve this purpose. Thus, in contrast to mAb delivery across the small intestinal epithelium, mAbs must be transcytosed using other receptor-mediated transcytosis systems to cross the endothelial cells at the BBB.

Transendothelium Based on Receptor-Mediated Transcytosis

Receptor-mediated transcytosis occurs across endothelial cells at the BBB using the insulin receptor (InsR) and transferrin receptor (TfR), as well as other receptors [9]. This indicates that substances conjugated with ligands that bind to such receptors can be delivered across the BBB [76]. TfR and anti-TfR Ab are often used as ligands for transendothelium substance delivery. When ligand-TfR affinity is moderate, the ligand is liberated from TfR by endosome maturation. Subsequently, free ligands are released into the brain through fusion between the basolateral membrane and endosome. On the other hand, when ligand-TfR affinity is high, ligand-TfR complexes are degraded in lysosomes without being released into the brain as a result of the sorting process. In an in vitro assay using SV40-immortalized adult rat brain endothelial cells (SV-ARBEC), among anti-TfR, rat bivalent Ab OX26 variants, namely OX2676 and OX26108 with medium affinity to TfR, were distributed in early endosomes and exhibited enhanced transcytosis, whereas OX265 with high affinity was distributed in late endosomes and lysosomes [77]. Moreover, in in vitro live imaging using bEND.3 cells, bispecific Ab against TfR with low affinity and γ-secretase (BACE1) did not reduce the TfR level, while that with high affinity reduced it by distributing to lysosomes and being degraded there together with TfR [78]. Interestingly, bispecific Ab against TfR and BACE1 intravenously administered in vivo in monkeys was reported to cross the BBB and reduce brain in an Aβ and TfR-dependent manner [79]. A similar system can be applied for bispecific Abs against TfR and tau species.

2.8.3. Plausible Design of mAbs to Clear Tau

In general, mAbs cannot enter the brain across the BBB. Thus, bispecific mAbs with Fc domain targeting not only tau species in the brain but also receptors inducing transcytosis at the BBB represent a promising molecular design (Figure 12). With respect to the intended trajectory: (i) intravenously administered well-designed bispecific mAbs could cross the BBB into the brain through receptor-mediated transcytosis using suitable receptors such as TfR, bind to arbitrary extracellular tau species, and be degraded with captured tau proteins in lysosomes after Fc receptor-mediated endocytosis into microglia (Figure 2); (ii) they can cross the BBB into the brain through receptor-mediated transcytosis using suitable receptors such as TfR, be internalized into neurons through Fc receptor-mediated endocytosis, bind to arbitrary cytosolic tau species after endosomal escape through unknown mechanisms, and be degraded by TRIM21-associated ubiquitin degradation (Figure 13). In particular cases, (iii) they can cross the BBB into the brain through receptor-mediated transcytosis using suitable receptors, such as TfR, bind to tau species, such as tau/pS422, exposed on lipid rafts of neuronal plasma membrane, be internalized into neurons through lipid raft-mediated endocytosis, and be degraded in lysosomes (Figure 14).

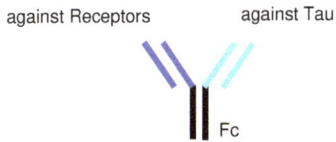

Figure 12. The structure of bispecific IgG against receptors and tau species.

The choice of pathological tau species for use as antigens remains elusive due to complex heterogeneity of tau. Therefore, anti-tau Abs targeting tau species, such as tau oligomers, need to be screened through repetitive in vivo experiments using animal models of AD.

2.8.4. Combination Therapies

The pathology of AD is widely considered to progress in a highly complex manner. Therefore, combination therapies represent potentially successful strategies for enhancing the therapeutic efficacy of AD treatment. This is supported by the fact that, to date, single-modality therapies have failed to show effectiveness against AD.

While senile plaques have been reported to be eliminated by active immunotherapy using AN-1792, dementia resulting from AD proceeded in this case, with no neurons firing there, according to Mach's principle of perception. In other words, nerve regeneration did not occur in response to treatment. Most likely, glial cells occupied the empty space after neuronal death. Based on these results, there is a need to pave the way for nerve regeneration in AD pathology. PD symptoms were reported to improve by injecting the fetal brain into the brains of PD patients aged 60 and younger [80]. Furthermore, umbilical cord matrix stem cell (UCMSC) transplantation was reported to improve the rotational behavior of PD model rats [81]. However, the sampling and use of fetal brain cells or UCMSCs is made difficult by their limited numbers and associated ethical issues. Mesenchymal stem cells (MSCs), which were first found in 2001, represent an alternative for differentiation into neurons. Autologous adipose-derived MSC therapy has been used for the treatment of several neurological diseases, including brain stem hemorrhage and cerebral infarction, and neurodegenerative diseases, such as amyotrophic lateral sclerosis (ALS), AD, PD, and neuropathy. In general, stem cells have the ability to spontaneously migrate to sites of injury, nidus, and regeneration [82], via the so-called homing process, and are able to cross the BBB after their intravenous administration.

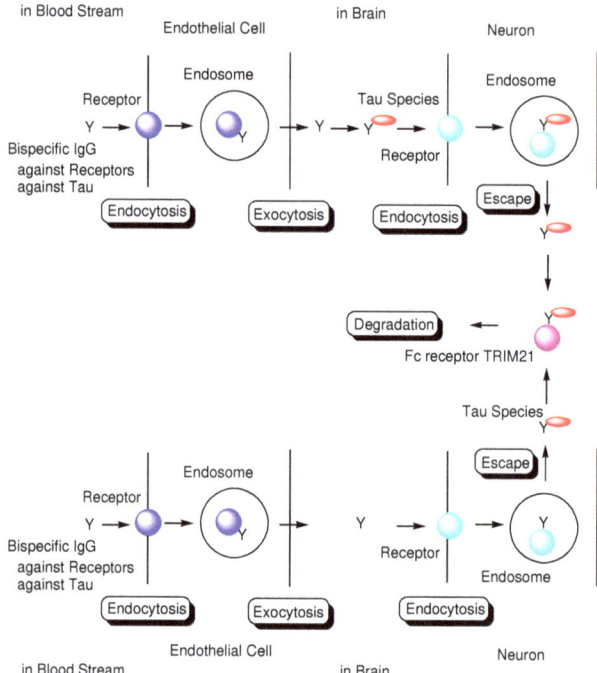

Figure 13. Tau degradation by the ubiquitin-proteasome pathway through Fc receptor-mediated endocytosis in neurons using bispecific Abs against tau and receptors. TRIM21 stands for tripartite motif-containing protein 21.

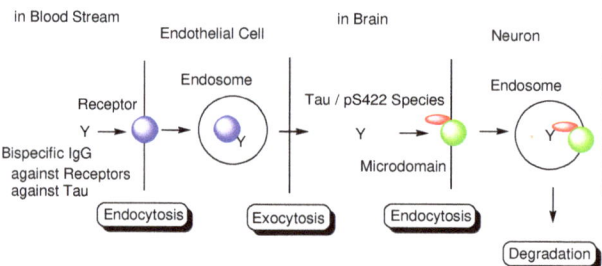

Figure 14. Tau/pS422 species lysosomal degradation through membrane microdomain-mediated endocytosis in neurons using bispecific Abs against tau/pS422 and receptors.

Even though tau oligomers of mild-to-moderate dementia patients are eliminated by anti-tau mAbs, Aβ oligomers may not only continue to injure neurons but also enhance the production of pathological tau oligomers as seeds, and must therefore also be eliminated. AN-1792-induced anti-Aβ Abs have been reported to eliminate senile plaques [16], although they did not eliminate all Aβ oligomers [17]. Aβ can be cleared by AN-1792-induced anti-

Aβ Abs outside the BBB via the dynamic equilibrium of Aβ between the brain and blood plasma [83]. Thus, Aβ-targeting vaccines may be effective for AD therapy.

Combination therapy using three agents, namely anti-tau oligomer and anti-TfR bispecific mAbs, AN-1792, and MSCs, could be an extraordinarily effective and economical method for the treatment of mild-to-moderate dementia in AD patients. During and after therapy, sustained recovery can be verified using magnetic resonance imaging (MRI) against Aβ and tau. When AN-1792 elicits acute meningoencephalitis, other Aβ-targeting vaccines can be utilized. Furthermore, low-molecular compounds, such as Hes1 dimer inhibitors for neural stem cell (NSC) differentiation [84] and histone deacetylase 3 (HDAC3) inhibitors [85] and SIRT2 inhibitors [86] for neurodegenerative diseases (Figure 15), can be used in combination with immunotherapy.

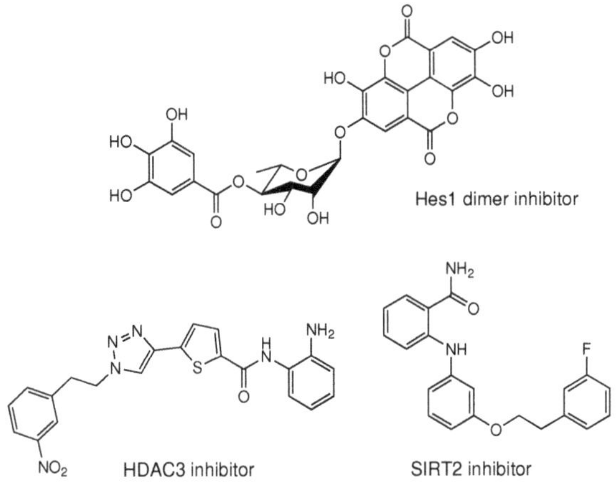

Figure 15. Structures of neurodegenerative disease modulators.

3. Conclusions

The development of drugs for the treatment of AD has been made difficult not only due to impermeability of drugs into the brain via the BBB [9], but also due to the complex mechanisms of AD pathogenesis, wherein the pathological mechanisms of Aβ and tau are known to play crucial roles. Almost all clinical trials using Aβ modulators have failed their respective stages, with aducanumab, anti-insoluble Aβ fibrils, and anti-soluble Aβ oligomer mAb being approved by the FDA in 2021. It has been revealed that the pathologies of Aβ and tau initially progress independently, only beginning to exert their influence on each other after some time. Subsequently, the pathology of AD reaches a point of no return [4]. NFTs composed of tau rather than senile plaques composed of Aβ are correlated with AD pathogenesis [5]. It has been suggested that once certain types of tau seeds are formed, AD pathology progresses via these seed species. Accordingly, the amyloid hypothesis has been modified based on the results of clinical trial and novel findings. Tau species are thought to spread from cell to cell and be duplicated based on seeds in a prion-like manner [25]. Thus, the elimination of toxic tau seed species using specific Abs represents a promising strategy for the treatment of AD. Nonetheless, although clinical trials using anti-tau Abs have been performed, none of these have managed to reach phase 3, due to the fact that the BBB impedes the entry of anti-tau Abs into the brain. Therefore, an alternative drug design needs to be developed. Intravenously administered bispecific Abs against tau and receptors that induce receptor-mediated transcytosis in capillary endothelial cells across the BBB may represent a solution to the aforementioned trajectory issues. Furthermore, as a tau elimination mechanism, (i) tau-Ab complexes may be internalized into microglia through FcR-mediated endocytosis and degraded in lysosomes (Figure 2); (ii) anti-tau Abs may be internalized into neurons through FcR-mediated endocytosis, capture cytosolic tau species after endosomal escape, and finally be degraded by the ubiquitin pathway after binding to TRIM21 as FcR and E3 ubiquitin ligase (Figure 13); (iii) Ab complexes with tau species, such as tau/pS422, which exist on lipid rafts of neuronal plasma membrane, may be internalized into neurons through lipid raft-mediated endocytosis and degraded in lysosomes (Figure 14). Salvation by FcRn in endothelial cells can lengthen the half-life of intravenously administered bispecific Abs.

The complexity of AD pathology is so high that single-modality therapies have been widely found to be ineffective. Therefore, combination therapies have been suggested to increase the therapeutic efficacy of AD treatments. The combination of bispecific Abs against tau and receptors at capillary endothelial cells, Aβ modulators, such as AN-1792 as vaccine, and stem cells, such as MSCs, via intravenous administration are potential candidates. Furthermore, low-molecular-weight compounds may be used in combination with these treatments. Aducanumab is known to cross the BBB by disturbing it. Thus, combination therapy using aducanumab, anti-tau Abs, and MSCs represents an alternative treatment. In the field of neuroscience, qualia are defined as sensory consciousness by which a person recalls "what a certain thing is like" in the brain. When dementia as a result of AD is treated via nerve cell regeneration, whether qualia are restored remains unclear, since they are formed through individual experiences. Nonetheless, medicinal chemists and pharmaceutical scientists hope to improve the quality of life of AD patients by creating innovative immunotherapy approaches using well-designed antibodies targeting AD-relevant tau species.

Funding: This research received no external funding.

Institutional Review Board Statement: Not applicable.

Informed Consent Statement: Not applicable.

Data Availability Statement: ClinicalTrials.gov (accessed on 25 December 2021) Identifier can be found at https://clinicaltrials.gov/ (accessed on 25 December 2021).

Acknowledgments: This review is just my opinion based on or inferred from available published articles and public knowledge. Thus, the intellectual property rights are not infringed upon.

Conflicts of Interest: The author declares no conflict of interest.

References

1. Stimulus package. *Nat. Med.* **2018**, *24*, 247. [CrossRef] [PubMed]
2. Pardridge, W.M. Blood-Brain Barrier and Delivery of Protein and Gene Therapeutics to Brain. *Front. Aging Neurosci.* **2020**, *11*, 373. [CrossRef] [PubMed]
3. Breijyeh, Z.; Karaman, R. Comprehensive Review on Alzheimer's Disease: Causes and Treatment. *Molecules* **2020**, *25*, 5789. [CrossRef] [PubMed]
4. Jack, C.R., Jr.; Knopman, D.S.; Jagust, W.J.; Petersen, R.C.; Weiner, M.W.; Aisen, P.S.; Shaw, L.M.; Vemuri, P.; Wiste, H.J.; Weigand, S.D.; et al. Tracking pathophysiological processes in Alzheimer's disease: An updated hypothetical model of dynamic biomarkers. *Lancet Neurol.* **2013**, *12*, 207–216. [CrossRef]
5. Bierer, L.M.; Hof, P.R.; Purohit, D.P.; Carlin, L.; Schmeidler, J.; Davis, K.L.; Perl, D.P. Neocortical neurofibrillary tangles correlate with dementia severity in Alzheimer's disease. *Arch. Neurol.* **1995**, *52*, 81–88. [CrossRef] [PubMed]
6. Tashima, T. Intriguing possibilities and beneficial aspects of transporter-conscious drug design. *Bioorg. Med. Chem.* **2015**, *23*, 4119–4131. [CrossRef]
7. Tashima, T. Intelligent substance delivery into cells using cell-penetrating peptides. *Bioorg. Med. Chem. Lett.* **2017**, *27*, 121–130. [CrossRef]
8. Tashima, T. Effective cancer therapy based on selective drug delivery into cells across their membrane using receptor-mediated endocytosis. *Bioorg. Med. Chem. Lett.* **2018**, *28*, 3015–3024. [CrossRef]
9. Tashima, T. Smart Strategies for Therapeutic Agent Delivery into Brain across the Blood-Brain Barrier Using Receptor-Mediated Transcytosis. *Chem. Pharm. Bull.* **2020**, *68*, 316–325. [CrossRef]
10. Tashima, T. Shortcut Approaches to Substance Delivery into the Brain Based on Intranasal Administration Using Nanodelivery Strategies for Insulin. *Molecules* **2020**, *25*, 5188. [CrossRef]
11. Tashima, T. Delivery of Orally Administered Digestible Antibodies Using Nanoparticles. *Int. J. Mol. Sci.* **2021**, *22*, 3349. [CrossRef] [PubMed]

12. Joseph Gaugler, J.; James, B.; Johnson, T.; Reimer, J.; Weuve, J. Alzheimer's disease facts and figures. *Alzheimer's Dement.* **2021**, *17*, 327–406. [CrossRef]
13. WHO. Dementia. Available online: https://www.who.int/news-room/fact-sheets/detail/dementia (accessed on 10 November 2021).
14. Kent, S.A.; Spires-Jones, T.L.; Durrant, C.S. The physiological roles of tau and Aβ: Implications for Alzheimer's disease pathology and therapeutics. *Acta Neuropathol.* **2020**, *140*, 417–447. [CrossRef] [PubMed]
15. Umeda, T.; Maekawa, S.; Kimura, T.; Takashima, A.; Tomiyama, T.; Mori, H. Neurofibrillary tangle formation by introducing wild-type human tau into APP transgenic mice. *Acta Neuropathol.* **2014**, *127*, 685–698. [CrossRef] [PubMed]
16. Holmes, C.; Boche, D.; Wilkinson, D.; Yadegarfar, G.; Hopkins, V.; Bayer, A.; Jones, R.W.; Bullock, R.; Love, S.; Neal, J.W.; et al. Long-term effects of Abeta42 immunisation in Alzheimer's disease: Follow-up of a randomised, placebo-controlled phase I trial. *Lancet* **2008**, *372*, 216–223. [CrossRef]
17. Maarouf, C.L.; Daugs, I.D.; Kokjohn, T.A.; Kalback, W.M.; Patton, R.L.; Luehrs, D.C.; Masliah, E.; Nicoll, J.A.R.; Sabbagh, M.N.; Beach, T.G.; et al. The biochemical aftermath of anti-amyloid immunotherapy. *Mol. Neurodegener.* **2010**, *5*, 39. [CrossRef]
18. Brunello, C.A.; Merezhko, M.; Uronen, R.-L.; Huttunen, H.J. Mechanisms of secretion and spreading of pathological tau protein. *Cell Mol. Life Sci.* **2020**, *77*, 1721–1744. [CrossRef]
19. Kopke, E.; Tung, Y.-C.; Shaikh, S.; Alonso, A.C.; Iqbal, K.; Grundke-Iqbal, I. Microtubule-associated protein tau. Abnormal phosphorylation of a non-paired helical filament pool in Alzheimer disease. *J. Biol. Chem.* **1993**, *268*, 24374–24384. [CrossRef]
20. Santacruz, K.; Lewis, J.; Spires, T.; Paulson, J.; Kotilinek, L.; Ingelsson, M.; Guimaraes, A.; De Ture, M.; Ramsden, M.; McGowan, E.; et al. Tau suppression in a neurodegenerative mouse model improves memory function. *Science* **2005**, *309*, 476–481. [CrossRef]
21. Kuchibhotla, K.V.; Wegmann, S.; Kopeikina, K.J.; Hawkes, J.; Rudinskiy, N.; Andermann, M.L.; Spires-Jones, T.L.; Bacskai, B.J.; Hyman, B.T. Neurofibrillary tangle-bearing neurons are functionally integrated in cortical circuits in vivo. *Proc. Natl. Acad. Sci. USA* **2014**, *111*, 510–514. [CrossRef]
22. Bittar, A.; Bhatt, N.; Kayed, R. Advances and considerations in AD tau-targeted immunotherapy. *Neurobiol. Dis.* **2020**, *134*, 104707. [CrossRef] [PubMed]
23. Kuzuhara, S.; Ihara, Y.; Toyokura, Y.; Shimada, H. A semiquantitative study on Alzheimer neurofibrillary tangles demonstrated immunohistochemically with anti-tau antibodies, in the brains of non-demented and demented old people. *No Shinkei = Brain Nerve* **1989**, *41*, 465–470.
24. Braak, H.; Braak, E. Frequency of stages of Alzheimer-related lesions in different age categories. *Neurobiol. Aging* **1997**, *18*, 351–357. [CrossRef]
25. Tarutani, A.; Miyata, H.; Nonaka, T.; Hasegawa, K.; Yoshida, M.; Saito, Y.; Murayama, S.; Robinson, A.C.; Mann, D.M.A.; Tomita, T.; et al. Human tauopathy-derived tau strains determine the substrates recruited for templated amplification. *Brain* **2021**, *144*, 2333–2348. [CrossRef] [PubMed]
26. Pernègre, C.; Duquette, A.; Leclerc, N. Tau Secretion: Good and Bad for Neurons. *Front. Neurosci.* **2019**, *13*, 649. [CrossRef] [PubMed]
27. Jiang, S.; Bhaskar, K. Degradation and Transmission of Tau by Autophagic-Endolysosomal Networks and Potential Therapeutic Targets for Tauopathy. *Front. Mol. Neurosci.* **2020**, *13*, 586731. [CrossRef] [PubMed]
28. Barini, E.; Plotzky, G.; Mordashova, Y.; Hoppe, J.; Rodriguez-Correa, E.; Julier, S.; LePrieult, F.; Mairhofer, I.; Mezler, M.; Biesinger, S.; et al. Tau in the brain interstitial fluid is fragmented and seeding–competent. *Neurobiol. Aging* **2021**, *109*, 64–77. [CrossRef]
29. Evans, L.D.; Wassmer, T.; Fraser, G.; Smith, J.; Perkinton, M.; Billinton, A.; Livesey, F.J. Extracellular Monomeric and Aggregated Tau Efficiently Enter Human Neurons through Overlapping but Distinct Pathways. *Cell Rep.* **2018**, *22*, 3612–3624. [CrossRef]
30. Puangmalai, N.; Bhatt, N.; Montalbano, M.; Sengupta, U.; Gaikwad, S.; Ventura, F.; McAllen, S.; Ellsworth, A.; Garcia, S.; Kayed, R. Internalization mechanisms of brain-derived tau oligomers from patients with Alzheimer's disease, progressive supranuclear palsy and dementia with Lewy bodies. *Cell Death Dis.* **2020**, *11*, 314. [CrossRef]
31. Christianson, H.C.; Belting, M. Heparan sulfate proteoglycan as a cell-surface endocytosis receptor. *Matrix Biol.* **2014**, *35*, 51–55. [CrossRef]
32. Zhu, H.-L.; Fernández, C.; Fan, J.-B.; Shewmaker, F.; Chen, J.; Minton, A.P.; Liang, Y. Quantitative characterization of heparin binding to Tau protein: Implication for inducer-mediated Tau filament formation. *J. Biol. Chem.* **2010**, *5*, 3592–3599. [CrossRef] [PubMed]
33. Giamblanco, N.; Fichou, Y.; Janot, J.-M.; Balanzat, E.; Han, S.; Balme, S. Mechanisms of Heparin-Induced Tau Aggregation Revealed by a Single Nanopore. *ACS Sens.* **2020**, *24*, 1158–1167. [CrossRef] [PubMed]
34. Rauch, J.N.; Luna, G.; Guzman, E.; Audouard, M.; Challis, C.; Sibih, Y.E.; Leshuk, C.; Hernandez, I.; Wegmann, S.; Hyman, B.T.; et al. LRP1 is a master regulator of tau uptake and spread. *Nature* **2020**, *580*, 381–385. [CrossRef] [PubMed]
35. Morozova, V.; Cohen, L.S.; Makki, A.E.-H.; Shur, A.; Pilar, G.; Idrissi, A.E.; Alonso, A.D. Normal and Pathological Tau Uptake Mediated by M1/M3 Muscarinic Receptors Promotes Opposite Neuronal Changes. *Front. Cell. Neurosci.* **2019**, *13*, 403. [CrossRef]
36. La-Rocque, S.D.; Moretto, E.; Butnaru, I.; Schiavo, G. Knockin' on heaven's door: Molecular mechanisms of neuronal tau uptake. *J. Neurochem.* **2021**, *156*, 563–588. [CrossRef] [PubMed]
37. Dujardin, S.; Bégard, S.; Caillierez, R.; Lachaud, C.; Delattre, L.; Carrier, S.; Loyens, A.; Galas, M.-C.; Bousset, L.; Melki, R.; et al. Ectosomes: A new mechanism for non-exosomal secretion of tau protein. *PLoS ONE* **2014**, *9*, e100760. [CrossRef]

38. Merezhko, M.; Brunello, C.A.; Yan, X.; Vihinen, H.; Jokitalo, E.; Uronen, R.-L.; Huttunen, H.J. Secretion of Tau via an Unconventional Non-vesicular Mechanism. *Cell Rep.* **2018**, *25*, 2027–2035. [CrossRef]
39. Debaisieux, S.; Rayne, F.; Yezid, H.; Beaumelle, B. The Ins and Outs of HIV-1 Tat. *Traffic* **2012**, *13*, 355–363. [CrossRef]
40. Steringer, J.P.; Nickel, W. A direct gateway into the extracellular space: Unconventional secretion of FGF2 through self-sustained plasma membrane pore. *Cell Dev. Biol.* **2018**, *83*, 3–7. [CrossRef]
41. Zurzolo, C. Tunneling nanotubes: Reshaping connectivity. *Curr. Opin. Cell Biol.* **2021**, *71*, 139–147. [CrossRef]
42. Gerson, J.E.; Sengupta, U.; Lasagna-Reeves, C.A.; Guerrero-Muñoz, M.J.; Troncoso, J.; Kayed, R. Characterization of tau oligomeric seeds in progressive supranuclear palsy. *Acta Neuropathol. Commun.* **2014**, *2*, 73. [CrossRef] [PubMed]
43. Pampuscenko, K.; Morkuniene, R.; Krasauskas, L.; Smirnovas, V.; Tomita, T.; Borutaite, V. Distinct Neurotoxic Effects of Extracellular Tau Species in Primary Neuronal-Glial Cultures. *Mol. Neurobiol.* **2021**, *58*, 658–667. [CrossRef] [PubMed]
44. Mondragón-Rodríguez, S.; Trillaud-Doppia, E.; Dudilot, A.; Bourgeois, C.; Lauzon, M.; Leclerc, N.; Boehm, J. Interaction of endogenous tau protein with synaptic proteins is regulated by N-methyl-D-aspartate receptor-dependent tau phosphorylation. *J. Biol. Chem.* **2012**, *287*, 32040–32053. [CrossRef] [PubMed]
45. Rudy, C.C.; Hunsberger, H.C.; Weitzner, D.S.; Reed, M.N. The Role of the Tripartite Glutamatergic Synapse in the Pathophysiology of Alzheimer's Disease. *Aging Dis.* **2015**, *6*, 131–148. [CrossRef]
46. Tovar, K.R.; Westbrook, G.L. The Incorporation of NMDA Receptors with a Distinct Subunit Composition at Nascent Hippocampal Synapses In Vitro. *J. Neurosci.* **1999**, *19*, 4180–4188. [CrossRef]
47. Angulo, M.C.; Kozlov, A.S.; Charpak, S.; Audinat, E. Glutamate Released from Glial Cells Synchronizes Neuronal Activity in the Hippocampus. *J. Neurosci.* **2004**, *2*, 6920–6927. [CrossRef]
48. Tovar, K.R.; McGinley, M.J.; Westbrook, G.L. Triheteromeric NMDA Receptors at Hippocampal Synapses. *J. Neurosci.* **2013**, *33*, 9150–9160. [CrossRef]
49. Castro-Alvarez, J.F.; Uribe-Arias, S.A.; Mejía-Raigosa, D.; Cardona-Gómez, G.P. Cyclin-dependent kinase 5, a node protein in diminished tauopathy: A systems biology approach. *Front. Aging Neurosci.* **2014**, *6*, 232. [CrossRef]
50. Matrone, C.; Petrillo, F.; Nasso, R.; Ferretti, G. Fyn Tyrosine Kinase as Harmonizing Factor in Neuronal Functions and Dysfunctions. *Int. J. Mol. Sci.* **2020**, *21*, 4444. [CrossRef]
51. Larson, M.; Sherman, M.A.; Amar, F.; Nuvolone, M.; Schneider, J.A.; Bennett, D.A.; Aguzzi, A.; Nuvolone, M.; Lesné, S.E. The Complex PrP^C-Fyn Couples Human Oligomeric Aβ with Pathological Tau Changes in Alzheimer's Disease. *J. Neurosci.* **2012**, *3*, 16857–16871. [CrossRef]
52. Goebel-Goody, S.M.; Davies, K.D.; Linger, R.M.A.; Freund, R.K.; Browning, M.D. Phospho-regulation of synaptic and extrasynaptic N-methyl-d-aspartate receptors in adult hippocampal slices. *Neuroscience* **2009**, *158*, 1446–1459. [CrossRef] [PubMed]
53. Ittner, L.M.; Ke, Y.D.; Delerue, F.; Bi, M.; Gladbach, A.; Eersel, J.V.; Wölfing, H.; Chieng, B.C.; Christie, M.J.; Napier, I.A.; et al. Dendritic function of tau mediates amyloid-beta toxicity in Alzheimer's disease mouse models. *Cell* **2010**, *142*, 387–397. [CrossRef] [PubMed]
54. Lopes, S.; Vaz-Silva, J.; Pinto, V.; Dalla, C.; Kokras, N.; Bedenk, B.; Natalie, M.; Czisch, M.; Almeida, O.F.X.; Sousa, N. Tau protein is essential for stress-induced brain pathology. *Proc. Natl. Acad. Sci. USA* **2016**, *113*, E3755–E3763. [CrossRef]
55. Miyamoto, T.; Stein, L.; Thomas, R.; Djukic, B.; Taneja, P.; Knox, J.; Vossel, K.; Mucke, L. Phosphorylation of tau at Y18, but not tau-fyn binding, is required for tau to modulate NMDA receptor-dependent excitotoxicity in primary neuronal culture. *Mol. Neurodegener.* **2017**, *12*, 41. [CrossRef]
56. Amar, F.; Sherman, M.A.; Rush, T.; Larson, M.; Boyle, G.; Chang, L.; Götz, J.; Buisson, A.; Lesné, S.E. The amyloid-β oligomer Aβ*56 induces specific alterations in neuronal signaling that lead to tau phosphorylation and aggregation. *Sci. Signal.* **2017**, *10*, eaal2021. [CrossRef] [PubMed]
57. Huang, Y.-R.; Liu, R.-T. The Toxicity and Polymorphism of β-Amyloid Oligomers. *Int. J. Mol. Sci.* **2020**, *21*, 4477. [CrossRef] [PubMed]
58. Ittner, A.; Ittner, L.M. Dendritic Tau in Alzheimer's Disease. *Neuron* **2018**, *99*, 13–27. [CrossRef] [PubMed]
59. Zhang, F.; Gannon, M.; Chen, Y.; Yan, S.; Zhang, S.; Feng, W.; Tao, J.; Sha, B.; Liu, Z.; Saito, T.; et al. β-amyloid redirects norepinephrine signaling to activate the pathogenic GSK3β/tau cascade. *Sci. Transl. Med.* **2020**, *12*, eaay1769. [CrossRef]
60. Wu, H.; Wei, S.; Huang, Y.; Chen, L.; Wang, Y.; Wu, X.; Zhang, Z.; Pei, Y.; Wang, D. Aβ monomer induces phosphorylation of Tau at Ser-214 through β2AR-PKA-JNK signaling pathway. *FASEB J.* **2020**, *34*, 5092–5105. [CrossRef] [PubMed]
61. Gibbons, G.S.; Kim, S.-J.; Wu, Q.; Riddle, D.M.; Leight, S.N.; Changolkar, L.; Xu, H.; Meymand, E.S.; O'Reilly, M.; Zhang, B.; et al. Conformation-selective tau monoclonal antibodies inhibit tau pathology in primary neurons and a mouse model of Alzheimer's disease. *Mol. Neurodegener.* **2020**, *15*, 64. [CrossRef] [PubMed]
62. Andersson, C.R.; Falsig, J.; Stavenhagen, J.B.; Christensen, S.; Kartberg, F.; Rosenqvist, N.; Finsen, B.; Pedersen, J.T. Antibody-mediated clearance of tau in primary mouse microglial cultures requires Fcγ-receptor binding and functional lysosomes. *Sci. Rep.* **2019**, *9*, 4658. [CrossRef] [PubMed]
63. Fuller, J.P.; Stavenhagen, J.B.; Teeling, J.L. New roles for Fc receptors in neurodegeneration-the impact on Immunotherapy for Alzheimer's Disease. *Front. Neurosci.* **2014**, *8*, 235. [CrossRef] [PubMed]
64. Zilkova, M.; Nolle, A.; Kovacech, B.; Kontsekova, E.; Weisova, P.; Filipcik, P.; Skrabana, R.; Prcina, M.; Hromadka, T.; Cehlar, O.; et al. Humanized tau antibodies promote tau uptake by human microglia without any increase of inflammation. *Acta Neuropathol. Commun.* **2020**, *8*, 74. [CrossRef] [PubMed]

65. Novak, P.; Schmidt, R.; Kontsekova, E.; Kovacech, B.; Smolek, T.; Katina, S.; Lubica Fialova, L.; Prcina, M.; Parrak, V.; Dal-Bianco, P.; et al. Fundamant: An interventional 72-week phase 1 follow-up study of AADvac1, an active immunotherapy against tau protein pathology in Alzheimer's disease. *Alzheimer's Res. Ther.* **2018**, *24*, 108. [CrossRef]
66. Novak, P.; Kovacech, B.; Katina, S.; Schmidt, R.; Scheltens, P.; Kontsekova, E.; Ropele, S.; Fialova, L.; Kramberger, M.; Paulenka-Ivanovova, N.; et al. Adamant: A placebo-controlled randomized phase 2 study of AADvac1, an active immunotherapy against pathological tau in Alzheimer's disease. *Nat. Aging* **2021**, *1*, 521–534. [CrossRef]
67. Mullard, A. Failure of first anti-tau antibody in Alzheimer disease highlights risks of history repeating. *Nat. Rev. Drug Discov.* **2021**, *20*, 3–5. [CrossRef]
68. Mader, S.; Brimberg, L. Aquaporin-4 Water Channel in the Brain and Its Implication for Health and Disease. *Cells* **2019**, *8*, 90. [CrossRef]
69. Noble, W.; Spires-Jones, T.L. Sleep well to slow Alzheimer's progression? *Science* **2019**, *363*, 813–814. [CrossRef]
70. Luo, W.; Liu, W.; Hu, X.; Hanna, M.; Caravaca, A.; Paul, S.M. Microglial internalization and degradation of pathological tau is enhanced by an anti-tau monoclonal antibody. *Sci. Rep.* **2015**, *5*, 11161. [CrossRef]
71. Collin, L.; Bohrmann, B.; Göpfert, U.; Oroszlan-Szovik, K.; Ozmen, L.; Grüninger, F. Neuronal uptake of tau/pS422 antibody and reduced progression of tau pathology in a mouse model of Alzheimer's disease. *Brain* **2014**, *137*, 2834–2846. [CrossRef]
72. Congdon, E.E.; Gu, J.; Sait, H.B.R.; Sigurdsson, E.M. Antibody uptake into neurons occurs primarily via clathrin-dependent Fcγ receptor endocytosis and is a prerequisite for acute tau protein clearance. *J. Biol. Chem.* **2013**, *288*, 35452–35465. [CrossRef] [PubMed]
73. McEwan, W.A.; Falcon, B.; Vaysburd, M.; Clift, D.; Oblak, A.L.; Ghetti, B.; Goedert, M.; James, L.C. Cytosolic Fc receptor TRIM21 inhibits seeded tau aggregation. *Proc. Natl. Acad. Sci. USA* **2017**, *114*, 74–579. [CrossRef] [PubMed]
74. Nation, D.A.; Sweeney, M.D.; Montagne, A.; Sagare, A.P.; D'Orazio, L.M.; Pachicano, M.; Sepehrband, F.; Nelson, A.R.; Buennagel, D.P.; Harrington, M.G.; et al. Blood–brain barrier breakdown is an early biomarker of human cognitive dysfunction. *Nat. Med.* **2019**, *25*, 270–276. [CrossRef] [PubMed]
75. Caram-Salas, N.; Boileau, E.; Farrington, G.K.; Garber, E.; Brunette, E.; Abulrob, A.; Stanimirovic, D. In vitro and in vivo methods for assessing FcRn-mediated reverse transcytosis across the blood-brain barrier. *Methods Mol. Biol.* **2011**, *763*, 383–401. [CrossRef] [PubMed]
76. Lajoie, J.M.; Shusta, E.V. Targeting receptor-mediated transport for delivery of biologics across the blood-brain barrier. *Annu. Rev. Pharmacol. Toxicol.* **2015**, *55*, 613–631. [CrossRef] [PubMed]
77. Haqqani, A.S.; Thom, G.; Burrell, M.; Delaney, C.E.; Brunette, E.; Baumann, E.; Sodja, C.; Jezierski, A.; Webster, C.; Stanimirovic, D.B. Intracellular sorting and transcytosis of the rat transferrin receptor antibody OX26 across the blood-brain barrier in vitro is dependent on its binding affinity. *J. Neurochem.* **2018**, *146*, 735–752. [CrossRef]
78. Bien-Ly, N.; Yu, Y.J.; Bumbaca, D.; Elstrott, J.; Boswell, C.A.; Zhang, Y.; Luk, W.; Lu, Y.; Dennis, M.S.; Weimer, R.M.; et al. Transferrin receptor (TfR) trafficking determines brain uptake of TfR antibody affinity variants. *J. Exp. Med.* **2014**, *211*, 233–244. [CrossRef]
79. Yu, J.J.; Atwal, J.K.; Zhang, Y.; Tong, R.K.; Wildsmith, K.R.; Tan, C.; Bien-Ly, N.; Hersom, M.; Maloney, J.A.; Meilandt, W.J.; et al. Therapeutic bispecific antibodies cross the blood-brain barrier in nonhuman primates. *Sci. Transl. Med.* **2014**, *6*, 261ra154. [CrossRef]
80. Lindvall, O.; Rehncrona, S.; Gustavii, B.; Brundin, P.; Astedt, B.; Widner, H.; Lindholm, T.; Björklund, A.; Leenders, K.L.; Rothwell, J.C.; et al. Fetal dopamine-rich mesencephalic grafts in Parkinson's disease. *Lancet* **1988**, *2*, 1483–1484. [CrossRef]
81. Weiss, M.L.; Medicetty, S.; Bledsoe, A.R.; Rachakatla, R.S.; Choi, M.; Merchav, S.; Luo, Y.; Rao, M.S.; Velagaleti, G.; Troyer, D. Human umbilical cord matrix stem cells: Preliminary characterization and effect of transplantation in a rodent model of Parkinson's disease. *Stem Cells* **2006**, *24*, 781–792. [CrossRef]
82. Liesveld, J.L.; Sharma, N.; Aljitawi, O.S. Stem cell homing: From physiology to therapeutics. *Stem Cells* **2020**, *38*, 1241–1253. [CrossRef] [PubMed]
83. DeMattos, R.B.; Bales, K.R.; Cummins, D.J.; Dodart, J.C.; Paul, S.M.; Holtzman, D.M. Peripheral anti-Aβ antibody alters CNS and plasma Aβ clearance and decreases brain Aβ burden in a mouse model of Alzheimer's disease. *Proc. Natl. Acad. Sci. USA* **2001**, *98*, 8850–8855. [CrossRef] [PubMed]
84. Arai, M.A. Target Protein-Oriented Isolations for Bioactive Natural Products. *Chem. Pharm. Bull.* **2021**, *69*, 503–515. [CrossRef] [PubMed]
85. Suzuki, T.; Kasuya, Y.; Itoh, Y.; Ota, Y.; Zhan, P.; Asamitsu, K.; Nakagawa, H.; Okamoto, T.; Miyata, N. Identification of Highly Selective and Potent Histone Deacetylase 3 Inhibitors Using Click Chemistry-Based Combinatorial Fragment Assembly. *PLoS ONE* **2013**, *14*, e68669. [CrossRef] [PubMed]
86. Suzuki, T.; Khan, M.N.A.; Sawada, H.; Imai, E.; Itoh, Y.; Yamatsuta, K.; Tokuda, N.; Takeuchi, J.; Seko, T.; Nakagawa, H.; et al. Design, synthesis, and biological activity of a novel series of human sirtuin-2-selective inhibitors. *J. Med. Chem.* **2012**, *55*, 5760–5773. [CrossRef] [PubMed]

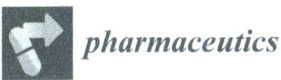

Review

Current Approaches to Monitor Macromolecules Directly from the Cerebral Interstitial Fluid

Marie-Laure Custers, Liam Nestor, Dimitri De Bundel, Ann Van Eeckhaut and Ilse Smolders *

Laboratory of Pharmaceutical Chemistry, Drug Analysis and Drug Information (FASC), Research Group Experimental Pharmacology (EFAR), Center for Neurosciences (C4N), Vrije Universiteit Brussel (VUB), Laarbeeklaan 103, 1090 Brussels, Belgium; marie-laure.custers@vub.be (M.-L.C.); liam.nestor@vub.be (L.N.); dimitri.de.bundel@vub.be (D.D.B.); aveeckha@vub.be (A.V.E.)
* Correspondence: ilse.smolders@vub.be

Abstract: Gaining insights into the pharmacokinetic and pharmacodynamic properties of lead compounds is crucial during drug development processes. When it comes to the treatment of brain diseases, collecting information at the site of action is challenging. There are only a few techniques available that allow for the direct sampling from the cerebral interstitial space. This review concerns the applicability of microdialysis and other approaches, such as cerebral open flow microperfusion and electrochemical biosensors, to monitor macromolecules (neuropeptides, proteins, . . .) in the brain. Microdialysis and cerebral open flow microperfusion can also be used to locally apply molecules at the same time at the site of sampling. Innovations in the field are discussed, together with the pitfalls. Moreover, the 'nuts and bolts' of the techniques and the current research gaps are addressed. The implementation of these techniques could help to improve drug development of brain-targeted drugs.

Keywords: microdialysis; cerebral open flow microperfusion; electrochemical biosensors; macromolecules

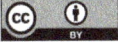

1. Introduction

Drug discovery and development processes are a lengthy, costly, uncertain, and thus challenging endeavor [1]. In this respect, designing medicines that specifically target the central nervous system (CNS) adds another layer of complexity. Apart from our still-limited understanding of the CNS, the presence of the blood–brain barrier (BBB) lies at the root of this problem [2].

Since the 1980s, when the first biological drug was approved by the Food and Drug Administration (FDA), the therapeutic landscape has drastically changed [3,4]. Although considerable progress has been made in the treatment of numerous cancers and autoimmune diseases using biologics, patients with neurological diseases cannot yet widely benefit from this revolution in drug development [5,6]. Due to the innate resistance of the BBB to the permeation of large molecules, concentrations of the biologics at the site of action are too low to achieve the desired therapeutic effect [2]. For instance, in June 2021, the FDA approved aducanumab, a first-of-its-kind disease-modifying drug used for the treatment of Alzheimer's Disease. The FDA approval was groundbreaking in the field of neurology, but highly debated. Moreover, in December 2021, aducanumab was eventually even rejected by the European Medicines Agency because the clinical benefits were ambiguous [5–7]. Apart from the rising levels of skepticism toward the validity of the classic amyloid cascade hypothesis, the poor clinical outcome of the biologic can possibly also be attributed to the lack of a brain-targeted drug delivery transport system following systemic administration [8].

Gaining insights into the pharmacokinetic and pharmacodynamic properties of lead compounds is crucial during drug development processes. When it comes to the treatment of brain diseases, collecting information at the site of action is challenging. Cerebrospinal fluid (CSF) concentrations do not necessarily reflect the real concentration in the brain parenchyma. Drug concentrations in the CSF give information regarding drug transport across the choroid plexus, which is the main component of the blood–CSF barrier, but such concentrations do not provide information concerning BBB transport. This misconception hinders progress in the development of drugs targeting the CNS, as explained by Pardridge [9]. Moreover, in recent years, the discovery of the glymphatic system, acting as a clearance pathway in the brain, stirred the debate about brain fluid dynamics even more [10–12]. Not only the influx but also the efflux mechanisms importantly impact the brain concentrations of (macro)molecules [13,14].

In fact, there are only a few techniques available that allow for the direct sampling from the cerebral interstitial space and thus provide insight into real concentrations in the brain parenchyma. Such techniques are microdialysis, cerebral open flow microperfusion (cOFM), and biosensors. While these techniques seem promising, they are not (yet) adopted into routine practice. A discussion on their strengths and limitations will be the main focus of this review. The juxtaposition of these three techniques will lead to a more comprehensive overview of recent developments and possibilities in this domain.

Apart from determining exogenous drug concentrations for pharmacokinetic and pharmacodynamic studies, a fundamental part of CNS drug development is the monitoring of endogenous molecules at the site of action to gain insights into the physiology of the brain and its disease processes. Initially, the above-mentioned techniques were developed to monitor neurotransmitters and other small molecules, but over the years, advances in the field have made it possible to monitor macromolecules (neuropeptides, proteins, ...) as well. As an example, microdialysis is used to determine cytokine levels [15], but also biomarkers such as amyloid-beta and tau have already been quantified in the cerebral interstitial fluid (ISF) both in mice [16–18] and in a clinical setting [19]. Moreover, the use of biosensors for the detection of the biomarker tau has been described as well [20]. A third feature of microdialysis and cOFM is the possibility to locally administer molecules at the site of sampling. This feature can be of interest, as the pharmacological effect (on neurotransmitter levels for example) of the compound under investigation can directly be determined upon its local application at the site of action [21].

Trastuzumab is a prime example of the applicability of these techniques. It is a therapeutic monoclonal antibody that binds to the juxtamembrane region of human epidermal growth factor receptor-2 (HER2) and is successfully used in patients suffering from HER2-overexpressing breast cancer [22]. It is the most used example of personalized medicine. Indeed, because only 30% of breast cancer patients express the HER2 protein, characterization of the molecular profile of patients is required to start treatment [22,23]. Trastuzumab is currently also being evaluated for treatment of patients with brain metastases. Its brain pharmacokinetic profile has been determined in rats and mice using both microdialysis and cOFM [24,25]. Biosensors could be an interesting approach in this regard as well, as they can be used to detect HER2 in cell or tumor lysates [26].

2. Technical and Historical Overview

2.1. Microdialysis

Microdialysis enables the continuous sampling of endogenous as well as exogenous compounds from the cerebral interstitial space using a probe with a semipermeable membrane. The probe is stereotactically implanted in the brain in the region of interest. A perfusion fluid, mimicking the ISF, often called artificial CSF, is perfused through the probe assembly using a controlled pulse-free syringe pump. At the outlet, the dialysate containing the substances of interest is collected without the need of a pull pump. The dialysate is collected fractionally and subsequently analyzed using a sensitive analytical method of choice. The underlying process for the exchange of substances is based on Fick's first law of passive diffusion. In addition to the concentration gradient and osmotic pressure, the molecular weight, hydrophobicity, and tertiary structure of the compound, as well as the cut-off and material of the membrane, play key roles in this process [27].

The foundation for the use of microdialysis in its present form, as described above, originates from the early 1960s. The first building blocks were laid by Gaddum [28] by the introduction of a push-pull cannula to collect substances directly from the brain. His work is based on a perfusion technique in subcutaneous tissue described by Fox and Hilton [29], although the cannula was positioned concentrically in the brain tissue to allow for more precise targeting. The development of this in vivo technique evolved from the different attempts to determine neurotransmitters by performing brain dissections followed by post-mortem analyses. Numerous technical problems surrounded these early experiments, such as inaccurate dissections, the validity and correlation of the measurements in post-mortem tissue to the in vivo values, and the fact that only a single measurement of a static moment could be determined [30]. Over the years, it became clear that the in vivo technique had limitations as well that led to numerous adaptations regarding the design of the push-pull cannula. The major bottleneck was the open flow system resulting in tissue damage [31]. To resolve this problem, a cannula was constructed containing a tip covered with a porous semipermeable membrane. This dialysis sac [32], or 'dialytrode' as it was called by Delgado et al. [33], was later replaced by a hollow fiber, namely the dialysis membrane [34]. This is the basic principle underlying microdialysis as still referred to nowadays. The major advantage of this innovation is that there is less damage and interference with the brain tissue as exposure of the brain tissue to the perfusate is avoided, making the technique more 'physiological' than the push-pull principle [31,34,35].

The main component of a microdialysis probe is its semi-permeable membrane. As brain microdialysis was historically applied to gain insight into neurotransmitter levels and other small molecules, cut-off values of the membrane typically ranged from 6 to 40 kDa. Interestingly, the molecular weight cut-off (MWCO) of the microdialysis probe does not reflect the actual pore size of the membrane. It gives information regarding the retention capabilities and thus the sampling efficiency for molecules of a certain size range. For example, a membrane with a 20 kDa MWCO will not allow 80–90% of molecules of that particular size to pass through [36]. Furthermore, there is an exponential decrease in the ability of molecules to pass the semipermeable membrane in relation to an increase in their molecular weight, making classical microdialysis even challenging for sampling molecules with a low molecular weight because of its low recovery rates and low dialysate concentration. Over the years, effort was put in developing probes with a higher cut-off to increase the utility of the technique [15,37–39]. At present, probes with cut-off values of 100 kDa–3 MDa are commercially available, allowing the exchange of macromolecules [37,38]. In these kinds of probes, the underlying process for the exchange of substances is primarily based on convection, meaning substances are carried across the membrane pores via bulk-flow together with the solution. Ultrafiltration and, thus, transmembrane pressure (hydrostatic pressure gradient across the membrane) are crucial in this process [39]. To control the fluidic path, thus preventing leakage of the perfusate into the brain parenchyma, a push-pull system is required (Figure 1a). Nevertheless, pressure fluctuations remain a hurdle. Takeda et al. circumvented this problem by introducing a vent hole at the head of the probe assembly (AtmosLM™, Eicom, Green Leaf Scientific, Dublin, Ireland). This vent hole allows for fast equalization of the pressure difference inside the probe with the atmospheric pressure [40].

Samples obtained with classic microdialysis do not require sample clean-up before analysis with liquid chromatography or capillary electrophoresis, as no large molecules are present, because of the low MWCO of the membrane. Because of the high MWCO, analysis of large pore microdialysis samples is generally more challenging [38].

Technically, the microdialysis probe construct consists of a guide cannula containing a healing dummy implanted in the brain above the region of interest. Before initiating the sampling experiments, the healing dummy is removed and replaced by the microdialysis probe. The membrane protrudes beneath the guide cannula as illustrated in Figure 2a.

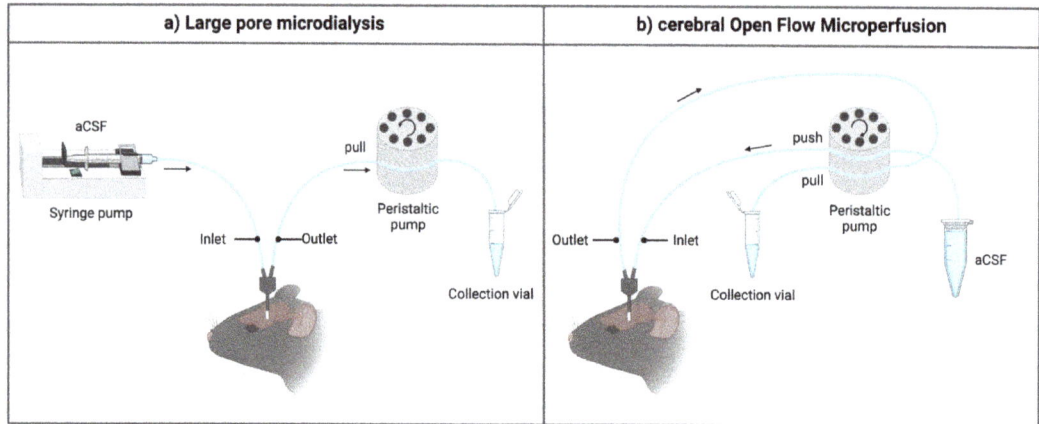

Figure 1. Schematic overview of the inlet and outlet tubings for the sampling techniques. (**a**) When using high-molecular-weight-cut-off microdialysis probes, a push-pull system is required to prevent loss of perfusion fluid through the large pores of the membrane. The setup generally contains a separate controlled pulse-free syringe pump and a peristaltic pull pump (e.g., using an AtmosLM™ or CMA ultra-high cut-off probe). For classical microdialysis, a pull pump is not used. (**b**) For the cerebral open flow microperfusion probe, a peristaltic push-pull microperfusion pump (MPP102 PC, Basi) can be used. Hereby, inflow and outflow can be controlled via the same pump head. Figure created with BioRender.com accessed on 6 April 2022. aCSF: artificial cerebrospinal fluid.

2.2. Cerebral Open Flow Microperfusion

Quite soon after its first introduction in the 1960s, the push-pull perfusion technique with its open flow system was put aside. As the use of a membrane has shown its limitations as well (see Section 3), Birngruber et al. went back to the roots and introduced in 2013 an advanced technique referred to as cOFM [41]. The two main features of the patented cOFM probe body design itself are (i) the replacement of the membrane by macroscopic openings and (ii) the biocompatible material (fluorinated ethylene propylene) it consists of [42]. The open structure of the device allows for sampling lipophilic (these tend to adsorb to the microdialysis membrane) and high-molecular-weight substances. The biocompatible material should make it possible to perform chronic sampling experiments as will be discussed in detail in Section 3.1 [43]. Historically, one of the main hurdles to prevent tissue damage by using the push-pull technique was to maintain the probe inlet flow generated by the push pump equal to the probe outlet flow generated by the pull pump [30,31]. This problem was solved by using a pair of high-precision syringe pumps [42]. These were later replaced by a peristaltic microperfusion pump (MPP102 PC, Basi) where inflow and outflow can be controlled via the same pump head (Figure 1b) [25,44].

Technically, the membrane-free cOFM probe body construct itself contains the open exchange area necessary to perform the sampling experiments and is implanted directly into the brain in (not above, as for the microdialysis guide) the region of interest, as illustrated in Figure 2b. It is recommended by the manufacturer to implant the probe body 14 days before initiating the sampling experiments [45]. This recovery period should ensure re-establishment of the BBB (for detailed discussion, see Section 3.1.1) and can be appraised as a third major feature of the probe design [41,42]. A healing dummy prevents tissue growing into the probe during this period. Sampling experiments can be initiated after 14 days by replacement of the healing dummy with a sampling insert [45].

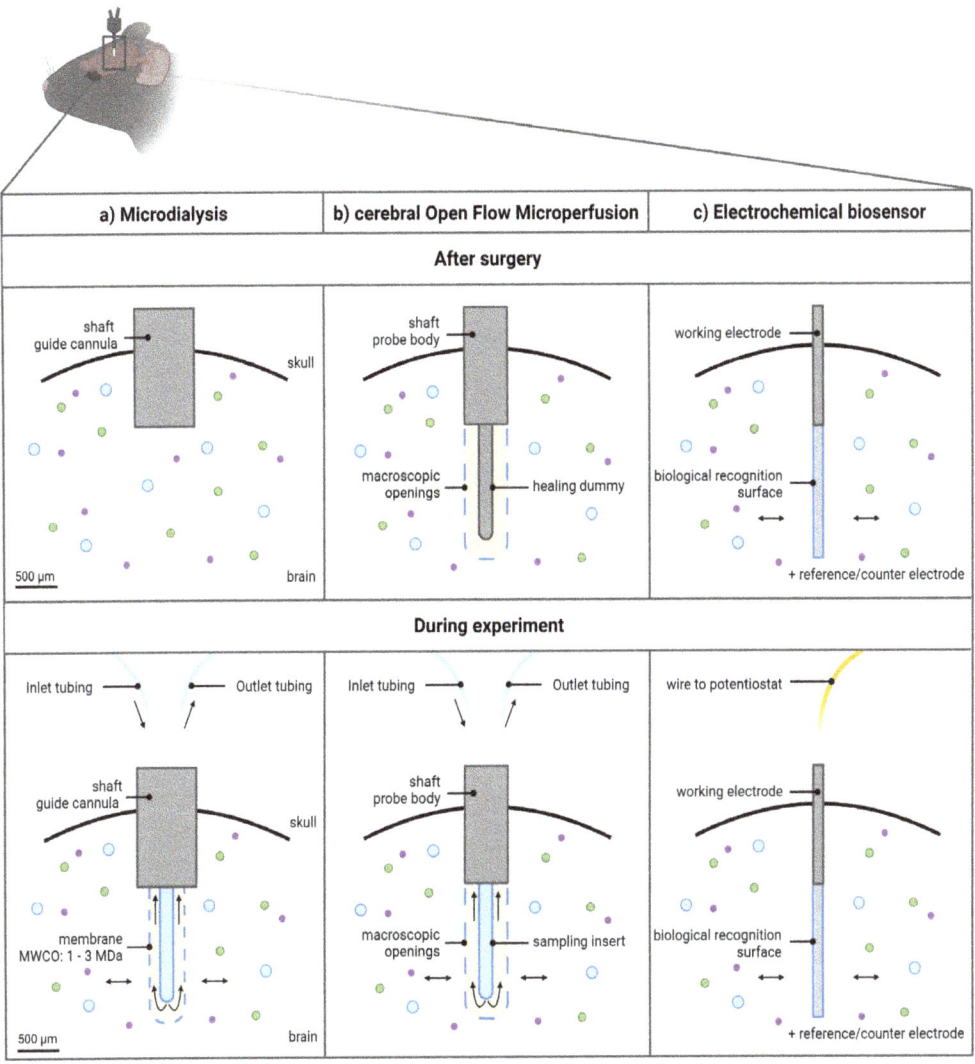

Figure 2. Schematic overview of the 3 approaches to monitor macromolecules directly from the cerebral interstitial fluid. (**a**) The microdialysis probe construct consists of a guide cannula containing a healing dummy implanted in the brain above the region of interest. Before initiating the experiments, the healing dummy is replaced by the probe connected to the tubings. The membrane protrudes beneath the guide cannula. Dimensions of the outer diameter of the shaft of the guide cannula and probe membrane are based on an AtmosLM™ probe. (**b**) The cerebral open flow microperfusion probe body construct/guide itself contains the open exchange area with macroscopic openings and is implanted directly into the brain in the region of interest. Before initiating the experiments, the healing dummy is replaced with the sampling insert connected to the tubings. (**c**) The electrochemical biosensor setup consists of the working electrode (cylinder type is shown), which is implanted in the brain region of interest, while the reference electrode can be implanted in the cortex and the counter electrode can be attached to an anchor screw placed in the skull (not shown). Scale bar indicates 500 µm. Figure created with BioRender.com accessed on 6 April 2022. MWCO: molecular weight cut-off.

2.3. Electrochemical Biosensors

While the two above-mentioned techniques rely on fluid sampling, a third technique, electrochemical biosensors, depends on the recognition of certain molecules directly in the cerebral ISF [46]. The principle of an electrochemical biosensor was first described by Clark and Lyons, in 1962 [47]. A typical biosensor consists of an immobilized, biological recognition element combined with a transducer that converts the biological reaction to a quantifiable signal. The biological recognition element is immobilized on the electrode surface. An electrochemical biosensor uses an electrochemical transducer to convert the signal, which is an electrical current in the case of an amperometric biosensor [48–50]. The measured electrical signal is a result of the redox current that is present at the surface of the electrode [51,52]. In this work, the focus is on electrochemical biosensors as this type of biosensor is not only used in fundamental scientific research [53] but also used in clinical practice. For example, the glucose biosensor has been used by diabetic patients for continuous glucose monitoring [50].

The first electrochemical biosensors were developed for the biosensing of molecules by the use of enzymes [50]. Enzymatic biosensors can be divided into three generations. In first-generation biosensors, an enzyme is used as the recognition element and the products used or produced in the enzymatic reaction are in relation to the concentration of the analyte of interest. Second-generation biosensors use electron carriers, while third-generation biosensors do not depend on a mediator but instead use direct electron transfer [51,52]. Enzymatic biosensors still make up the majority of implantable biosensors [54,55]. Apart from enzymes as the biological recognition element, aptamers, antibodies, or antigens can also be used [49,56] to (specifically) recognize the analyte of interest. Nevertheless, interference can be expected by other (small) electroactive compounds. A selective membrane layer/polymer is often used to prevent interference [57,58].

The best examples for the in vivo use of this elegant technique are the glucose biosensor [50] and the assessment of several endogenous small brain molecules such as glutamate [53,59,60] or other molecules [61,62]. While the use of biosensors to establish drug concentrations in the brain is limited, there are examples of biosensors that have been developed for the determination of disease biomarkers [63–65] useful for personalized medicine [23,26,66]. Nowadays, biosensors are also being developed for the measurement of large molecules, such as for the detection of tau protein as the biomarker for neurodegenerative diseases [63] or for the detection of hepatitis C virus for diagnostic purposes [67–69]. However, the latter are mostly being developed for ex vivo use in biological samples and not yet routinely in vivo. For example, several groups have described the development of a tau protein biosensor, of which an overview can be found in the review by Ameri et al. [20]. The aggregation of tau protein is associated with neurodegeneration and Alzheimer's disease [17,63]. While the aggregated tau is usually seen in later stages of the disease, it can be of interest to identify soluble tau oligomers during the early stages of the disease. The applicability of biosensors for this purpose is shown in an in vitro setting by Esteves-Villanueva et al. [63]. Another example is the development of an electrochemical biosensor for the determination of the HER2 receptor in cell or tumor lysates, which is the target of the aforementioned trastuzumab monoclonal antibody against cancer and requires characterization of HER2 [26,66].

Typically, in an in vivo setting, a three-electrode system is used: (i) the working electrode (which is the biosensor), (ii) the reference electrode, and (iii) a counter electrode [67,69,70]. Specifically, to monitor extracellular concentrations in the brain tissue, the working electrode(s) is (are) implanted in the brain region of interest (Figure 2c), while the reference electrode can be implanted in the cortex and the counter electrode can be attached to an anchor screw placed in the skull [71].

3. Strengths and Limitations

With thousands of publications [27], it can be said that microdialysis is well-established as a technique to gain direct insight into the brain environment. As a consequence, its strengths and limitations are generally well defined, yet controversy still exists in the literature. The three main topics dominating this discussion are the integrity of the BBB, inflammation of the brain tissue surrounding the probe (membrane), and the low recovery rates and associated sticking to the different parts of the setup. cOFM is developed in response to these concerns and attempts to overcome microdialysis' limitations, although the main principle of the two techniques (and thus its main strengths and limitations) remains the same. On the contrary, while there are some identical advantages and disadvantages between the sampling techniques and electrochemical biosensors, biosensors possess a number of interesting other features (e.g., better spatial/temporal resolution) depending on the aim of the study. Moreover, the use of both techniques can be complementary as they rely on a different principle for the assessment of analyte concentrations. An overview is given in Table 1 and the different topics are explained in detail in the following subsections.

Table 1. Overview of strengths and limitations influencing the possible applications of the three techniques.

	Large Pore Microdialysis	cOFM	Biosensors
Timeframe			
- Start	After 16–24 h	After 14 days	Upon equilibration
- Duration	48–72 h	Up to 30 days	2–3 weeks
Recovery	Limited due to membrane	Macroscopic openings	Recognition element
- Membrane	Aspecific adsorption	Not applicable	Not applicable
Spatial resolution	±500 µm OD		±50–125 µm OD
	Depending on length probe: mm		Cylinder vs. disc
Temporal resolution	minutes		(milli)seconds
Sample analysis	(Bio-)analytical technique		Not applicable
Analyte range	Omics screening possible		Limited
Others	Local administration of molecules possible		-

cOFM: cerebral open flow microperfusion, OD: outer diameter.

3.1. Timeframe to Perform Experiments

When designing a study, the following should be taken into account with regard to the timeframe of the conducted experiments: (i) the recovery period after implantation of the devices in the brain to ensure the integrity of the BBB before initiating an experiment, as well as (ii) the length of the experiment depending on biofouling on the surfaces of the device leading to deviating results.

3.1.1. Blood–Brain Barrier Integrity

All three techniques are commonly referred to as being minimally invasive, although it is clear that the surgical implantation of the probe/electrode has its consequences [72]. Therefore, a recovery and equilibration period should be considered prior to starting the experiments. The literature is not conclusive regarding the integrity of the BBB [41,73–80]. Moreover, manuals available with the different commercialized microdialysis probes do not even provide information about this.

As seen in Figure 2a, the microdialysis probe membrane protrudes beneath the guide cannula. Hence, additional injury is caused when the probe itself is inserted in the brain. Consequently, inserting the microdialysis probe just before the start of the sampling procedure does not provide sufficient recovery time. For example, in Sumbria et al. [73], the integrity of the BBB following microdialysis probe implantation was assessed by determining the extravasation of fluorescent markers, both with a low (sodium fluorescein) and high (Evans Blue) molecular weight, around the probe tract after intravenous administration. The results show an increased extravasation immediately after implantation, but not after 1.5 h or 24 h [73]. In Caljon et al. [74], experiments were started after a 16 h recovery period following microdialysis probe implantation. BBB integrity was assessed using Evans Blue and ^{99m}Tc-Sestamibi, revealing no significant extravasation [74], thus all indicating only acute damage immediately after implantation [73,74,77,78,81,82]. Other studies have shown that a biphasic response in BBB permeability occurs, with an increase immediately after probe implantation and a second increase 1–2 days after [75,76,79]. In contrast, Groothuis et al. [75] showed that BBB function is disrupted during at least 28 days after implantation.

cOFM was introduced as a new in vivo technique for measuring substance transport across the intact BBB [41]. The main difference with the microdialysis probe construct is that the cOFM guide cannula contains the open exchange area and is directly implanted in the brain in the region of interest. It was shown that up until 9 days after cOFM probe implantation, the Evans Blue extravasation was still significantly higher than in a negative control, although it decreased to 15%. Therefore, a recovery period of 14 days is recommended by the manufacturer prior to starting cOFM experiments in order to assure BBB integrity [41]. When using a microdialysis probe, the latter is impossible, as is explained in Section 3.1.2. Immediately before cOFM sampling, the healing dummy is replaced by the sampling insert, creating limited new damage according to the manufacturer as the cOFM probe body is implanted in the region of interest and the sampling insert is exactly in-line with the previously implanted guide. The probe is flushed at a high flow (typically 2 min at 5 µL/min) and a 1 h run-in phase is taken into account as an equilibration period [45]. In Custers et al. [44], serotonin and γ-aminobutyric acid levels were determined 2 h and 20–24 h after sampling insert replacement to gain insight into possible disturbance of the brain environment, demonstrating that the 1 h run-in phase does not suffice. The BBB is probably disrupted again after insertion of the sampling insert and flushing with the perfusate as it is in direct contact with the brain tissue (because of the absence of a membrane). Most cOFM studies in the literature are performed under anesthesia, which restricts the duration of the sampling experiment itself and makes a longer run-in phase impossible [41,43,45,80,83,84]. In an awake setup, the equilibration period can and should be prolonged [25,44].

Biosensors offer a benefit by the increased spatial resolution and reduction in implantation trauma, as the outer diameter of the implanted device is smaller compared to the sampling probes, as seen in Figure 2 and Table 1. There is no consensus on when cerebral biosensor experiments can be initiated after implantation. The signal can be continuously monitored from the moment just after implantation, although it is important to wait for the baseline to stabilize before initiating an experiment. For example, some groups start measuring minutes after implantation [53,59], while others wait a few hours [71], although the latter strongly depends on the type of electrode that is used and the experimental setup (awake vs. under anesthesia) [85]. Hence, this equilibration period is based on the sensor rather than on brain homeostasis and the integrity of the BBB.

3.1.2. Inflammation

Apart from the recovery/equilibration period before experiment initiation, deciding on the duration of the experimental sampling duration is equally challenging. The key factor limiting the application time and functionality of the techniques is the immunological reaction of the body following implantation of the foreign object and the associated biofouling on its surface [27,72,76,86].

When implanted for too long, the microdialysis membrane becomes clogged (resulting in decreased recovery rates) due to the formation of glial scar tissue and adhesion of molecules onto the membrane. Therefore, it is typically recommended to perform microdialysis experiments for a maximum of 72 h [27,87]. However, chronic microdialysis experiments have also been described in literature [88–91].

cOFM attempted to overcome this issue by introducing the membrane-free probe and improving the biocompatibility of the probe body using fluorinated ethylene propylene. The study of Birngruber et al. shows no formation of a continuous glial scar up to 30 days after probe implantation in the rat brain [43]. Hence, an advantage of cOFM over microdialysis is the notion that intermittent sampling in a chronic setting should theoretically be more feasible, although abundant literature on this application is not yet available. Commercialized equipment for microdialysis experiments mainly use a guide cannula and probe shaft made of stainless steel (Eicom, Green Leaf Scientific, Dublin, Ireland; CMA Microdialysis AB, Kista, Sweden). A replacement of the metallic material with a guide cannula using a better biocompatible material such as polyether imide/fused silica (Microbiotech/se AB, Stockholm, Sweden) or polyamide/polyurethane (CMA Microdialysis AB) could markedly reduce the immune response as well. There is little reason to believe that fluorinated ethylene propylene can offer better biocompatibility than the other polymers [92], although the presence of the membrane remains a limiting factor. To the extent of our knowledge, no clear comparison exists in the literature between the different available commercial and custom-made microdialysis probe types, although abundant literature is available regarding the inflammatory response. The study of Custers et al. shows that if both a microdialysis probe (AtmosLM™, stainless steel) and cOFM probe are used within their recommended timeframe, the inflammatory response is comparable [44]. Birngruber et al. compared the cOFM probe with a CMA 12 microdialysis probe that consists of a metal-free, biocompatible guide cannula and probe shaft according to the manual (although not specified in the manuscript) [43]. Surprisingly, this study demonstrates a markedly increased astrocytic and microglial reaction for the implanted microdialysis probe 15 days after implantation compared to the cOFM probe [43]. This emphasizes that further research is needed.

Another important factor to consider is the perfusate as there is no consensus on its composition. To minimize an inflammatory response, the physiology of the cerebral ISF should be mimicked, and the solution should be filtered or sterilized. The addition of other components such as bovine serum albumin (BSA) and dextran, which are needed in the context of aspecific adsorption and osmotic pressure, may adversely affect the inflammatory response [44].

In the field of implantable electrochemical biosensors, attention is also paid to avoid biofouling. As is the case with the sampling techniques, the duration of use of these biosensors is also limited as biofouling hampers analyte diffusion toward the biorecognition element, which results in lower sensitivity. Another important point is the inactivation or degradation of the biological recognition element [54,55,93–95]. It is well-known that compounds adhere on the surface of the electrode, although efforts are made to limit this. These efforts include the use of naturally occurring or bio-mimicking materials such as chitosan, collagen, and gelatin, but also hydrophilic, superhydrophobic, and drug-eluting materials can be used. Their mechanism of action is, for example, based on the regulation of the host immune response and making the biosensor surface thermodynamically unfavorable for biofouling [55]. For example, in the study of Brown et al. [96], it is shown that exposure of the Nafion®-coated platinum sensor to proteins and lipids in an in vitro setting resulted in a decrease in sensitivity up to 24 h, after which levels stabilized. These results were confirmed in vivo up to 8 days after implantation [96]. Generally, chronic in vivo cerebral biosensor experiments are performed for a maximum of 2–3 weeks, although this strongly depends on the sensor used [71,96–98].

In summary, regarding microdialysis, it is typically recommended to initiate experiments 16–24 h after probe implantation [73,74], based on BBB integrity, with a maximal duration of 48–72 h [87,99,100], based on the formation of glial scar tissue around the probe that hampers the exchange of molecules [27,76]. Regarding cOFM, experiments can be initiated 14 days after probe implantation [41,80], based on BBB integrity, with a minimal duration of 30 days [43], based on the formation of glial scar tissue [45]. There is no consensus on the timeframe to perform cerebral biosensor experiments. However, the signal can be continuously monitored from the moment upon baseline stabilization after implantation, with a maximum duration of 2–3 weeks, although the latter strongly depends on the type of sensors that are used [71,98].

3.2. Recovery Rates

Apart from biofouling, multiple other factors determine the recovery rate of the compound of interest. A first factor determining the recovery rate in microdialysis is the MWCO of the membrane. Furthermore, in addition to lipophilic small molecules, macromolecules such as peptides and proteins tend to adsorb to the membrane. An overview of the modification strategies of the microdialysis membrane surface to reduce aspecific adsorption is given by Van Wanseele et al. [38]. For example, the AN69 membrane offers great potential for reducing aspecific adsorption of peptides [101]. However, next to adsorption of the compound of interest to the probe membrane, sticking can also occur at other parts of the microdialysis setup. Adding BSA to the perfusate to block aspecific binding is commonly used as a main solution together with the use of low-binding tubings. Furthermore, an in vitro adsorption test should be performed prior to in vivo experiments. As for cOFM, the inner lumen of the probe is coated with polytetrafluoroethylene as an additional measure to decrease adsorption [102,103].

The study of Altendorfer-Kroath et al. [83] comparing a 20 kDa microdialysis probe with a cOFM probe, but also the study of Custers et al. [44] comparing a 1 MDa microdialysis probe with a cOFM probe, shows discrepancies between in vitro recovery/adsorption tests compared to the in vivo obtained results. In both studies, the cOFM probe performs better in vitro compared to the microdialysis probe, although this advantage almost completely disappears in an in vivo setting. As problems with ultrafiltration and osmolarity are minimized because of the optimized design of the probe/pump and perfusate, we believe tortuosity of the brain parenchyma can provide a possible answer for this discrepancy [44,104]. To estimate absolute ISF concentrations, for both techniques, in vivo recovery should be determined as well. Typical methods to do so are the no-net-flux approach, the extrapolation-to-zero flow, and the recovery by gain/loss method [27]. Although, in practice, relative concentrations are often used.

To the extent of our knowledge, three studies are available in the literature comparing cOFM with AtmosLM™ to sample macromolecules, namely trastuzumab [25], a brain-penetrating nanobody [44], and tau [18]. Their findings on recovery rates of the macromolecules with the two techniques differ substantially. In the study of Le Prieult et al., 10-fold higher ISF trastuzumab levels were found with cOFM compared to microdialysis when not corrected for in vivo recovery. They also showed that the use of either in vitro or in vivo recovery has a substantial impact on absolute concentrations [25]. In the study of Custers et al., with both techniques, equivalent levels (uncorrected) of a brain-penetrating nanobody were found [44]. The study of Barini et al. shows that ISF sampled by cOFM increased the seeding propensity of tau in the HEK293-tau biosensor cell assay more than ISF sampled through the microdialysis probe. They examined whether this was due to the differential recovery of tau or differential sampling of tau species. Tau levels were significantly higher in AtmosLM™ ISF than in cOFM ISF, although the overall composition of tau fragments was unaffected by the sampling procedure. They hypothesized that the enhanced ability to trigger tau aggregation may require additional ISF components that are only present in cOFM ISF [18]. Because of these divergent results and conclusions, it is clear that there is a need for additional comparative studies with macromolecules of different classes.

Despite in vitro calibrations of the biosensors, the activity of an enzyme is dependent on the environment it is used in. Hence, the activity of the enzyme can be different in vivo versus in vitro and absolute concentrations remain an estimate [54]. In in vivo measurements, baseline currents are measured and changes in this current indicate a change in analyte concentration. Hence, results can be reported as the measured current compared to the baseline current [53,59] but also as concentrations [105]. Both methods of reporting offer a great insight into the change in extracellular concentration of the analyte of interest over time.

3.3. Spatiotemporal Resolution

The spatial resolution of a microdialysis and cOFM probe is comparable as the outer diameter is around 500 µm for both and the membrane/open exchange length is typically 1–4 mm depending on the species and target of interest. As a decreased outer probe diameter leads to increased spatial resolution [106], biosensors offer the best spatial resolution out of the three techniques. The outer diameter of a biosensor is typically between 50 and 125 µm, although strongly depending on the type of sensor. Moreover, apart from the cylinder-type biosensors where the biological recognition surface is similar to the membrane/open exchange length, disc-type biosensors have their biological recognition surface located only at the tip of the electrode. These compact disc-type biosensors offer the opportunity to specifically target a brain subregion such as the CA1 region of the hippocampus [54,107].

For microdialysis and cOFM, the limiting factor determining the temporal resolution is the desired sample volume. It depends on the flow rate and associated recovery that, in turn, depends on the subsequent analytical method and is generally minimally in the minutes range [108]. Generally, for cOFM, a flow rate of 0.3–1 µL/min is recommended. Higher flow rates are avoided to prevent tissue damage and analyte depletion in the vicinity of the probe (especially for macromolecules with low concentrations at the site of action) [45]. Lower flow rates are avoided because of the temporal resolution. As for microdialysis, common flow rates are 0.3–2 µL/min [27], because the membrane acts as a protection layer for the brain tissue. On the contrary, biosensors have an optimal temporal resolution in the (milli)seconds range [109,110]. The latter is mainly dependent on the diffusion of the analyte through the membrane layer/polymer [111].

3.4. Sample Analysis

Samples obtained with microdialysis or cOFM require a subsequent sensitive analytical method for their analysis. This is not the case for biosensors, which are an analysis method themselves, and the concentration of the analyte is in relation to the obtained current [51].

For the sampling techniques, the information that can be obtained is only as good as the subsequent analytical method. An analytical method requiring a high sample volume, because of a high limit of detection, has great implications on the temporal resolution of the technique. Moreover, because of low recovery rates for some molecules, an ideal analytical method should be sensitive, have a low limit of detection/limit of quantification, and thus require low sample volumes in addition to being validated by the applicable standards [108]. Analytical methods that are mostly used and are extremely well fitted for the analysis of microdialysates are miniaturized liquid chromatography or capillary electrophoresis coupled to mass spectrometry [112–115], although other detection methods can be suitable. Especially, the use of capillary electrophoresis coupled to mass spectrometry could be interesting because it generally requires very low sample volumes and can thus improve temporal resolution [112,116].

Nevertheless, chronic sampling combined with a high temporal resolution can lead to a great number of samples. Despite the fact that analytical methods are being developed with a short run time, it can become labor-intensive to analyze all these samples. We believe that the use of biosensors has an advantage for chronic sampling, as subsequent sample analysis is not necessary. However, with biosensors, only a limited number of molecules can be monitored simultaneously. In this regard, the use of sampling methods offers a big advantage by enabling the monitoring of a large range of different molecules, for example, in a proteomic screening [117].

Samples collected with large pore microdialysis or cOFM contain, in addition to the analyte of interest, more, other interfering compounds such as proteins, enzymes, and triglycerides compared to classical microdialysis. As a result, these samples cannot be analyzed with the abovementioned methods without doing a sample clean-up [38]. Hence, another possibility is the use of biological assays such as an enzyme-linked immunosorbent assay (ELISA) or single-molecule array (Simoa) where sample pretreatment is a less important factor. Both techniques offer great sensitivity; however, they are expensive and generally require a high sample volume, negatively influencing the temporal resolution [118]. Furthermore, an assay based on LOCI™ (Luminescent Oxygen Channelling Immunoassay) technology can be explored, such as an AlphaLISA™ or AlphaScreen™. The benefit in these kinds of biological assays is that they are quick (require no wash-steps) and very sensitive, allowing detection down to the attomolar (10^{-18}) level combined with small sample volumes (<10 µL) [119,120]. However, the small sample volume can impact the validity of the assay.

4. Overview of Macromolecules Sampled from the ISF

In Table 2, examples of macromolecules determined in the cerebral ISF using microdialysis or cOFM are given.

Table 2. Examples of macromolecules sampled from the cerebral interstitial fluid.

	Microdialysis		cOFM	
Neuropeptides and proteins	Cytokines	[40,80,121–135]	Cytokines	[80]
	TNF-alpha	[40,126]	TNF-alpha	[80]
	Neuromedins	[114]	Leptin	[84]
	Substance P	[136]	Tau	[18]
	Hormones	[137–139]	Antibodies	[25]
	Matrix metalloproteinases	[134,135,140–142]	Nanobodies	[44]
	Growth factors	[123–125,128,130,131,135]		
	S100B	[143,144]		
	Apolipoprotein E	[145]		
	Amyloid beta	[16,19,40,146–148]		
	Tau	[17–19,146,147,149]		
	Neurofilaments	[19,150]		
	Antibodies	[24,25]		
	Nanobodies	[44,74]		
Others	microRNAs	[151]	PEGylated liposomal doxorubicin	[152]
	Prostaglandin E2	[153,154]		

Most studies to date that have used microdialysis and cOFM to sample macromolecules concern protein structures. A first class comprises neuropeptides such as hormones [84,137,138], substance P [136], and the neuromedins [114]. From a biochemical point of view, neuropeptides can be situated in the gray zone between small molecules and proteins. With an approximate length of 3–100 amino-acid residues, they are smaller than regular proteins (up to 2000 amino-acid residues) and up to 50 times bigger than the neurotransmitters sampled with classical microdialysis [38,155]. Their quantification in the ISF poses a challenge because of their concentrations in the femto- to picomolar range and sticking behavior to the different parts of the sampling setup. Furthermore, the sampling of larger proteins such as inflammation mediators [40,80,121–135] and many markers for neurodegeneration [16–19,40,146–150] but also growth factors [123–125,128,130,131,135] and matrix metalloproteinases [134,135,140–142] have been described. Due to their involvement in several neurological disorders, the investigation of their concentration-dependent role at the site of action in the (patho)physiological processes has received attention. Another hot topic is the quantification of nanobodies [44,74] and antibodies [24,25] in the cerebral ISF. Finally, two studies have appeared that sampled liposomes [152], as well as microRNAs [151]. The insight into ISF concentrations of these latter macromolecules is of high interest for the treatment of neurological disorders, thinking, for example, about the potential implementation of monoclonal antibodies as biologics (with or without the use of a shuttling moiety), but RNA therapeutics could also be of interest in this context.

To the extent of our knowledge, electrochemical biosensors are not yet used for in vivo monitoring of macromolecules in the cerebral ISF.

5. Innovations in the Field from a Legal Perspective

A research gap exists in the literature regarding the patented innovations for the approaches to monitor macromolecules directly from the cerebral ISF. A search on the term 'microdialysis' in the European online database Espacenet, developed by the European Patent Office, yields 3925 hits [156]. The invention of the microdialysis probe as described by Ungerstedt et al. [34] can be seen as the prior art for all the following patents within this field. His invention was patented in 1984 [157] and assigned to CMA Microdialysis AB, one of the major players on the commercial market, as an application in 1993 [158]. Since then, there have been several adaptations made. We believe the current state-of-the-art for sampling macromolecules can be represented by the cOFM probe, invented by Birngruber and Altendorfer-Kroath and patented as a 'Catheter having a healing dummy' [41,159,160], and the AtmosLM™ microdialysis probe invented by Nishino et al. [40,161]. However, numerous other inventions have been patented. For example, a patent exists for performing a proteomic study using push-pull microdialysis combined with a MetaQuant probe [162,163]. Stenken and Sellati hold a patent for the sampling of peptides and proteins (e.g., cytokines) in the cerebral ISF using antibody-coated microspheres to enhance recovery [15,164,165]. Regarding biosensors, the patented electrochemical device of Clark in 1959 can be considered the prior art for all innovations within this domain [166]. An overview of all the innovations on the market related to the monitoring of macromolecules in the cerebral ISF would present an excellent guide for researchers within the field.

6. Conclusions

The concept of the sampling techniques and biosensors emerged around the same time and they have evolved simultaneously for the past 60 years, depending on the goals of the experiment. Compared to the thousands of microdialysis papers dominating the literature during the past decades, since 2013, a dozen articles using cOFM are published. The latest review comparing cOFM to microdialysis does not present a complete picture, because the open flow system is compared with classical microdialysis probes having a low MWCO [167], although large pore microdialysis is promising as well [37]. Since 2021, three studies were published for the first time comparing a cOFM probe with a large pore microdialysis probe to sample macromolecules [18,25,44]. Regarding electrochemical biosensors, a large body of literature exists as well, although it seems to have had less of a breakthrough in an in vivo setting in the domain of neuroscience compared to microdialysis.

In our opinion, there is no outstanding technique that can replace the others for brain neurochemical monitoring, as they all have their strengths and limitations. The choice of technique should depend on the goal of the study and should consider all factors. In the context of brain-targeted drug delivery, while monitoring, special caution should be taken regarding the integrity of the BBB, and the use of an appropriate control is crucial. Furthermore, statements about 'real' concentrations should be considered carefully as it is challenging to determine absolute concentrations in vivo. In conclusion, we strongly believe that the implementation of these techniques leads to a better understanding of the physiology of the brain, is of high importance for pharmacokinetic and pharmacodynamic studies of novel brain-targeted drug candidates, and can thus help to improve the drug discovery and development processes of drugs targeting the CNS.

Author Contributions: Conceptualization, M.-L.C., L.N., A.V.E. and I.S.; writing—original draft preparation, M.-L.C. and L.N.; writing—review and editing, M.-L.C., L.N., D.D.B., A.V.E. and I.S.; supervision, D.D.B., A.V.E. and I.S.; funding acquisition, M.-L.C., D.D.B., A.V.E. and I.S. All authors have read and agreed to the published version of the manuscript.

Funding: Marie-Laure Custers and Liam Nestor are researchers at the Vrije Universiteit Brussel. This review is supported by the Scientific Fund Willy Gepts of the UZ Brussel (WFWG2021), the Research Foundation Flanders (S007918N; 1528219N), and the strategic research program of the Vrije Universiteit Brussel (SRP49).

Institutional Review Board Statement: Not applicable.

Informed Consent Statement: Not applicable.

Data Availability Statement: Not applicable.

Conflicts of Interest: The authors declare no conflict of interest.

Abbreviations

BBB, Blood–brain barrier; BSA, Bovine serum albumin; CNS, Central nervous system; cOFM, Cerebral open flow microperfusion; CSF, Cerebrospinal fluid; FDA, Food and Drug Administration; HER2, Human epidermal growth factor receptor-2; ISF, Interstitial fluid; MWCO, Molecular weight cut-off; OD, Outer diameter.

References

1. Kola, I.; Landis, J. Can the Pharmaceutical Industry Reduce Attrition Rates? *Nat. Rev. Drug Discov.* **2004**, *3*, 711–715. [CrossRef] [PubMed]
2. Qosa, H.; Volpe, D.A. The Development of Biological Therapies for Neurological Diseases: Moving on from Previous Failures. *Expert Opin. Drug Discov.* **2018**, *13*, 283–293. [CrossRef] [PubMed]
3. Kinch, M.S. An Overview of FDA-Approved Biologics Medicines. *Drug Discov. Today* **2015**, *20*, 393–398. [CrossRef] [PubMed]
4. Liu, J.K.H. The History of Monoclonal Antibody Development-Progress, Remaining Challenges and Future Innovations. *Ann. Med. Surg.* **2014**, *3*, 113–116. [CrossRef]
5. Gklinos, P.; Papadopoulou, M.; Stanulovic, V.; Mitsikostas, D.D.; Papadopoulos, D. Monoclonal Antibodies as Neurological Therapeutics. *Pharmaceuticals* **2021**, *14*, 92. [CrossRef]
6. Kaplon, H.; Chenoweth, A.; Crescioli, S.; Reichert, J.M. Antibodies to Watch in 2022. *MAbs* **2022**, *14*, 2014296. [CrossRef]
7. EMA Refusal of the Marketing Authorisation for Aduhelm (Aducanumab). Available online: https://www.ema.europa.eu/en/documents/smop-initial/refusal-marketing-authorisation-aduhelm-aducanumab_en.pdf (accessed on 28 February 2022).
8. Pardridge, W.M. Treatment of Alzheimer's Disease and Blood–Brain Barrier Drug Delivery. *Pharmaceuticals* **2020**, *13*, 394. [CrossRef]
9. Pardridge, W.M. CSF, Blood-Brain Barrier, and Brain Drug Delivery. *Expert Opin. Drug Deliv.* **2016**, *13*, 963–975. [CrossRef]
10. Abbott, N.J.; Pizzo, M.E.; Preston, J.E.; Janigro, D.; Thorne, R.G. The Role of Brain Barriers in Fluid Movement in the CNS: Is There a 'Glymphatic' System? *Acta Neuropathol.* **2018**, *135*, 387–407. [CrossRef]
11. Mestre, H.; Mori, Y.; Nedergaard, M. The Brain's Glymphatic System: Current Controversies. *Trends Neurosci.* **2020**, *43*, 458–466. [CrossRef]
12. Kaur, J.; Fahmy, L.M.; Davoodi-Bojd, E.; Zhang, L.; Ding, G.; Hu, J.; Zhang, Z.; Chopp, M.; Jiang, Q. Waste Clearance in the Brain. *Front. Neuroanat.* **2021**, *15*, 665803. [CrossRef] [PubMed]
13. van Lessen, M.; Shibata-Germanos, S.; van Impel, A.; Hawkins, T.A.; Rihel, J.; Schulte-Merker, S. Intracellular Uptake of Macromolecules by Brain Lymphatic Endothelial Cells during Zebrafish Embryonic Development. *Elife* **2017**, *6*, e25932. [CrossRef] [PubMed]
14. Strazielle, N.; Ghersi-Egea, J.F. Physiology of Blood-Brain Interfaces in Relation to Brain Disposition of Small Compounds and Macromolecules. *Mol. Pharm.* **2013**, *10*, 1473–1491. [CrossRef] [PubMed]
15. Ao, X.; Stenken, J.A. Microdialysis Sampling of Cytokines. *Methods* **2006**, *38*, 331–341. [CrossRef]
16. Cirrito, J.R.; May, P.C.; O'Dell, M.A.; Taylor, J.W.; Parsadanian, M.; Cramer, J.W.; Audia, J.E.; Nissen, J.S.; Bales, K.R.; Paul, S.M.; et al. In Vivo Assessment of Brain Interstitial Fluid with Microdialysis Reveals Plaque-Associated Changes in Amyloid-β Metabolism and Half-Life. *J. Neurosci.* **2003**, *23*, 8844–8853. [CrossRef]
17. Yamada, K.; Cirrito, J.R.; Stewart, F.R.; Jiang, H.; Finn, M.B.; Holmes, B.B.; Binder, L.I.; Mandelkow, E.M.; Diamond, M.I.; Lee, V.M.Y.; et al. In Vivo Microdialysis Reveals Age-Dependent Decrease of Brain Interstitial Fluid Tau Levels in P301S Human Tau Transgenic Mice. *J. Neurosci.* **2011**, *31*, 13110–13117. [CrossRef]

18. Barini, E.; Plotzky, G.; Mordashova, Y.; Hoppe, J.; Rodriguez-Correa, E.; Julier, S.; LePrieult, F.; Mairhofer, I.; Mezler, M.; Biesinger, S.; et al. Tau in the Brain Interstitial Fluid Is Fragmented and Seeding–Competent. *Neurobiol. Aging* **2022**, *109*, 64–77. [CrossRef]
19. Magnoni, S.; Esparza, T.J.; Conte, V.; Carbonara, M.; Carrabba, G.; Holtzman, D.M.; Zipfel, G.J.; Stocchetti, N.; Brody, D.L. Tau Elevations in the Brain Extracellular Space Correlate with Reduced Amyloid-β Levels and Predict Adverse Clinical Outcomes after Severe Traumatic Brain Injury. *Brain* **2012**, *135*, 1268–1280. [CrossRef]
20. Ameri, M.; Shabaninejad, Z.; Movahedpour, A.; Sahebkar, A.; Mohammadi, S.; Hosseindoost, S.; Ebrahimi, M.S.; Savardashtaki, A.; Karimipour, M.; Mirzaei, H. Biosensors for Detection of Tau Protein as an Alzheimer's Disease Marker. *Int. J. Biol. Macromol.* **2020**, *162*, 1100–1108. [CrossRef]
21. Légat, L.; Smolders, I.; Dupont, A.G. AT1 Receptor Mediated Hypertensive Response to Ang II in the Nucleus Tractus Solitarii of Normotensive Rats Involves NO Dependent Local GABA Release. *Front. Pharmacol.* **2019**, *10*, 460. [CrossRef]
22. Wang, Z. Personalized Medicine for HER2 Positive Breast Cancer. *Breast Cancer Manag.* **2015**, *4*, 237–240. [CrossRef]
23. Issa, A.M. Personalized Medicine and the Practice of Medicine in the 21st Century. *McGill J. Med.* **2007**, *10*, 53–57. [CrossRef] [PubMed]
24. Chang, H.Y.; Morrow, K.; Bonacquisti, E.; Zhang, W.Y.; Shah, D.K. Antibody Pharmacokinetics in Rat Brain Determined Using Microdialysis. *MAbs* **2018**, *10*, 843–853. [CrossRef] [PubMed]
25. Le Prieult, F.; Barini, E.; Laplanche, L.; Schlegel, K.; Mezler, M. Collecting Antibodies and Large Molecule Biomarkers in Mouse Interstitial Brain Fluid: A Comparison of Microdialysis and Cerebral Open Flow Microperfusion. *MAbs* **2021**, *13*, 1918819. [CrossRef]
26. Mucelli, S.P.; Zamuner, M.; Tormen, M.; Stanta, G.; Ugo, P. Nanoelectrode Ensembles as Recognition Platform for Electrochemical Immunosensors. *Biosens. Bioelectron.* **2008**, *23*, 1900–1903. [CrossRef]
27. Hammarlund-udenaes, M. Microdialysis as an Important Technique in Systems Pharmacology—A Historical and Methodological Review. *AAPS J.* **2017**, *19*, 1294–1303. [CrossRef]
28. Gaddum, J. Push-Pull Cannulae. *J. Physiol.* **1961**, *155*, 46–47. [CrossRef]
29. Fox, B.Y.R.H.; Hilton, S.M. Bradykinin Formation in Human Skin as a Factor in Heat Vasodilatation. *J. Appl. Physiol.* **1958**, *142*, 219–232. [CrossRef]
30. Myers, R.D. Development of Push-Pull Systems for Perfusion of Anatomically Distinct Regions of the Brain of the Awake Animal. *Ann. N. Y. Acad. Sci.* **1986**, *473*, 21–41. [CrossRef]
31. Myers, R.D.; Adell, A.; Lankford, M.F. Simultaneous Comparison of Cerebral Dialysis and Push-Pull Perfusion in the Brain of Rats: A Critical Review. *Neurosci. Biobehav. Rev.* **1998**, *22*, 371–387. [CrossRef]
32. Bito, L.; Davson, H.; Levin, E.; Murray, M.; Snider, N. The Concentrations of Free Amino Acids and Other Electrolytes in Cerebrospinal Fluid, in Vivo Dialysate of Brain, and Blood Plasma of the Dog. *J. Neurochem.* **1966**, *13*, 1057–1067. [CrossRef] [PubMed]
33. Delgado, J.M.; DeFeudis, F.V.; Roth, R.H.; Ryugo, D.K.; Mitruka, B.M. Dialytrode for Long Term Intracerebral Perfusion in Awake Monkeys. *Arch. Int. Pharmacodyn. Ther.* **1972**, *198*, 9–21. [PubMed]
34. Ungerstedt, U.; Herrera-Marschitz, M.; Jungnelius, U.; Stahle, L.; Tossman, U.; Zetterström, T. *Dopamine Synaptic Mechanisms Reflected in Studies Combining Behavioural Recordings and Brain Dialysis*; Pergamon Press Ltd.: Oxford, UK, 1982.
35. Ungerstedt, U.; Pyock, C. Functional Correlates of Dopamine Neurotransmission. *Bull. Schweiz. Akad. Med. Wiss.* **1974**, *30*, 44–55. [PubMed]
36. Chu, J.; Koudriavtsev, V.; Hjort, K.; Dahlin, A.P. Fluorescence Imaging of Macromolecule Transport in High Molecular Weight Cut-off Microdialysis. *Anal. Bioanal. Chem.* **2014**, *406*, 7601–7609. [CrossRef]
37. Jadhav, S.B.; Khaowroongrueng, V.; Derendorf, H. Microdialysis of Large Molecules. *J. Pharm. Sci.* **2016**, *105*, 3233–3242. [CrossRef]
38. Van Wanseele, Y.; De Prins, A.; De Bundel, D.; Smolders, I.; Van Eeckhaut, A. Challenges for the in Vivo Quantification of Brain Neuropeptides Using Microdialysis Sampling and LC-MS. *Bioanalysis* **2016**, *8*, 1965–1985. [CrossRef]
39. Chu, J.; Hjort, K.; Larsson, A.; Dahlin, A.P. Impact of Static Pressure on Transmembrane Fluid Exchange in High Molecular Weight Cut off Microdialysis. *Biomed. Microdevices* **2014**, *16*, 301–310. [CrossRef]
40. Takeda, S.; Sato, N.; Ikimura, K.; Nishino, H.; Rakugi, H.; Morishita, R. Novel Microdialysis Method to Assess Neuropeptides and Large Molecules in Free-Moving Mouse. *Neuroscience* **2011**, *186*, 110–119. [CrossRef]
41. Birngruber, T.; Ghosh, A.; Perez-Yarza, V.; Kroath, T.; Ratzer, M.; Pieber, T.R.; Sinner, F. Cerebral Open Flow Microperfusion: A New in Vivo Technique for Continuous Measurement of Substance Transport across the Intact Blood-Brain Barrier. *Clin. Exp. Pharmacol. Physiol.* **2013**, *40*, 864–871. [CrossRef]
42. Birngruber, T.; Sinner, F. Cerebral Open Flow Microperfusion (COFM) an Innovative Interface to Brain Tissue. *Drug Discov. Today Technol.* **2016**, *20*, 19–25. [CrossRef]
43. Birngruber, T.; Ghosh, A.; Hochmeister, S.; Asslaber, M.; Kroath, T.; Pieber, T.R.; Sinner, F. Long-Term Implanted COFM Probe Causes Minimal Tissue Reaction in the Brain. *PLoS ONE* **2014**, *9*, e90221. [CrossRef] [PubMed]
44. Custers, M.-L.; Wouters, Y.; Jaspers, T.; De Bundel, D.; Dewilde, M.; Van Eeckhaut, A.; Smolders, I. Applicability of Cerebral Open Flow Microperfusion and Microdialysis to Quantify a Brain-Penetrating Nanobody in Mice. *Anal. Chim. Acta* **2021**, *1178*, 338803. [CrossRef] [PubMed]

45. Hummer, J.; Altendorfer-Kroath, T.; Birngruber, T. Cerebral Open Flow Microperfusion to Monitor Drug Transport Across the Blood-Brain Barrier. *Curr. Protoc. Pharmacol.* **2019**, *85*, e60. [CrossRef] [PubMed]
46. Zhang, Y.; Jiang, N.; Yetisen, A.K. Brain Neurochemical Monitoring. *Biosens. Bioelectron.* **2021**, *189*, 113351. [CrossRef]
47. Clark, L.C.; Lyons, C. Electrode Systems for Continuous Monitoring in Cardiovascular Surgery. *Ann. N. Y. Acad. Sci.* **1962**, *102*, 29–45. [CrossRef]
48. Naresh, V.; Lee, N. A Review on Biosensors and Recent Development of Nanostructured Materials-Enabled Biosensors. *Sensors* **2021**, *21*, 1109. [CrossRef]
49. Leca-Bouvier, B.; Blum, L.J. Biosensors for Protein Detection: A Review. *Anal. Lett.* **2005**, *38*, 1491–1517. [CrossRef]
50. Yoo, E.H.; Lee, S.Y. Glucose Biosensors: An Overview of Use in Clinical Practice. *Sensors* **2010**, *10*, 4558–4576. [CrossRef]
51. Rocchitta, G.; Spanu, A.; Babudieri, S.; Latte, G.; Madeddu, G.; Galleri, G.; Nuvoli, S.; Bagella, P.; Demartis, M.I.; Fiore, V.; et al. Enzyme Biosensors for Biomedical Applications: Strategies for Safeguarding Analytical Performances in Biological Fluids. *Sensors* **2016**, *16*, 780. [CrossRef]
52. Murugaiyan, S.B.; Ramasamy, R.; Gopal, N.; Kuzhandaivelu, V. Biosensors in Clinical Chemistry: An Overview. *Adv. Biomed. Res.* **2014**, *3*, 67. [CrossRef]
53. Scofield, M.D.; Boger, H.A.; Smith, R.J.; Hao, L.; Haydon, P.G.; Kalivas, P.W. Gq-DREADD Selectively Initiates Glial Glutamate Release and Inhibits Cue-Induced Cocaine Seeking. *Biol. Psychiatry* **2015**, *78*, 441–451. [CrossRef] [PubMed]
54. Kotanen, C.N.; Moussy, F.G.; Carrara, S.; Guiseppi-Elie, A. Implantable Enzyme Amperometric Biosensors. *Biosens. Bioelectron.* **2012**, *35*, 14–26. [CrossRef] [PubMed]
55. Xu, J.; Lee, H. Anti-Biofouling Strategies for Long-Term Continuous Use of Implantable Biosensors. *Chemosensors* **2020**, *8*, 66. [CrossRef]
56. Bhalla, N.; Jolly, P.; Formisano, N.; Estrela, P. Introduction to Biosensors. *Essays Biochem.* **2016**, *60*, 1–8. [CrossRef]
57. Deng, H.; Shen, W.; Gao, Z. An Interference-Free Glucose Biosensor Based on an Anionic Redox Polymer-Mediated Enzymatic Oxidation of Glucose. *ChemPhysChem* **2013**, *14*, 2343–2347. [CrossRef]
58. Peng, Y.; Wei, C.W.; Liu, Y.N.; Li, J. Nafion Coating the Ferrocenylalkanethiol and Encapsulated Glucose Oxidase Electrode for Amperometric Glucose Detection. *Analyst* **2011**, *136*, 4003–4007. [CrossRef]
59. Ganesana, M.; Trikantzopoulos, E.; Maniar, Y.; Lee, S.T.; Venton, B.J. Development of a Novel Micro Biosensor for in Vivo Monitoring of Glutamate Release in the Brain. *Biosens. Bioelectron.* **2019**, *130*, 103–109. [CrossRef]
60. Johnston, M.V.; Ammanuel, S.; O'Driscoll, C.; Wozniak, A.; Naidu, S.; Kadam, S.D. Twenty-Four Hour Quantitative-EEG and in-Vivo Glutamate Biosensor Detects Activity and Circadian Rhythm Dependent Biomarkers of Pathogenesis in Mecp2 Null Mice. *Front. Syst. Neurosci.* **2014**, *8*, 118. [CrossRef]
61. Lowry, J.P.; Miele, M.; O'Neill, R.D.; Boutelle, M.G.; Fillenz, M. An Amperometric Glucose-Oxidase/Poly(o-Phenylenediamine) Biosensor for Monitoring Brain Extracellular Glucose: In Vivo Characterisation in the Striatum of Freely-Moving Rats. *J. Neurosci. Methods* **1998**, *79*, 65–74. [CrossRef]
62. Cordeiro, C.A.; de Vries, M.G.; Ngabi, W.; Oomen, P.E.; Cremers, T.I.F.H.; Westerink, B.H.C. In Vivo Continuous and Simultaneous Monitoring of Brain Energy Substrates with a Multiplex Amperometric Enzyme-Based Biosensor Device. *Biosens. Bioelectron.* **2015**, *67*, 677–686. [CrossRef]
63. Esteves-Villanueva, J.O.; Trzeciakiewicz, H.; Martic, S. A Protein-Based Electrochemical Biosensor for Detection of Tau Protein, a Neurodegenerative Disease Biomarker. *Analyst* **2014**, *139*, 2823–2831. [CrossRef] [PubMed]
64. Carneiro, P.; Loureiro, J.; Delerue-Matos, C.; Morais, S.; do Carmo Pereira, M. Alzheimer's Disease: Development of a Sensitive Label-Free Electrochemical Immunosensor for Detection of Amyloid Beta Peptide. *Sens. Actuators B Chem.* **2017**, *239*, 157–165. [CrossRef]
65. Azimzadeh, M.; Rahaie, M.; Nasirizadeh, N.; Ashtari, K.; Naderi-Manesh, H. An Electrochemical Nanobiosensor for Plasma MiRNA-155, Based on Graphene Oxide and Gold Nanorod, for Early Detection of Breast Cancer. *Biosens. Bioelectron.* **2016**, *77*, 99–106. [CrossRef] [PubMed]
66. Stanta, G. Electrochemical Nanobiosensors and Protein Detection. *Eur. J. Nanomed.* **2008**, *1*, 33–36. [CrossRef]
67. Antipchik, M.; Korzhikova-Vlakh, E.; Polyakov, D.; Tarasenko, I.; Reut, J.; Öpik, A.; Syritski, V. An Electrochemical Biosensor for Direct Detection of Hepatitis C Virus. *Anal. Biochem.* **2021**, *624*, 114196. [CrossRef]
68. Ilkhani, H.; Farhad, S. A Novel Electrochemical DNA Biosensor for Ebola Virus Detection. *Anal. Biochem.* **2018**, *557*, 151–155. [CrossRef]
69. Peng, Y.; Pan, Y.; Sun, Z.; Li, J.; Yi, Y.; Yang, J. An Electrochemical Biosensor for Sensitive Analysis of the SARS-CoV-2 RNA. *Biosens. Bioelectron.* **2021**, *186*, 113309. [CrossRef]
70. Velho, G.; Froguel, P.; Sternberg, R.; Thevenot, D.R.; Reach, G. In Vitro and In Vivo Stability of Electrode Potentials in Needle-Type Glucose Sensors. Influence of Needle Material. *Diabetes* **1989**, *38*, 164–171. [CrossRef]
71. Reid, C.H.; Finnerty, N.J. An Electrochemical Investigation into the Effects of Local and Systemic Administrations of Sodium Nitroprusside in Brain Extracellular Fluid of Mice. *Bioelectrochemistry* **2020**, *132*, 107441. [CrossRef]
72. Khan, A.S.; Michael, A.C. Invasive Consequences of Using Micro-Electrodes and Microdialysis Probes in the Brain. *TrAC-Trends Anal. Chem.* **2003**, *22*, 503–508. [CrossRef]
73. Sumbria, R.K.; Klein, J.; Bickel, U. Acute Depression of Energy Metabolism after Microdialysis Probe Implantation Is Distinct from Ischemia-Induced Changes in Mouse Brain. *Neurochem. Res.* **2011**, *36*, 109–116. [CrossRef] [PubMed]

74. Caljon, G.; Caveliers, V.; Lahoutte, T.; Stijlemans, B.; Ghassabeh, G.H.; Van Den Abbeele, J.; Smolders, I.; De Baetselier, P.; Michotte, Y.; Muyldermans, S.; et al. Using Microdialysis to Analyse the Passage of Monovalent Nanobodies through the Blood-Brain Barrier. *Br. J. Pharmacol.* **2012**, *165*, 2341–2353. [CrossRef] [PubMed]
75. Groothuis, D.R.; Ward, S.; Schlageter, K.E.; Itskovich, A.C.; Schwerin, S.C.; Allen, C.V.; Dills, C.; Levy, R.M. Changes in Blood-Brain Barrier Permeability Associated with Insertion of Brain Cannulas and Microdialysis Probes. *Brain Res.* **1998**, *803*, 218–230. [CrossRef]
76. De Lange, E.C.M.; Danhof, M.; De Boer, A.G.; Breimer, D.D. Methodological Considerations of Intracerebral Microdialysis in Pharmacokinetic Studies on Drug Transport across the Blood-Brain Barrier. *Brain Res. Rev.* **1997**, *25*, 27–49. [CrossRef]
77. Benveniste, H.; Drejer, J.; Schousboe, A.; Diemer, N.H. Regional Cerebral Glucose Phosphorylation and Blood Flow After Insertion of a Microdialysis Fiber Through the Dorsal Hippocampus in the Rat. *J. Neurochem.* **1987**, *49*, 729–734. [CrossRef]
78. Mitala, C.M.; Wang, Y.; Borland, L.M.; Jung, M.; Shand, S.; Watkins, S.; Weber, S.G.; Michael, A.C. Impact of Microdialysis Probes on Vasculature and Dopamine in the Rat Striatum: A Combined Fluorescence and Voltammetric Study. *J. Neurosci. Methods* **2008**, *174*, 177–185. [CrossRef]
79. Morgan, M.E.; Singhal, D.; Anderson, B.D. Quantitative Assessment of Blood-Brain Barrier Damage during Microdialysis. *J. Pharmacol. Exp. Ther.* **1996**, *277*, 1167–1176.
80. Ghosh, A.; Birngruber, T.; Sattler, W.; Kroath, T.; Ratzer, M.; Sinner, F.; Pieber, T.R. Assessment of Blood-Brain Barrier Function and the Neuroinflammatory Response in the Rat Brain by Using Cerebral Open Flow Microperfusion (COFM). *PLoS ONE* **2014**, *9*, e98143. [CrossRef]
81. Tossman, U.; Ungerstedt, U. Microdialysis in the Study of Extracellular Levels of Amino Acids in the Rat Brain. *Acta Physiol. Scand.* **1986**, *128*, 9–14. [CrossRef]
82. Benveniste, H.; Drejer, J.; Schousboe, A.; Diemer, N.H. Elevation of the Extracellular Concentrations of Glutamate and Aspartate in Rat Hippocampus During Transient Cerebral Ischemia Monitored by Intracerebral Microdialysis. *J. Neurochem.* **1984**, *43*, 1369–1374. [CrossRef]
83. Altendorfer-Kroath, T.; Schimek, D.; Eberl, A.; Rauter, G.; Ratzer, M.; Raml, R.; Sinner, F.; Birngruber, T. Comparison of Cerebral Open Flow Microperfusion and Microdialysis When Sampling Small Lipophilic and Small Hydrophilic Substances. *J. Neurosci. Methods* **2019**, *311*, 394–401. [CrossRef] [PubMed]
84. Kleinert, M.; Kotzbeck, P.; Altendorfer-Kroath, T.; Birngruber, T.; Tschöp, M.H.; Clemmensen, C. Time-Resolved Hypothalamic Open Flow Micro-Perfusion Reveals Normal Leptin Transport across the Blood–Brain Barrier in Leptin Resistant Mice. *Mol. Metab.* **2018**, *13*, 77–82. [CrossRef] [PubMed]
85. Hamdan, S.K.; Zain, Z.M. In Vivo Electrochemical Biosensor for Brain Glutamate Detection: A Mini Review. *Malays. J. Med. Sci.* **2014**, *21*, 11–25.
86. Benveniste, H.; Diemer, N.H. Cellular Reactions to Implantation of a Microdialysis Tube in the Rat Hippocampus. *Acta Neuropathol.* **1987**, *74*, 234–238. [CrossRef]
87. Hascup, E.R.; af Bjerkén, S.; Hascup, K.N.; Pomerleau, F.; Huettl, P.; Strömberg, I.; Gerhardt, G.A. Histological Studies of the Effects of Chronic Implantation of Ceramic-Based Microelectrode Arrays and Microdialysis Probes in Rat Prefrontal Cortex. *Brain Res.* **2009**, *1291*, 12–20. [CrossRef]
88. Meller, S.; Brandt, C.; Theilmann, W.; Klein, J.; Löscher, W. Commonalities and Differences in Extracellular Levels of Hippocampal Acetylcholine and Amino Acid Neurotransmitters during Status Epilepticus and Subsequent Epileptogenesis in Two Rat Models of Temporal Lobe Epilepsy. *Brain Res.* **2019**, *1712*, 109–123. [CrossRef]
89. Osborne, P.G.; O'Connor, W.T.; Kehr, J.; Ungerstedt, U. In Vivo Characterisation of Extracellular Dopamine, GABA and Acetylcholine from the Dorsolateral Striatum of Awake Freely Moving Rats by Chronic Microdialysis. *J. Neurosci. Methods* **1991**, *37*, 93–102. [CrossRef]
90. Orłowska-Majdak, M. Microdialysis of the Brain Structures: Application in Behavioral Research on Vasopressin and Oxytocin. *Acta Neurobiol. Exp.* **2004**, *64*, 177–188.
91. Korf, J.; Venema, K. Amino Acids in Rat Striatal Dialysates: Methodological Aspects and Changes After Electroconvulsive Shock. *J. Neurochem.* **1985**, *45*, 1341–1348. [CrossRef]
92. FDA Use of International Standard ISO 10993-1, "Biological Evaluation of Medical Devices—Part 1: Evaluation and Testing within a Risk Management Process". Available online: https://www.fda.gov/regulatory-information/search-fda-guidance-documents/use-international-standard-iso-10993-1-biological-evaluation-medical-devices-part-1-evaluation-and (accessed on 15 March 2022).
93. Lin, P.-H.; Li, B.-R. Antifouling Strategies in Advanced Electrochemical Sensors and Biosensors. *Analyst* **2020**, *145*, 1110–1120. [CrossRef]
94. Xu, C.; Wu, F.; Yu, P.; Mao, L. In Vivo Electrochemical Sensors for Neurochemicals: Recent Update. *ACS Sens.* **2019**, *4*, 3102–3118. [CrossRef] [PubMed]
95. Tan, C.; Robbins, E.M.; Wu, B.; Cui, X.T. Recent Advances in In Vivo Neurochemical Monitoring. *Micromachines* **2021**, *12*, 208. [CrossRef]
96. Brown, F.O.; Finnerty, N.J.; Lowry, J.P. Nitric Oxide Monitoring in Brain Extracellular Fluid: Characterisation of Nafion®-Modified Pt Electrodes In Vitro and In Vivo. *Analyst* **2009**, *134*, 2012. [CrossRef] [PubMed]

97. Reid, C.H.; Finnerty, N.J. Long Term Amperometric Recordings in the Brain Extracellular Fluid of Freely Moving Immunocompromised NOD SCID Mice. *Sensors* **2017**, *17*, 419. [CrossRef] [PubMed]
98. Morales-Villagrán, A.; Medina-Ceja, L.; López-Pérez, S.J. Simultaneous Glutamate and EEG Activity Measurements during Seizures in Rat Hippocampal Region with the Use of an Electrochemical Biosensor. *J. Neurosci. Methods* **2008**, *168*, 48–53. [CrossRef]
99. Clapp-Lilly, K.L.; Roberts, R.C.; Duffy, L.K.; Irons, K.P.; Hu, Y.; Drew, K.L. An Ultrastructural Analysis of Tissue Surrounding a Microdialysis Probe. *J. Neurosci. Methods* **1999**, *90*, 129–142. [CrossRef]
100. Grabb, M.C.; Sciotti, V.M.; Gidday, J.M.; Cohen, S.A.; Van Wylen, D.G.L. Neurochemical and Morphological Responses to Acutely and Chronically Implanted Brain Microdialysis Probes. *J. Neurosci. Methods* **1998**, *82*, 25–34. [CrossRef]
101. Thomas, M.; Moriyama, K.; Ledebo, I. AN69: Evolution of the World's First High Permeability Membrane. In *High-Performance Membrane Dialyzers*; Karger: Basel, Switzerland, 2011; Volume 173, pp. 119–129, ISBN 9783805598132.
102. Birngruber, T. *Development of a Continuous Sampling System for Monitoring Transport across the Intact Blood-Brain Barrier*; Graz University of Technology: Graz, Austria, 2013.
103. Pieber, T.; Birngruber, T.; Bodenlenz, M.; Höfferer, C.; Mautner, S.; Tiffner, K.; Sinner, F. Open Flow Microperfusion: An Alternative Method to Microdialysis? In *AAPS Advances in the Pharmaceutical Sciences Series*; Springer: New York, NY, USA, 2013; pp. 283–302, ISBN 9781461448143.
104. Nicholson, C.; Phillips, J.M. Ion Diffusion Modified by Tortuosity and Volume Fraction in the Extracellular Microenvironment of the Rat Cerebellum. *J. Physiol.* **1981**, *321*, 225–257. [CrossRef]
105. Kealy, J.; Bennett, R.; Woods, B.; Lowry, J.P. Real-Time Changes in Hippocampal Energy Demands during a Spatial Working Memory Task. *Behav. Brain Res.* **2017**, *326*, 59–68. [CrossRef]
106. Thelin, J.; Jörntell, H.; Psouni, E.; Garwicz, M.; Schouenborg, J.; Danielsen, N.; Linsmeier, C.E. Implant Size and Fixation Mode Strongly Influence Tissue Reactions in the CNS. *PLoS ONE* **2011**, *6*, e16267. [CrossRef]
107. Xiao, T.; Wu, F.; Hao, J.; Zhang, M.; Yu, P.; Mao, L. In Vivo Analysis with Electrochemical Sensors and Biosensors. *Anal. Chem.* **2017**, *89*, 300–313. [CrossRef] [PubMed]
108. Cooley, J.C.; Ducey, M.W.; Regel, A.R.; Nandi, P.; Lunte, S.M.; Lunte, C.E. Analytical Considerations for Microdialysis Sampling. In *AAPS Advances in the Pharmaceutical Sciences Series*; Springer: New York, NY, USA, 2013; pp. 35–66, ISBN 9781461448150.
109. Weltin, A.; Kieninger, J.; Urban, G.A. Microfabricated, Amperometric, Enzyme-Based Biosensors for In Vivo Applications. *Anal. Bioanal. Chem.* **2016**, *408*, 4503–4521. [CrossRef] [PubMed]
110. Perry, M.; Li, Q.; Kennedy, R.T. Review of Recent Advances in Analytical Techniques for the Determination of Neurotransmitters. *Anal. Chim. Acta* **2009**, *653*, 1–22. [CrossRef] [PubMed]
111. Thevenot, D.; Toth, K.; Durst, R.; Wilson, G. Electrochemical Biosensors: Recommended Definitions and Classification. *Biosens. Bioelectron.* **2001**, *16*, 121–131. [CrossRef]
112. Phetsanthad, A.; Vu, N.Q.; Yu, Q.; Buchberger, A.R.; Chen, Z.; Keller, C.; Li, L. Recent Advances in Mass Spectrometry Analysis of Neuropeptides. *Mass Spectrom. Rev.* **2021**, e21734. [CrossRef]
113. Zhou, Y.; Mabrouk, O.S.; Kennedy, R.T. Rapid Preconcentration for Liquid Chromatography–Mass Spectrometry Assay of Trace Level Neuropeptides. *J. Am. Soc. Mass Spectrom.* **2013**, *24*, 1700–1709. [CrossRef]
114. Maes, K.; Béchade, G.; Van Schoors, J.; Van Wanseele, Y.; Van Liefferinge, J.; Michotte, Y.; Harden, S.N.; Chambers, E.E.; Claereboudt, J.; Smolders, I.; et al. An Ultrasensitive Nano UHPLC–ESI–MS/MS Method for the Quantification of Three Neuromedin-like Peptides in Microdialysates. *Bioanalysis* **2015**, *7*, 605–619. [CrossRef]
115. Zestos, A.G.; Kennedy, R.T. Microdialysis Coupled with LC-MS/MS for In Vivo Neurochemical Monitoring. *AAPS J.* **2017**, *19*, 1284–1293. [CrossRef]
116. van Mever, M.; Segers, K.; Drouin, N.; Guled, F.; Van der Heyden, Y.; Van Eeckhaut, A.; Hankemeier, T.; Ramautar, R. Direct Profiling of Endogenous Metabolites in Rat Brain Microdialysis Samples by Capillary Electrophoresis-Mass Spectrometry with on-Line Preconcentration. *Microchem. J.* **2020**, *156*, 104949. [CrossRef]
117. Maurer, M.H.; Berger, C.; Wolf, M.; Fütterer, C.D.; Feldmann, R.E.; Schwab, S.; Kuschinsky, W. The Proteome of Human Brain Microdialysate. *Proteome Sci.* **2003**, *1*, 7. [CrossRef]
118. Rissin, D.M.; Kan, C.W.; Campbell, T.G.; Howes, S.C.; Fournier, D.R.; Song, L.; Piech, T.; Patel, P.P.; Chang, L.; Rivnak, A.J.; et al. Single-Molecule Enzyme-Linked Immunosorbent Assay Detects Serum Proteins at Subfemtomolar Concentrations. *Nat. Biotechnol.* **2010**, *28*, 595–599. [CrossRef] [PubMed]
119. PerkinElmer AlphaLISA and AlphaScreen No-Wash Assays. Available online: https://www.perkinelmer.com/nl/lab-products-and-services/application-support-knowledgebase/alphalisa-alphascreen-no-wash-assays/alphalisa-alphascreen-no-washassays-main.html (accessed on 18 November 2020).
120. PerkinElmer Principles of AlphaScreen™. Available online: https://resources.perkinelmer.com/lab-solutions/resources/docs/APP_AlphaScreen_Principles.pdf (accessed on 2 March 2022).
121. Helmy, A.; Guilfoyle, M.R.; Carpenter, K.L.; Pickard, J.D.; Menon, D.K.; Hutchinson, P.J. Recombinant Human Interleukin-1 Receptor Antagonist in Severe Traumatic Brain Injury: A Phase II Randomized Control Trial. *J. Cereb. Blood Flow Metab.* **2014**, *34*, 845–851. [CrossRef] [PubMed]

122. Helmy, A.; Guilfoyle, M.R.; Carpenter, K.L.; Pickard, J.D.; Menon, D.K.; Hutchinson, P.J. Recombinant Human Interleukin-1 Receptor Antagonist Promotes M1 Microglia Biased Cytokines and Chemokines Following Human Traumatic Brain Injury. *J. Cereb. Blood Flow Metab.* **2016**, *36*, 1434–1448. [CrossRef] [PubMed]
123. Hillman, J.; Åneman, O.; Persson, M.; Andersson, C.; Dabrosin, C.; Mellergård, P. Variations in the Response of Interleukins in Neurosurgical Intensive Care Patients Monitored Using Intracerebral Microdialysis. *J. Neurosurg.* **2007**, *106*, 820–825. [CrossRef] [PubMed]
124. Mellergård, P.; Åneman, O.; Sjögren, F.; Pettersson, P.; Hillman, J. Changes in Extracellular Concentrations of Some Cytokines, Chemokines, and Neurotrophic Factors after Insertion of Intracerebral Microdialysis Catheters in Neurosurgical Patients. *Neurosurgery* **2008**, *62*, 151–158. [CrossRef] [PubMed]
125. Mellergård, P.; Sjögren, F.; Hillman, J. The Cerebral Extracellular Release of Glycerol, Glutamate, and FGF2 Is Increased in Older Patients Following Severe Traumatic Brain Injury. *J. Neurotrauma* **2012**, *29*, 112–118. [CrossRef]
126. Hanafy, K.A.; Grobelny, B.; Fernandez, L.; Kurtz, P.; Connolly, E.S.; Mayer, S.A.; Schindler, C.; Badjatia, N. Brain Interstitial Fluid TNF-α after Subarachnoid Hemorrhage. *J. Neurol. Sci.* **2010**, *291*, 69–73. [CrossRef]
127. Wang, X.; Lennartz, M.R.; Loegering, D.J.; Stenken, J.A. Interleukin-6 Collection through Long-Term Implanted Microdialysis Sampling Probes in Rat Subcutaneous Space. *Anal. Chem.* **2007**, *79*, 1816–1824. [CrossRef]
128. Winter, C.D.; Iannotti, F.; Pringle, A.K.; Trikkas, C.; Clough, G.F.; Church, M.K. A Microdialysis Method for the Recovery of IL-1β, IL-6 and Nerve Growth Factor from Human Brain In Vivo. *J. Neurosci. Methods* **2002**, *119*, 45–50. [CrossRef]
129. Hillman, J.; Åneman, O.; Anderson, C.; Sjögren, F.; Säberg, C.; Mellergård, P. A Microdialysis Technique for Routine Measurement of Macromolecules in the Injured Human Brain. *Neurosurgery* **2005**, *56*, 1264–1270. [CrossRef]
130. Duo, J.; Stenken, J.A. In Vitro and In Vivo Affinity Microdialysis Sampling of Cytokines Using Heparin-Immobilized Microspheres. *Anal. Bioanal. Chem.* **2011**, *399*, 783–793. [CrossRef] [PubMed]
131. Winter, C.D. Raised Parenchymal Interleukin-6 Levels Correlate with Improved Outcome after Traumatic Brain Injury. *Brain* **2004**, *127*, 315–320. [CrossRef] [PubMed]
132. Sarrafzadeh, A.; Schlenk, F.; Gericke, C.; Vajkoczy, P. Relevance of Cerebral Interleukin-6 After Aneurysmal Subarachnoid Hemorrhage. *Neurocrit. Care* **2010**, *13*, 339–346. [CrossRef] [PubMed]
133. Hutchinson, P.J.; O'Connell, M.T.; Rothwell, N.J.; Hopkins, S.J.; Nortje, J.; Carpenter, K.L.H.; Timofeev, I.; Al-Rawi, P.G.; Menon, D.K.; Pickard, J.D. Inflammation in Human Brain Injury: Intracerebral Concentrations of IL-1 α, IL-1 β, and Their Endogenous Inhibitor IL-1ra. *J. Neurotrauma* **2007**, *24*, 1545–1557. [CrossRef] [PubMed]
134. Roberts, D.J.; Jenne, C.N.; Léger, C.; Kramer, A.H.; Gallagher, C.N.; Todd, S.; Parney, I.F.; Doig, C.J.; Yong, V.W.; Kubes, P.; et al. Association between the Cerebral Inflammatory and Matrix Metalloproteinase Responses after Severe Traumatic Brain Injury in Humans. *J. Neurotrauma* **2013**, *30*, 1727–1736. [CrossRef]
135. Marcus, H.J.; Carpenter, K.L.H.; Price, S.J.; Hutchinson, P.J. In Vivo Assessment of High-Grade Glioma Biochemistry Using Microdialysis: A Study of Energy-Related Molecules, Growth Factors and Cytokines. *J. Neurooncol.* **2010**, *97*, 11–23. [CrossRef]
136. Yamamoto, K.; Asano, K.; Tasaka, A.; Ogura, Y.; Kim, S.; Ito, Y.; Yamatodani, A. Involvement of Substance P in the Development of Cisplatin-Induced Acute and Delayed Pica in Rats. *Br. J. Pharmacol.* **2014**, *171*, 2888–2899. [CrossRef]
137. Kutlu, S.; Aydin, M.; Alcin, E.; Ozcan, M.; Bakos, J.; Jezova, D.; Yilmaz, B. Leptin Modulates Noradrenaline Release in the Paraventricular Nucleus and Plasma Oxytocin Levels in Female Rats: A Microdialysis Study. *Brain Res.* **2010**, *1317*, 87–91. [CrossRef]
138. Frost, S.I.; Keen, K.L.; Levine, J.E.; Terasawa, E. Microdialysis Methods for In Vivo Neuropeptide Measurement in the Stalk-Median Eminence in the Rhesus Monkey. *J. Neurosci. Methods* **2008**, *168*, 26–34. [CrossRef]
139. Ide, S.; Hara, T.; Ohno, A.; Tamano, R.; Koseki, K.; Naka, T.; Maruyama, C.; Kaneda, K.; Yoshioka, M.; Minami, M. Opposing Roles of Corticotropin-Releasing Factor and Neuropeptide Y within the Dorsolateral Bed Nucleus of the Stria Terminalis in the Negative Affective Component of Pain in Rats. *J. Neurosci.* **2013**, *33*, 5881–5894. [CrossRef]
140. Guilfoyle, M.R.; Carpenter, K.L.H.; Helmy, A.; Pickard, J.D.; Menon, D.K.; Hutchinson, P.J.A. Matrix Metalloproteinase Expression in Contusional Traumatic Brain Injury: A Paired Microdialysis Study. *J. Neurotrauma* **2015**, *32*, 1553–1559. [CrossRef] [PubMed]
141. Roberts, D.J.; Jenne, C.N.; Léger, C.; Kramer, A.H.; Gallagher, C.N.; Todd, S.; Parney, I.F.; Doig, C.J.; Yong, V.W.; Kubes, P.; et al. A Prospective Evaluation of the Temporal Matrix Metalloproteinase Response after Severe Traumatic Brain Injury in Humans. *J. Neurotrauma* **2013**, *30*, 1717–1726. [CrossRef] [PubMed]
142. Sarrafzadeh, A.; Copin, J.-C.; Bengualid, D.J.; Turck, N.; Vajkoczy, P.; Bijlenga, P.; Schaller, K.; Gasche, Y. Matrix Metalloproteinase-9 Concentration in the Cerebral Extracellular Fluid of Patients during the Acute Phase of Aneurysmal Subarachnoid Hemorrhage. *Neurol. Res.* **2012**, *34*, 455–461. [CrossRef] [PubMed]
143. Sen, J.; Belli, A.; Petzold, A.; Russo, S.; Keir, G.; Thompson, E.J.; Smith, M.; Kitchen, N. Extracellular Fluid S100B in the Injured Brain: A Future Surrogate Marker of Acute Brain Injury? *Acta Neurochir.* **2005**, *147*, 897–900. [CrossRef]
144. Afinowi, R.; Tisdall, M.; Keir, G.; Smith, M.; Kitchen, N.; Petzold, A. Improving the Recovery of S100B Protein in Cerebral Microdialysis: Implications for Multimodal Monitoring in Neurocritical Care. *J. Neurosci. Methods* **2009**, *181*, 95–99. [CrossRef]
145. Ulrich, J.D.; Burchett, J.M.; Restivo, J.L.; Schuler, D.R.; Verghese, P.B.; Mahan, T.E.; Landreth, G.E.; Castellano, J.M.; Jiang, H.; Cirrito, J.R.; et al. In Vivo Measurement of Apolipoprotein E from the Brain Interstitial Fluid Using Microdialysis. *Mol. Neurodegener.* **2013**, *8*, 13. [CrossRef]

146. Herukka, S.-K.; Rummukainen, J.; Ihalainen, J.; von und zu Fraunberg, M.; Koivisto, A.M.; Nerg, O.; Puli, L.K.; Seppälä, T.T.; Zetterberg, H.; Pyykkö, O.T.; et al. Amyloid-β and Tau Dynamics in Human Brain Interstitial Fluid in Patients with Suspected Normal Pressure Hydrocephalus. *J. Alzheimer's Dis.* **2015**, *46*, 261–269. [CrossRef]
147. Marklund, N.; Blennow, K.; Zetterberg, H.; Ronne-Engström, E.; Enblad, P.; Hillered, L. Monitoring of Brain Interstitial Total Tau and Beta Amyloid Proteins by Microdialysis in Patients with Traumatic Brain Injury. *J. Neurosurg.* **2009**, *110*, 1227–1237. [CrossRef]
148. Brody, D.L.; Magnoni, S.; Schwetye, K.E.; Spinner, M.L.; Esparza, T.J.; Stocchetti, N.; Zipfel, G.J.; Holtzman, D.M. Amyloid-β Dynamics Correlate with Neurological Status in the Injured Human Brain. *Science* **2008**, *321*, 1221–1224. [CrossRef]
149. Helbok, R.; Schiefecker, A.; Delazer, M.; Beer, R.; Bodner, T.; Pfausler, B.; Benke, T.; Lackner, P.; Fischer, M.; Sohm, F.; et al. Cerebral Tau Is Elevated after Aneurysmal Subarachnoid Haemorrhage and Associated with Brain Metabolic Distress and Poor Functional and Cognitive Long-Term Outcome. *J. Neurol. Neurosurg. Psychiatry* **2015**, *86*, 79–86. [CrossRef]
150. Petzold, A.; Tisdall, M.M.; Girbes, A.R.; Martinian, L.; Thom, M.; Kitchen, N.; Smith, M. In Vivo Monitoring of Neuronal Loss in Traumatic Brain Injury: A Microdialysis Study. *Brain* **2011**, *134*, 464–483. [CrossRef] [PubMed]
151. Bache, S.; Rasmussen, R.; Rossing, M.; Hammer, N.R.; Juhler, M.; Friis-Hansen, L.; Nielsen, F.C.; Møller, K. Detection and Quantification of MicroRNA in Cerebral Microdialysate. *J. Transl. Med.* **2015**, *13*, 149. [CrossRef] [PubMed]
152. Birngruber, T.; Raml, R.; Gladdines, W.; Gatschelhofer, C.; Gander, E.; Ghosh, A.; Kroath, T.; Gaillard, P.J.; Pieber, T.R.; Sinner, F. Enhanced Doxorubicin Delivery to the Brain Administered through Glutathione PEGylated Liposomal Doxorubicin (2B3-101) as Compared with Generic Caelyx,®/Doxil®—A Cerebral Open Flow Microperfusion Pilot Study. *J. Pharm. Sci.* **2014**, *103*, 1945–1948. [CrossRef] [PubMed]
153. Umbrain, V.J.; Lauwers, M.-H.; Shi, L.; Smolders, I.; Michotte, Y.; Poelaert, J. Comparison of the Effects of Intrathecal Administration of Levobupivacaine and Lidocaine on the Prostaglandin E 2 and Glutamate Increases in Cerebrospinal Fluid: A Microdialysis Study in Freely Moving Rats. *Br. J. Anaesth.* **2009**, *102*, 540–545. [CrossRef]
154. Nakamura, Y.; Sakaguchi, T.; Tamai, I.; Nakanishi, T. Quantification of Prostaglandin E2 Concentration in Interstitial Fluid from the Hypothalamic Region of Free-Moving Mice. *Bio Protoc.* **2019**, *9*, e3324. [CrossRef]
155. Hökfelt, T.; Bartfai, T.; Bloom, F. Neuropeptides: Opportunities for Drug Discovery. *Lancet Neurol.* **2003**, *2*, 463–472. [CrossRef]
156. European Patent Office. Espacenet-Patent Search. Available online: https://worldwide.espacenet.com/patent/search?q=microdialysis (accessed on 4 May 2022).
157. Ungerstedt, C.U. Sonde de Dialyse. Patent FR2537000A1, 8 June 1984.
158. Ungerstedt, C.U. Dialysis Probe. U.S. Patent 4,694,832, 22 September 1987.
159. Birngruber, T.; Altendorfer-Kroath, T. Catheter Having a Healing Dummy. International Patent WO 2012/156478 A1, 22 November 2011.
160. Birngruber, T.; Altendorfer-Kroath, T. Catheter Having a Healing Dummy. U.S. Patent 9,656,018 B2, 23 May 2017.
161. Nishino, H.; Ikimura, K.; Tekda, S.; Sato, N.; Morishita, R. Dialysis Probe. U.S. Patent 2011/0259811 A1, 27 October 2011.
162. Cremers, T.I.F.H.; de Vries, M.G.; Huinink, K.D.; van Loon, J.P.; Hart, M.V.D.; Ebert, B.; Westerink, B.H.C.; De Lange, E.C.M. Quantitative Microdialysis Using Modified Ultraslow Microdialysis: Direct Rapid and Reliable Determination of Free Brain Concentrations with the MetaQuant Technique. *J. Neurosci. Methods* **2009**, *178*, 249–254. [CrossRef]
163. Cremers, T.I.F.H. Use of Push Pull Microdialysis in Combination with Shotgun Proteomics for Analyzing the Proteome in Extracellular Space of Brain. International Patent WO2017174557A2, 12 October 2017.
164. Stenken, J.A.; Sellati, T.J. Method and Kit for Enhancing Extraction and Quantification of Target Molecules Using Microdialysis. U.S. Patent US 2004/0248181 A1, 9 December 2004.
165. Ao, X.; Sellati, T.J.; Stenken, J.A. Enhanced Microdialysis Relative Recovery of Inflammatory Cytokines Using Antibody-Coated Microspheres Analyzed by Flow Cytometry. *Anal. Chem.* **2004**, *76*, 3777–3784. [CrossRef]
166. Clark, L.C. Electrochemical Device for Chemical Analysis. U.S. Patent 2,913,386, 17 November 1959.
167. Stangler, L.A.; Kouzani, A.; Bennet, K.E.; Dumee, L.; Berk, M.; Worrell, G.A.; Steele, S.; Burns, T.C.; Howe, C.L. Microdialysis and Microperfusion Electrodes in Neurologic Disease Monitoring. *Fluids Barriers CNS* **2021**, *18*, 52. [CrossRef]

www.ingramcontent.com/pod-product-compliance
Lightning Source LLC
LaVergne TN
LVHW070452100526
838202LV00014B/1710

MDPI
St. Alban-Anlage 66
4052 Basel
Switzerland
Tel. +41 61 683 77 34
Fax +41 61 302 89 18
www.mdpi.com

Pharmaceutics Editorial Office
E-mail: pharmaceutics@mdpi.com
www.mdpi.com/journal/pharmaceutics

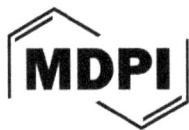